# Mastering DMEK and PDEK

# Springer Nature More Media App

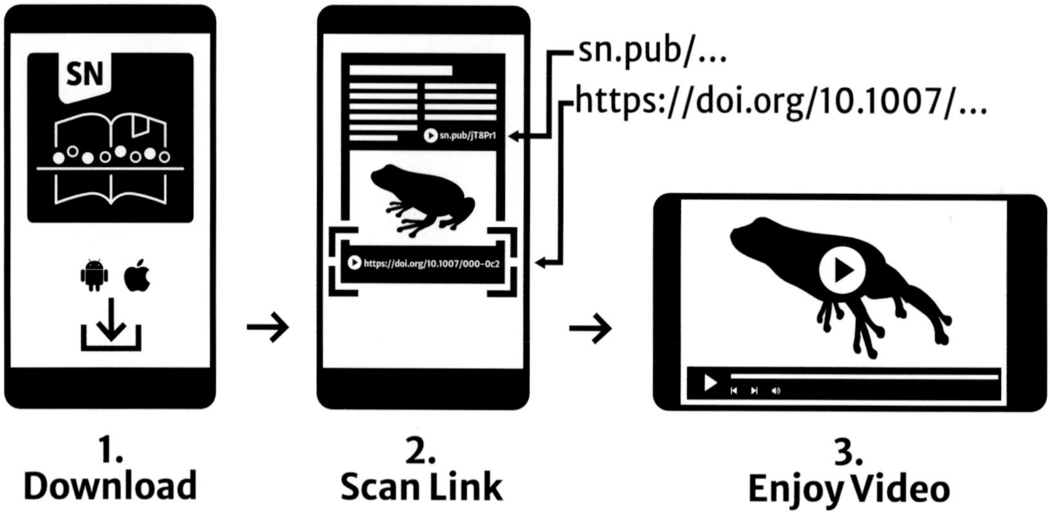


Support: customerservice@springernature.com

Soosan Jacob
Editor

# Mastering DMEK and PDEK

## Thin Membrane Endothelial Keratoplasty

Second Edition

Springer

*Editor*
Soosan Jacob
Director and Chief, Dr. Agarwal's
Refractive and Cornea Foundation
Senior Consultant, Cataract
and Glaucoma Services, Dr. Agarwal's
Eye Hospital
Chennai, India

This work contains media enhancements, which are displayed with a "play" icon. Material in the print book can be viewed on a mobile device by downloading the Springer Nature "More Media" app available in the major app stores. The media enhancements in the online version of the work can be accessed directly by authorized users.

ISBN 978-981-97-3468-9 ISBN 978-981-97-3469-6 (eBook)
https://doi.org/10.1007/978-981-97-3469-6



This Springer imprint is published by the registered company Springer Nature Singapore Pte Ltd.
The registered company address is: 152 Beach Road, #21-01/04 Gateway East, Singapore 189721, Singapore

*To my one and only daughter, the love of my life—Riya*
*Shine bright like the diamond that you are!*

# Foreword

For nearly a century, penetrating keratoplasty was the gold standard for corneal transplantation. However, with innovative thinking and creative techniques, in just the last 25–30 years, some of the leading minds in corneal surgery have completely changed the paradigm for corneal transplantation. Thanks to the contributions of many of these leaders in the field, today, a patient with endothelial dysfunction can have targeted therapy for their condition, with a much more rapid recovery. Just in the last decade, endothelial keratoplasty has evolved from DSEK to UT-DSEK to DMEK and PDEK and now to even DSO. The world's literature is jam-packed with study after study on these various evolving techniques for treating endothelial dysfunction, each with their own conclusions. But how can we use these studies to help us do the best surgical procedure for the right patient?

*This Video Textbook on Mastering DMEK and PDEK: Thin Membrane Endothelial Keratoplasty* is the answer. In this indispensable resource, Master surgeon Dr. Soosan Jacob has compiled a well-organized and exceptionally practical and useful reference that provides everything a corneal surgeon would need in order to choose the appropriate endothelial procedure for each patient. Beautifully illustrated with abundant color photographs and videos of each of these topics, this book focuses on thin membrane endothelial keratoplasty (TMEK), a term coined by Dr. Jacob to refer to DMEK and PDEK, and also gives a brief look forwards into newer evolving techniques. Both the novice and the experienced surgeon will benefit from the detailed explanations from leading authorities in the field. Dr. Jacob has assembled a smartly organized line up of topics that begin with the history of endothelial keratoplasty and then patient selection for keratoplasty. Graft preparation of the various types of EK is discussed, followed by challenging situations for the various types of grafts, and then their complications and postoperative management. Other related procedures that are being done or investigated are also discussed, and a systematic review of the literature on the clinical outcomes of all of the different types of EK is even included: exactly what the surgeon needs to help decide on the type of procedures to offer.

As a highly decorated figure in the field of ophthalmology, Dr. Soosan Jacob is widely regarded as a foremost leader, an award-winning innovator, and a trailblazer. Her ability to bring her ideas to fruition has changed the way we practice, and this book is just one example of her pioneering spirit. The world already recognizes Dr. Jacob as a master surgeon and renowned educator, and with this book, she melds these two aspects of her world reputation into a resource that will instruct corneal surgeons around the globe on how to harness current techniques and technologies to best treat our patients with endothelial dysfunction.

Department of Ophthalmology and Scheie Eye Institute
University of Pennsylvania Perelman School of Medicine
Philadelphia, PA, USA

Bennie H. Jeng
Harold G. Scheie

# Preface

The landscape of corneal surgeries is constantly evolving—sometimes through subtle refinements, at other times with groundbreaking advancements. As techniques and technologies improve, what was once considered the gold standard is continually being redefined. Medicine, by its very nature, is dynamic, and as surgeons, we strive to achieve outcomes that bring us ever closer to the pristine normalcy of the cornea.

Over the years, anterior and posterior lamellar keratoplasty have set new benchmarks, becoming the standard of care. Among these, endothelial keratoplasty has emerged as the first choice whenever endothelial replacement is required. In 2012, Descemet stripping automated endothelial keratoplasty (DSAEK) surpassed penetrating keratoplasty in terms of corneal graft utilization in the USA. However, the trend has since shifted toward thinner grafts, with ultra-thin DSAEK, Descemet's membrane endothelial keratoplasty (DMEK), and pre-Descemet's endothelial keratoplasty (PDEK) leading the way.

DMEK and PDEK both involve the transplantation of ultra-thin membranous grafts, typically ranging from 15 to 30 μm in thickness. Their surgical techniques and clinical outcomes align closely, setting them apart from DSAEK and ultra-thin DSAEK. Recognizing this, I introduce the term **thin membrane endothelial keratoplasty (TMEK)** to collectively describe endothelial keratoplasties utilizing these thin, membranous grafts, which are optically and anatomically superior but can exhibit rapid and sometimes chaotic movement within the anterior chamber. TMEK techniques provide faster recovery, superior visual outcomes, and multiple other intra- and post-operative advantages. However, many corneal surgeons remain hesitant to adopt them, often perceiving these techniques as complex and demanding a steep learning curve.

This **second edition on endothelial keratoplasty** focuses on **TMEK**, filling a crucial gap in the literature, as no existing book comprehensively covers membranous EK. This guide aims to assist both novice surgeons embarking on their TMEK journey and experienced surgeons seeking a refresher—offering a structured approach to mastering these techniques with confidence and minimal setbacks. My hope is that this book serves as a road map, making the path forward more accessible.

I am deeply grateful to the many individuals who have supported me in bringing this book to life. I extend my heartfelt thanks to all my co-authors, who generously contributed their time, insights, and expertise; my friends and colleagues for their unwavering encouragement; and my assistant, **Arun Kumar**, whose organizational support prevented me from being overwhelmed. Special thanks to **Naren Aggarwal, Jagjeet Kaur Saini, and Ejaz Ahmad** from Springer for their invaluable help in ensuring this book meets the highest standards. I am also profoundly indebted to my mentors, **Drs. Amar** and **Athiya Agarwal**, for their unwavering guidance and encouragement.

My deepest appreciation goes to my patients, from whom I have learned invaluable lessons, and to my teachers, who selflessly shared their wisdom and skill. Finally, I am forever grateful to my family—my parents, **Mary Jacob** and **Lt. Col. Jacob Mathai,** whose values have shaped me; my siblings, **Alex and Asha**, for their steadfast support; my husband, best friend, confidant, and sounding board, **Dr. Abraham Oomman**, and my children, **Ashwin and Riya**, who love and tolerate me despite my idiosyncrasies.

Above all, with deepest faith, I place my trust in God, who has guided me thus far and whom I know will continue to lead me forward.

> **"Great things in this world depend not so much on where we stand but in which direction we are moving."**—*Oliver Wendell Holmes*

Chennai, India Soosan Jacob

# Contents

# About the Editor

**Soosan Jacob** MS, FRCS, DNB, MNAMS serves as the Director and Chief, Dr. Agarwal's Refractive and Cornea Foundation (DARCF) and Senior Consultant, Cataract and Glaucoma Services, Dr. Agarwal's Group of Eye Hospitals, Chennai, India. She is a noted speaker, widely respected for her innovative techniques and management of complex surgical scenarios.

She has been ranked among the top 20 (17th) ophthalmologists worldwide in the prestigious Power List of Ophthalmologists 2024, published by "The Ophthalmologist," a leading publication in the field (https://powerlist.theophthalmologist.com/) and is one of only three women on this list. She has also been previously listed on the Power Lists 2022 and 2021 of the top 100 most influential people in the world of ophthalmology (https://bit.ly/38IbZ2c, https://bit.ly/37RftPI) and the top 100 most influential women ophthalmologists in the world (https://bit.ly/2OqESpQ, https://bit.ly/3fOflwF). She has been featured as one of the five of the most influential female figures in ophthalmology at a virtual roundtable (https://bit.ly/3oPPaO8) and has been included in the KOL influencers list of 50 notable global figures in ophthalmology by Media MICE, another leading and influential ophthalmic publication in consecutive years. In addition, she is listed consecutively in Stanford's 2020, 2021, 2022, 2023, and 2024 lists of top 2% scientists from around the world (published by Elsevier). She has close to 30,000 followers on her various social media handles.

She is the recipient of the following prestigious international awards: JRS (Journal of Refractive Surgery) Waring Medal for Editorial excellence; ISRS (International Society of Refractive Surgery) Kritzinger Memorial Award (the first Indian and the first woman internationally to receive this award); ISRS Founder's Award (the first Indian to receive this award); Innovator's Award (Connecticut Society of Eye Physicians); ESCRS (European Society of Cataract and Refractive Surgery) John Henahan Award for Young Ophthalmologist; AAO (American Academy of Ophthalmology) International Ophthalmologist Education Award; AAO International Scholar Award; AAO Achievement Award; AAO Senior Achievement Award; AAO Secretariat Award; ASCRS (American Society of Cataract and Refractive Surgery) Top-Gun Instructor Award; Bruce Jackson Oration (Canadian Ophthalmological Society); Harold Stein Innovator Lecture (Canadian Ophthalmological Society); Ronald G. Michels Lectureship (Wilmer Eye Institute, Johns Hopkins University); Sally Letson Oration (Sally Letson Symposium, Canada); Vesna Morela Innovational Lecture (Ljubljana Refractive Society,

Slovenia); and inaugural Hermann von Helmholtz Lecture (6th biennial Heidelberg Helmholtz meeting) and is also a two-time recipient of the ASCRS Golden Apple Award and also the prestigious Indian awards: IIRSI (Intraocular Implant and Refractive Society of India) Special Gold Medal; UKSOS Gold Medal (Uttarakhand); AM Gokhale Award and Oration (Pune Ophthalmic Society); Dr. TN Gopinathan Menon Memorial Oration Award and Gold Medal (Cochin Ophthalmic Club); Dr. PR Mondal Memorial Oration Award (Ophthalmic Society of West Bengal); the Silver Jubilee Ishwarchandra Oration Award (Vidarbha Ophthalmic Society); Diva Eye Institute Oration (All Gujarat Ophthalmological Society); and TNOA SS Badrinath SOA SN Alumni Award of Honor. In addition, she has won more than 50 prestigious international awards for her surgical videos as well as Best Paper of Session awards on her innovations and challenging cases at prestigious international conferences in the United States and Europe.

She is President-Elect and Secretary, ISRS (International Society of Refractive Surgery); past Chair of the Multimedia Editorial Board, ISRS; Associate Editor, Journal of Refractive Surgery; Associate Editor, Journal of Refractive Surgery Case Reports; Section Editor (Refractive Surgery), EyeNet (American Academy of Ophthalmology); Executive Committee Member, ISRS; Executive Committee Member, Global Education and Research Society of Ophthalmology (GERSO); Council Board Member of GERSO (the first woman member on the GERSO council and one of the initial members who helped shape its aims and objectives); Chair of the Cornea Committee, GERSO; and is on the editorial board of Indian Journal of Ophthalmology; EyeNet (AAO); EuroTimes; IJKECD; Ocular Surgery News, Asia Pacific; Glaucoma Today; Cataract and Refractive Surgery Today, Europe; Medical Hypothesis in Optometry; the Tamil Nadu Ophthalmic Association-JOSR; and Ophthalmology and Therapy.

She conducts courses and delivers lectures at numerous national and international conferences. She has delivered keynote lectures at various international and national conferences. She has also been invited to teach her techniques and innovations, twice by the Bascom Palmer Eye Institute, Miami, USA, which is the number one ranked eye institute in the world, the Wilmer Eye Institute-Johns Hopkins University, Yale University, and also by many other hospitals, including the King Khaled Eye Specialist Hospital, Riyadh; Jules Gonin Eye Institute, Switzerland; the Sao Geraldo Hospital, Brazil, and many others. She has been the Program Director for the International Society of Refractive Surgery (ISRS) Symposium at the ESCRS, Paris 2019, as well as the Program Coordinator for the Asia-Pacific for the Refractive Surgery Program at the World Ophthalmology Congress, Cape Town 2020.

She has authored more than 130 peer-reviewed publications (bit.ly/2GfduD0), more than 200 chapters in 34 textbooks, and is editor for 17 ophthalmology textbooks and a reviewer for many prestigious journals. She has helped shape scientific sessions of important events by holding key positions, such as Program Director, ISRS Symposium, ESCRS 2019, Paris; Member, Refractive Surgery Program Committee, World Ophthalmology

Conference, 2020, Cape Town, South Africa; Executive Committee Member, GERSO; Chair, Cornea Committee GERSO, among others.

She has a special interest in cutting-edge cataract, cornea, glaucoma, complex anterior segment reconstruction, and refractive surgery. Her innovations, many of which have won international awards, include anterior segment transplantation, where cornea, sclera, artificial iris, pupil, and IOL are transplanted en bloc for anterior staphyloma; suprabrow single-stab incision ptosis surgery to enhance postoperative cosmesis; turnaround techniques for false channel dissection during Intacs implantation; the glued endo-capsular ring, glued capsular hook, and the paper clip capsule stabilizer for subluxated cataracts; stab incision glaucoma surgery (SIGS) as a guarded filtration surgery technique; contact lens-assisted crosslinking (CACXL) for safely crosslinking thin keratoconic corneas; endo-illuminator-assisted DMEK (E-DMEK), air pump-assisted PDEK, and host Descemetic scaffolding for easier and better surgical results; PrEsbyopic Allogenic Refractive Lenticule (PEARL) Inlay for treating presbyopia; corneal allogeneic intrastromal ring segment (CAIRS), customized CAIRS, and custom-shaped CAIRS for keratoconus and other corneal ectasias; the Jacob modified technique for pre-Descemetic DALK as a primary treatment for acute hydrops; sutureless SMILE lenticule-assisted resurfacing with interface tattooing for limbal dermoid; temporary pupillary scaffolding for positive vitreous pressure in penetrating keratoplasty; the white ring sign; and the sequential segmental terminal lenticular side cut dissection for safe and effective lenticule extraction in SMILE surgery. She has proposed a new classification of Descemet's membrane detachments into rhegmatogenous, tractional, bullous, and complex detachments, with a suitable treatment algorithm and a new technique of relaxing descemetotomy for bullous and tractional Descemet's detachment.

Her surgeries and surgical techniques have often been the editor's choice in prestigious international ophthalmic websites (AAO/ONE network, ISRS, Eyetube, etc.). She has two popular bimonthly columns, "Complications in Cataract and Refractive Surgery" and "Everything You Want to Know About" in the prestigious EuroTimes magazine published by ESCRS. She has her own surgical educational YouTube channel: Dr. Soosan Jacob, with more than 10,000 subscribers (goo.gl/9STje0). Her video blog, "Journey Into the Eye: A Surgeon's Video Blog," in the prestigious Ocular Surgery News, USA, and her Facebook pages also feature her surgical videos. Dr. Jacob is senior faculty for training postgraduate, fellowship, and overseas doctors.

Her life and work have been featured on the Ocular Surgery News cover page (bit.ly/2P8tWsY), "5Q" interview (the prestigious Cataract and Refractive Surgery Today (CRST): bit.ly/2DcT3Gp), "Sound Off" column (CRSToday: https://bit.ly/2VKRV3T), "One Day in the Life of…" (CRST: bit.ly/2IyBIR1; bit.ly/2UxR6yW), and "Around the World" column (MillennialEye: bit.ly/2GdmqZS), and she is also the first researcher internationally to be interviewed in the prestigious CRST "Researcher's Column" (bit.ly/2X9iKPC). In addition, her work has been featured extensively in the print version as well as through video interviews by EyeWorld, EyeNet AAO, EuroTimes, Ophthalmology Times, OSN-Healio, CRST, Glaucoma Today, Ophthalmologist, Review of Ophthalmology, and others. She is active academically on Facebook (www.facebook.com/soosan.jacob.1; www.facebook.com/drsoosanjacob/), LinkedIn (in.linkedin.com/in/soosan-jacob-b028411), Twitter (@drsoosanjacob), and Instagram (https://www.instagram.com/dr.soosanjacob/). She can be contacted at dr_soosanj@hotmail.com.

# 1 Thin Membrane Endothelial Keratoplasty (TMEK): An Introduction

Soosan Jacob

Posterior lamellar keratoplasty evolved from Deep Lamellar Endothelial Keratoplasty (DLEK) to Descemet's Stripping Endothelial Keratoplasty (DSEK), Descemet's Stripping Automated Endothelial Keratoplasty (DSAEK), and then further to the currently preferred techniques—ultra-thin DSAEK, Descemet's Membrane Endothelial Keratoplasty (DMEK), and Pre-Descemet's Endothelial Keratoplasty (PDEK) [1–3].

Of the newer and thinner grafts, DMEK [4–7] and PDEK [8–15] are somewhat similar in both appearance and graft dynamics within the anterior chamber during the stage of graft unrolling.

**Thin Membrane Endothelial Keratoplasty (TMEK)** is a new term coined by the author (SJ) to refer to endothelial keratoplasty using the ultra-thin membranous DMEK and PDEK grafts. These are composed of endothelium transferred on the Descemet's membrane (DM) alone (DMEK which is about 15 microns in thickness) or on a bed of the pre-Descemet's layer (PDL) and DM (PDEK which is about 25–30 microns thick). Though DMEK and PDEK have significant differences, they also have various similarities which allow them to be clubbed together as TMEK.

S. Jacob (✉)
Dr. Agarwal's Refractive and Cornea Foundation, Chennai, India

Dr. Agarwal's Eye Hospital and Eye Research Centre, Chennai, India

Visual recovery is fast for both DMEK and PDEK—patients gaining corneal clarity as fast as day 1 and being able to see as soon as the bubble absorbs. This is slower than DSAEK and ultra-thin DSAEK both of which take longer. The visual outcome of DMEK and PDEK is also better than DSAEK since the amount of extra tissue that is implanted is less. The induced refractive error and the hyperopic shift are therefore lesser than with DSAEK [16–19]. In a similar manner, the risk of rejection is more with DSAEK than with TMEK grafts.

Surgically, the PDEK graft and the DMEK graft behave very similar to each other in the manner in which they roll into a scroll. In both grafts, the roll is with the Descemet's side facing inwards and in both, the graft dynamics and behavior while it floats in the AC before and while being unrolled is similar. Graft loading, injection, determination of side, and unrolling are all done in the same manner for DMEK and PDEK grafts. The learning curve for both DMEK and PDEK surgery is more difficult than DSAEK though the resilient nature of the PDEK graft, its better graft handle ability and tear resistance makes it easier to perform than DMEK.

PDEK and DMEK differ from each other in some ways as well. Younger donor tissue can be used for PDEK while for DMEK, older tissue is preferred. The use of younger donor tissue can allow a higher initial endothelial cell transfer in PDEK.



S. Jacob (ed.), *Mastering DMEK and PDEK*, https://doi.org/10.1007/978-981-97-3469-6_1

Also, while the DMEK graft is flimsy and tears soon, the PDEK graft is resilient and does not tear easily. This makes DMEK surgery tougher in complex cases such as in vitrectomized eyes, deep anterior chambers, glaucoma valves, aniridia eyes, etc. whereas PDEK and DSAEK can be performed with ease in such complex eyes. In both DMEK and PDEK, however, graft loss may occur during preparation and this risk is higher than with the risk of graft loss in DSAEK.

## References


1. Jacob S. Mastering endothelial keratoplasty, vol. 1. Springer India; 2016.
2. Eye Bank Association of America. 2012 Eye banking statistical report. Washington, DC: Eye Bank Association of America; 2013.
3. Gain P, Jullienne R, et al. Global survey of corneal transplantation and eye banking. JAMA Ophthalmol. 2016;134(2):167–73.
4. Melles GR, Eggink FA, Lander F, et al. A surgical technique for posterior lamellar keratoplasty. Cornea. 1998;17:618–26.
5. Melles GRJ, Lander F, van Dooren BTH, et al. Preliminary clinical results of posterior lamellar keratoplasty through a sclerocorneal pocket incision. Ophthalmology. 2000;107:1850–7.
6. Melles GR, Ong TS, Ververs B, et al. Descemet membrane endothelial keratoplasty (DMEK). Cornea. 2006;25:987–90.
7. Melles GRJ, Ong TS, Ververs B, et al. Preliminary clinical results of Descemet membrane endothelial keratoplasty. Am J Ophthalmol. 2008;145:222–7.
8. Dua HS, et al. Human corneal anatomy redefined. A novel pre-Descemet's layer (Dua's layer). Ophthalmology. 2013;120(9):P1778–85.
9. Dua HS, Said DG. Clinical evidence of the pre-Descemets layer (Dua's layer) in corneal pathology. Eye (Lond). 2016;30(8):1144–5.
10. Agarwal A, Dua HS, Jacob S, et al. Pre-Descemet's endothelial keratoplasty (PDEK). Br J Ophthalmol. 2014;98(9):1181–5.
11. Tsatsos M, Mironidou M, Jacob S, et al. Factors influencing corneal predescemetic endothelial keratoplasty (PDEK) graft creation: It's all in a bubble. Hell J Nucl Med. 2019;22(Suppl 2):42–6.
12. Agarwal A, et al. Young donor-graft assisted endothelial keratoplasty (PDEK/DMEK) with epithelial debridement for chronic pseudophakic bullous keratopathy. Can J Ophthalmol. 2017;52(5):519–26.
13. Jacob S, Agarwal A, et al. Endoilluminator-assisted transcorneal illumination for Descemet membrane endothelial keratoplasty: enhanced intraoperative visualization of the graft in corneal decompensation secondary to pseudophakic bullous keratopathy. J Cataract Refract Surg. 2014;40(8):1332–6.
14. Jacob S, et al. Air pump-assisted graft centration, graft edge unfolding, and graft Uncreasing in young donor graft pre-Descemet endothelial Keratoplasty. Cornea. 2017;36(8):1009–13.
15. Jacob S, et al. Native means of graft stabilization: host descemetic scaffolding and wound scaffolding to decrease the risk for graft detachment in DMEK and PDEK. J Cataract Refract Surg. 2019;45(8):1059–63.
16. Price FW Jr, Price MO. Descemet's stripping with endothelial keratoplasty in 50 eyes: a refractive neutral corneal transplant. J Refract Surg. 2005;21:339–45.
17. Gorovoy MS. Descemet-stripping automated endothelial keratoplasty. Cornea. 2006;25:886–9.
18. Lee WB, Jacobs DS, Musch DC, et al. Descemet's stripping endothelial keratoplasty: safety and outcomes. A report by the American Academy of Ophthalmology. Ophthalmology. 2009;116:1818–30.
19. Daoud YJ, Munro AD, Delmonte DD, et al. Effect of cornea donor graft thickness on the outcome of Descemet stripping automated endothelial keratoplasty surgery. Am J Ophthalmol. 2013;156(5):860–6.

# 2 History of Lamellar Keratoplasty

Sujatha Mohan and Bina John

## 2.1 Early History of Corneal Transplantation

The history of corneal transplantation can be traced as far back as the second century AD when the Greek physician Galen (130–200 AD) proposed abrasio cor'naea (precursor of superficial keratectomy) as a means of restoring corneal transparency [1]. From then to the seventeenth century can be called "the Dark Ages" of corneal transplantation when there were no reports regarding any significant progress as far as corneal experimentation and research are concerned. In the eighteenth century, the French surgeon Guillame Pellier de Quengsy published a monograph where he suggested that an opaque cornea could be replaced by a transparent material to restore vision [2].

The blinding Egyptian Ophthalmia (trachoma) of the early nineteenth century led to experiments with corneal transplantation from the initial work of Samuel Bigger who did the first successful allograft in a pet gazelle in the year 1837 [3] and Richard Kissam who replaced a young Irishman's opaque cornea with a xenograft from a pig in the year 1838 [4]. The rest of the nineteenth century saw divided opinions among ophthalmologists between those who favored allografts to xenografts and between lamellar and full-thickness keratoplasties.

The first successful human allograft transplantation was performed in 1905 by Edward Zirm who transplanted a donor cornea from the enucleated eye of an 11 year old with penetrating injury to a patient with bilateral alkali burns [5]. The Russian ophthalmologist Vladimir Filatov (1875–1956) was the first to suggest the use of cadaver eyes for corneal transplants [6].

Penetrating keratoplasty (PKP) has been the gold standard for corneal transplantation from then till the end of the twentieth century. But, PKP with its attendant problems of intraoperative complications secondary to the open sky technique and postoperative problems including glaucoma, uveitis, cataract, cystoid macular edema (CME), surface irregularity, and astigmatism led to research into a suitable alternative to PKP, leading to the beginnings of lamellar keratoplasty which is now slowly replacing PKP as the surgery of choice in patients with corneal opacities (Figs. 2.1 and 2.2).

S. Mohan (✉) · B. John
Rajan Eye Care Hospital Pvt Ltd, Chennai, India


S. Jacob (ed.), *Mastering DMEK and PDEK*, https://doi.org/10.1007/978-981-97-3469-6_2

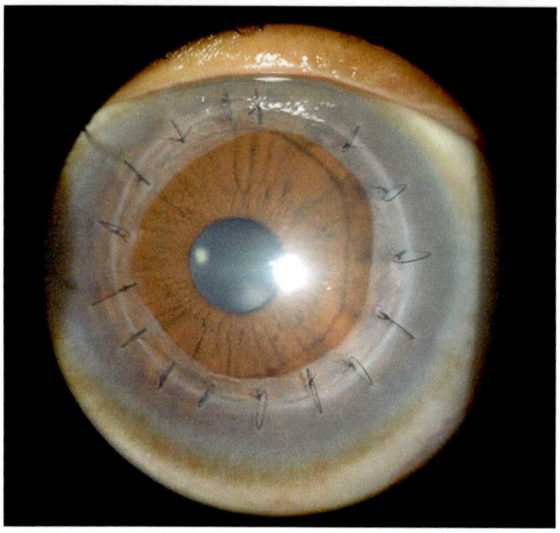

Fig. 2.1 Full-thickness penetrating keratoplasty. (Fig Courtesy Dr. Soosan Jacob, Dr. Agarwal's Eye Hospital, Chennai, India)

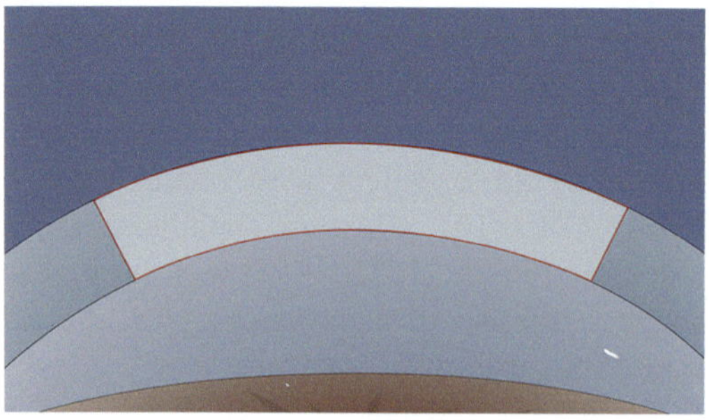

Fig. 2.2 Penetrating keratoplasty: illustration showing a full-thickness donor graft used to replace a full-thickness trephination from the host cornea. (Fig Courtesy Dr. Soosan Jacob, Dr. Agarwal's Eye Hospital, Chennai, India)

## 2.2 Lamellar Keratoplasty (LK)

Lamellar keratoplasty where selective transplantation of diseased layers of the cornea is done while retaining healthy tissue can be either anterior or posterior lamellar keratoplasty in which either the anterior or posterior corneal layers are transplanted depending on the site of corneal pathology.

### 2.2.1 Anterior Lamellar Keratoplasty

Anterior lamellar keratoplasty (ALK) involves removal of diseased corneal tissue leaving behind healthy stroma, Descemet's membrane

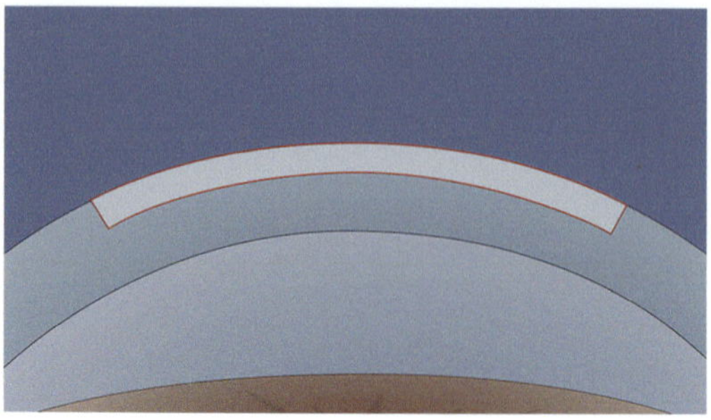

Fig. 2.3 Superficial anterior lamellar keratoplasty (SALK): illustration showing a SALK graft used to replace the affected anterior 30–50% of the host cornea. (Fig Courtesy Dr. Soosan Jacob, Dr. Agarwal's Eye Hospital, Chennai, India)

(DM), or endothelium. ALK is indicated for disorders with a healthy endothelium such as keratoconus (KC), superficial scars, and anterior corneal dystrophies. Anterior lamellar keratoplasty can be superficial anterior lamellar keratoplasty (SALK) or deep anterior lamellar keratoplasty (DALK).

**SALK:** Performed when the anterior 30–50% of the cornea is affected and replaced with a similar amount of donor tissue. Stroma-to-stroma interface may however lead to degradation of visual acuity over time (Fig. 2.3) [7].

**DALK:** In DALK where the recipient cornea is dissected into the DM, the stroma-DM interface is reported to have better visual results (Figs. 2.4 and 2.5) [8, 9].

ALK has several advantages over PK in that donor corneal requirements are not as stringent as for PK [10], endothelial graft rejection is eliminated [11], suture removal and discontinuation of topical steroids can be done earlier and it also avoids the complications of an intraocular procedure [12]. Comparing PK with modern ALK did not see much difference with respect to post op refractive error and BCVA if residual stromal bed is minimal but intra op complications like DM perforation forcing a conversion to PK, incomplete or irregular dissection, increased surgical time due to technical challenges and post op complications like interface haze, interface neovascularization, and pupillary block are some of the complications associated with LK [12].

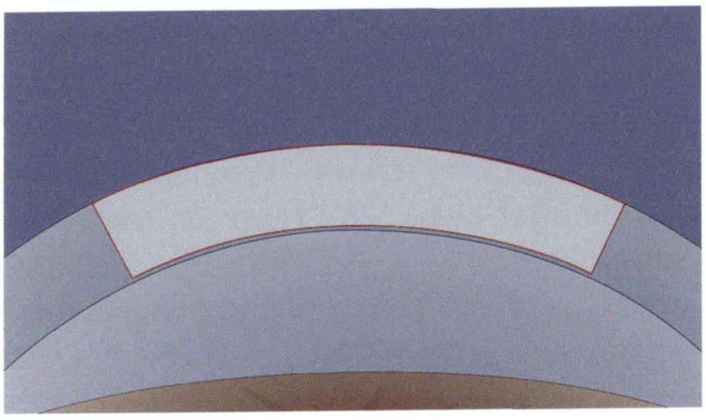

**Fig. 2.4** Deep anterior lamellar keratoplasty: illustration showing the recipient cornea dissected up to the pre-Descemet's layer and replaced with a donor graft stripped of Descemet's membrane. (Fig Courtesy Dr. Soosan Jacob, Dr. Agarwal's Eye Hospital, Chennai, India)

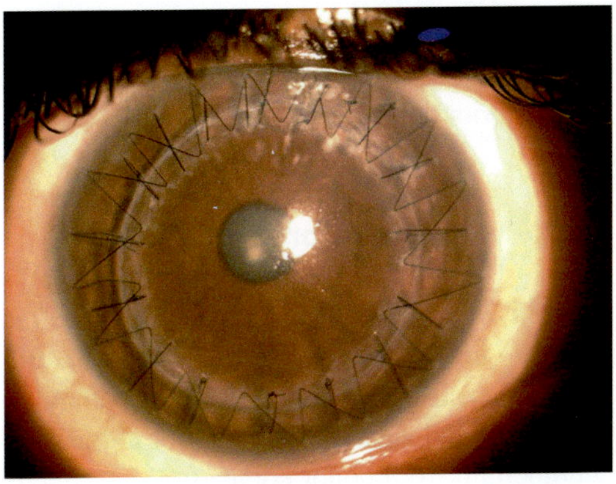

**Fig. 2.5** Deep anterior lamellar keratoplasty (DALK): post-operative slit lamp image of a DALK graft. (Fig Courtesy Dr. Soosan Jacob, Dr. Agarwal's Eye Hospital, Chennai, India)

### 2.2.2 Posterior Lamellar Keratoplasty

Posterior lamellar keratoplasty involves replacing the host's endothelium with healthy donor tissue in patients affected by Fuchs endothelial dystrophy (Fig. 2.6), aphakic or pseudophakic bullous keratopathy.

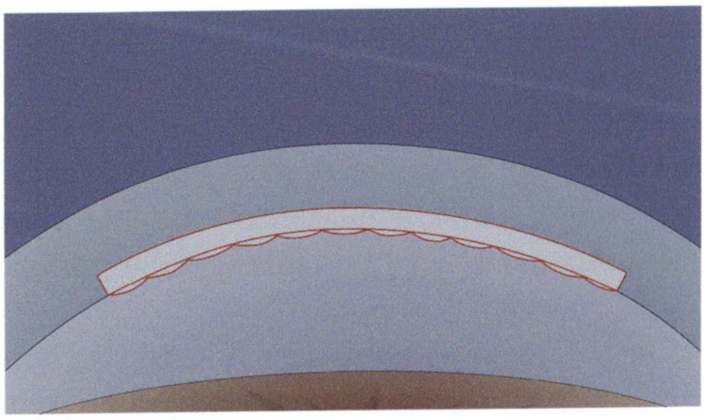

**Fig. 2.6** Posterior lamellar keratoplasty: illustration showing placement of a self-adherent sutureless 6 mm donor graft after excising a 6 mm posterior corneal stromal disc from the central posterior lamella. (Fig Courtesy Dr. Soosan Jacob, Dr. Agarwal's Eye Hospital, Chennai, India)

## 2.3 Early History of Lamellar Keratoplasty

The German professor Arthur Von Hippel (1841–1916) advocated lamellar xenografts as far back as the end of the nineteenth century [1]. Von Hippel in 1877 used a trephine to prepare a human donor corneal graft of the same size and shape as the defect in the recipient cornea, which was left sutureless and kept in place only by pressure of the eyelids [13]. Eleven years later von Hippel presented his new technique of circumscribed lamellar keratoplasty where he replaced a partial thickness disc of the host's leucomatous cornea with a full-thickness xenograft from a dog. Hippel claimed that this technique which was easier to perform than full-thickness keratoplasty and where complications of vitreous loss and displacement of other intraocular structures such as the lens was less when compared to full-thickness procedures resulted in complete healing at the end of 3 weeks with improvement in vision [13]. His outstanding experimental and clinical work showed that corneal endothelium and Descemet's membrane should remain intact if a corneal graft has to succeed. Experiments in which partial thickness of the cornea was removed with a clockwork mechanical trephine and replaced with a full-thickness donor graft were attempted with good results as far back as the late nineteenth century.

In 1892, Fuchs reported on 30 lamellar grafts from rabbits, dogs, and human eyes with disappointing results [14]. Further modifications of lamellar keratoplasty were published in 1908 by Plange, who inserted oval full-thickness corneal grafts, like the face of a watch, into a corneal stromal pocket and in 1910 by Lohlein, who used conjunctival flaps of the donor for securing a full-thickness corneal transplant [13]. The mid-twentieth century saw a revival of lamellar keratoplasty with better clinical results from many corneal surgeons around the world including Barraquer in Columbia, Arruga in Spain, Rycroft in England, and Franceschetti in Switzerland [15].

LK has evolved over time with attempts [16–27] to achieve precision of depth and smoothness of both donor and recipient tissue to facilitate a smooth interface and optimize visual outcomes with the help of automation and sophisticated microsurgical instruments. The technical difficulties of LK and the suboptimal visual outcomes when compared to PK have led to numerous innovations in technique to overcome these draw backs. Lamellar corneal surgeries have undergone considerable evolution from the initial surgical attempts and the history of anterior and posterior lamellar keratoplasties will be discussed separately.

## 2.4 History of Posterior Lamellar Keratoplasty

Over the past few decades, the concept of selective replacement of the posterior cornea has transformed corneal transplantation. PK which was the standard of care for posterior corneal pathology has been replaced by endothelial keratoplasty (EK) due to the advantages which EK offers. These include minimal changes of the corneal surface with less induced astigmatism promoting rapid visual recovery, prevention of the potential complications of open sky surgery, preservation of corneal sensation, and a tectonically stronger globe [28]. However, one of the drawbacks of EK is the endothelial cell loss which occurs during donor preparation, insertion, and attachment [29]. There has been a constant evolution of techniques to minimize the endothelial cell loss and provide long-term visual clarity to the graft.

## 2.5 History of Endothelial Keratoplasty

There have been 2 approaches to EK, an anterior and posterior approach.

### 2.5.1 Anterior Approach

First EK was performed by Charles Tillet in 1956 [30] who made a partial thickness posterior stromal flap, excised the central recipient pathological cornea and sutured the posterior cornea and endothelium from donor cornea to the recipient. Results were however not successful due to endothelial damage and poor donor recipient adhesion.

Innovations to the anterior approach included a scleral–limbal approach to EK, first described by Ko et al. in animal studies 1993 which preserved the integrity of the corneal surface but used sutures to attach the posterior graft [31] and a microkeratome used by Barraquer [32] to create a hinged anterior flap. The anterior corneal approach did not however gain wide acceptance due to altered corneal topography related to use of sutures and flap problems.

### 2.5.2 Posterior Approach

**Posterior Lamellar Keratoplasty**: The current success of EK is due to the pioneering work of Melles in the late 1990s [33] after his experiments with cat, monkey, and cadaver eyes. He introduced the concept of a self-adherent sutureless 6 mm donor graft introduced through an 8 mm limbal incision after excising a 6 mm posterior corneal stromal disc from the central posterior lamella using a flat trephine and scissors, followed by placement of an air bubble into the AC which facilitated adherence of the graft to the host cornea. The limbal incision and absence of surface sutures allowed rapid visual recovery with normal topography and good tectonic strength.

**Deep Lamellar Endothelial Keratoplasty**: In 1999, Terry modified the technique with the help of an artificial anterior chamber which allowed use of donor sclerocorneal buttons rather than whole globes and also use of cohesive viscoelastics to help in recipient tissue resection and donor endothelial cell protection which he named as deep lamellar endothelial keratoplasty(DLEK) [34]. The 8-mm incisions were then reduced to 5 mm to help decrease astigmatism which required folding of the donor lenticule but both PLK and DLEK did not gain popularity due to the extensive manual lamellar dissection required for both donor lenticule and posterior corneal tissue removal (Fig. 2.7).

**Descemet's Stripping Endothelial Keratoplasty (DSEK)**: Melles introduced Descemetorhexis in 2004 [35], which involved stripping of the DM from the recipient which made the posterior lamellar dissection easier and faster to do allowing a smoother recipient bed. The term DSEK was coined by Price after modifications to the procedure [36]. This decreases the possibility of complications in the recipient like anterior perforation and premature posterior perforation. One of the main drawbacks of DSEK is an increased dislocation rate compared with PLK due to the smoother interface. In DSEK, the lamellar dissection of the donor tissue is performed manually which gives rise to inconsistent depth dissection.

**Descemets Stripping Automated Endothelial Keratoplasty (DSAEK)**: Microkeratome for automated smooth resection of the donor cornea in order to ensure a smooth interface introduced by Gorovoy paved the way for DSAEK [37]. It reduces the risk of perforation and is more consistent and easier to do. DSAEK was however associated with the complications of primary graft failure and dislocation of the donor tissue (Figs. 2.8 and 2.9).

**Descemet's Membrane Endothelial Keratoplasty (DMEK)**: DMEK was introduced in 2006 by Melles [38] where only the DM and endothelial cells are transplanted and has come a long way in a few short years despite initial concerns about its technical difficulty. The perceived advantages of DMEK include faster rehabilitation and precise anatomic reconstruc-

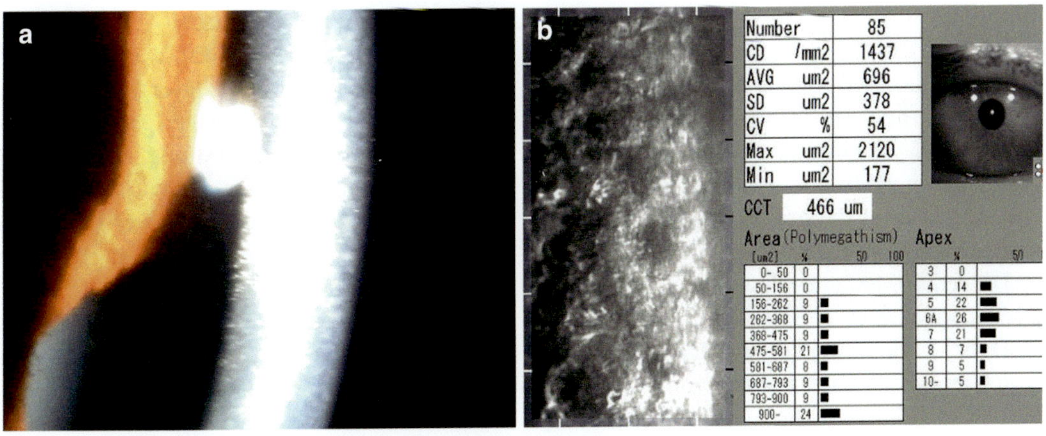


**Fig. 2.7** (**a**) Slit lamp image showing altered specular reflex in a patient with Fuch's dystrophy; (**b**) a quantitative as well as qualitative decline seen on specular microscopy in the same patient. (Fig Courtesy Dr. Soosan Jacob, Dr. Agarwal's Eye Hospital, Chennai, India)

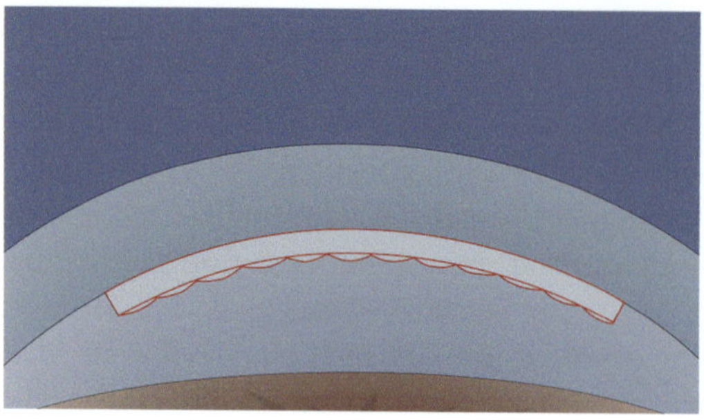

**Fig. 2.8** Descemet's stripping automated endothelial keratoplasty (DSAEK): illustration showing a donor graft consisting of stroma, Descemet's membrane, and endothelium created with an automated microkeratome transplanted on to the recipient cornea after stripping the host Descemet's membrane. (Fig Courtesy Dr. Soosan Jacob, Dr. Agarwal's Eye Hospital, Chennai, India)

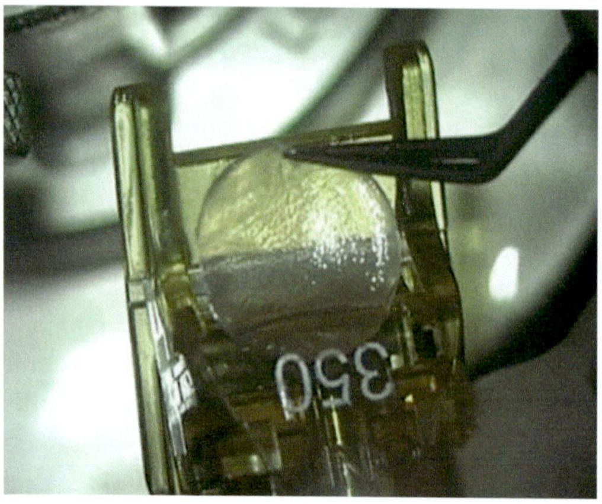

**Fig. 2.9** Descemet's stripping automated endothelial keratoplasty (DSAEK): creation of a DSAEK graft. (Fig Courtesy Dr. Soosan Jacob, Dr. Agarwal's Eye Hospital, Chennai, India)

tion of the diseased cornea, decreased incidence of rejection, and steroid induced OHT since the patients can be weaned off steroids earlier. Challenge in DMEK is donor manipulation in the AC to unroll the graft and position it correctly (Figs. 2.10 and 2.11).

**DMAEK**: McCauley described a variation of DMEK which uses a microkeratome [39].

**Hybrid variation of DMEK—DMEK-S** which retains an outer rim of stroma with bare DM in the center of the donor, described by Studeny [40] combines the visual benefits of DMEK with the ease of tissue handling of DSEK.

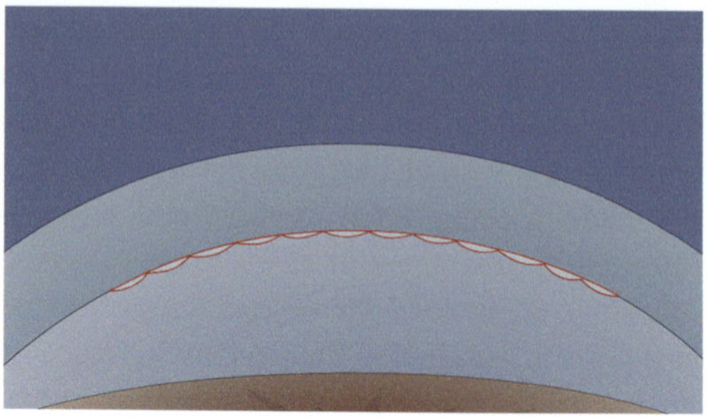

**Fig. 2.10** Descemet's membrane endothelial keratoplasty: illustration showing the recipient cornea stripped of DM. Donor tissue consisting of DM with endothelial cells is transplanted. (Fig Courtesy Dr. Soosan Jacob, Dr. Agarwal's Eye Hospital, Chennai, India)

**Ultra-thin DSAEK** using a double pass cut with the microkeratome. It refers to grafts between 40 and 100 microns thick, thereby acting as a bridge between DSAEK and DMEK.

**Discovery of the Pre-Descemet's Layer or Dua's Layer**: Dua et al. in (2013) proposed the existence of a new fourth layer of the cornea that had not been previously described [41]. This lies between the corneal stroma and the Descemet's membrane and is a tough layer that is impervious to air. It was detected during experiments injecting air into donor corneo-scleral rims which resulted in formation of three types of big bubbles—Types 1, 2, and 3. Though controversial at the time, the pre-Descemet's layer has led to the description of the pre-Descemet's endothelial keratoplasty (PDEK).

**PDEK (Pre-Descemet's Endothelial Keratoplasty)**: In PDEK [42], a composite of pre-Descemet's layer (Dua's layer) with the DM and endothelium is transplanted subsequent to removal of the recipients DM ***and*** also provides near anatomical restoration without any induced refraction and offers advantages over DMEK in tissue handling and unfolding in the eye (Figs. 2.12 and 2.13).

**DMET (Descemet's Membrane Endothelial Transfer)**: DMET [43] involves performing a usual 9 mm Descemetorhexis followed by injection of the Descemet's membrane into the anterior chamber. The scroll is anchored at one end to the incision, and the rest is left free floating. The suggested mechanism of action of the sur-

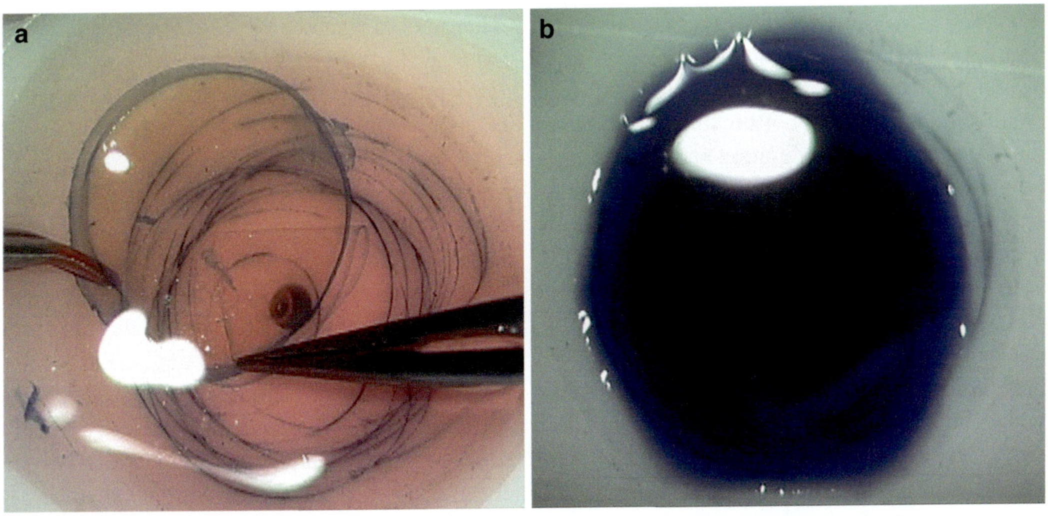


**Fig. 2.11** Descemet's membrane endothelial keratoplasty: (**a**) DMEK graft stripped from a punched out donor cornea; (**b**) the graft is stained with Trypan blue. (Fig Courtesy Dr. Soosan Jacob, Dr. Agarwal's Eye Hospital, Chennai, India)

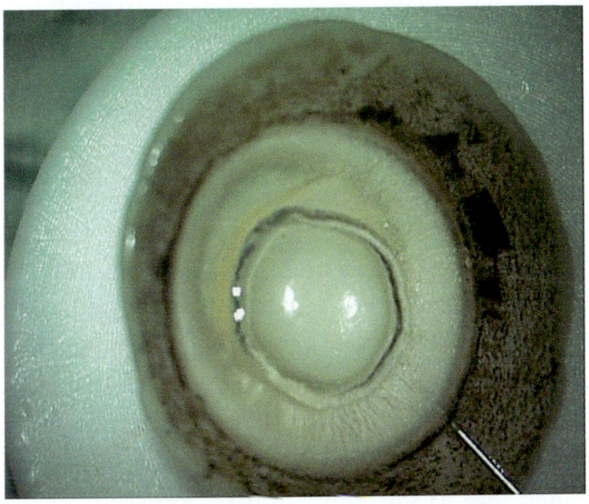

**Fig. 2.12** Pre-Descemet's endothelial keratoplasty: PDEK graft is seen. (Fig Courtesy Dr. Soosan Jacob, Dr. Agarwal's Eye Hospital, Chennai, India)

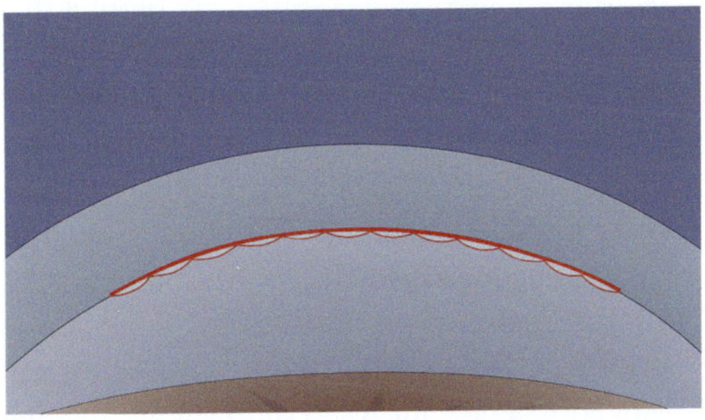

**Fig. 2.13** Pre-Descemet's endothelial keratoplasty (PDEK): illustration showing a composite of pre-Descemet's layer (Dua's layer), Descemet's membrane and endothelium transplanted after stripping Descemet's membrane—endothelium complex from the host. (Fig Courtesy Dr. Soosan Jacob, Dr. Agarwal's Eye Hospital, Chennai, India)

gery is that an area of contact between the host stroma and the implanted Descemet's membrane is sufficient to regain corneal clarity as it this is thought to stimulate host peripheral endothelial cells. Corneal clarity is thought to be finally regained from endothelial cell migration and proliferation of both donor and host endothelial cells. The surgery is therefore much simpler and faster as there is no need for unrolling, centering or floating up the graft. The absence of air tamponade also decreases complications such as pupillary block.

**DWEK (Descemetorhexis Without Endothelial Keratoplasty) or DSO (Descemet's Stripping Only)**: This procedure is done for Fuch's endothelial dystrophy and creates a central, circular Descemetorhexis of about 4 mm in size using a reverse Sinskey hook [44]. The central DM is then peeled away. This removes central guttata. The central corneal edema then resolves with time secondary to migration and regeneration of peripheral endothelial cells. The removal of guttata by itself can result in a decrease in light scatter, improved contrast sensitivity and visual acuity in these patients. It also does away with complications such as graft rejection, graft failure, graft dislocation, and graft availability if the procedure is combined with endothelial keratoplasty. Rho kinase inhibitors may be added to help migration and proliferation of endothelial cells. Delayed clearance of edema may force a subsequent surgery with endothelial transplantation.

**Quarter Descemet's Membrane Endothelial Keratoplasty**: Quarter DMEK [45] shares one donor cornea between four recipient eyes. This helps widen the donor pool, especially in places where donor cornea of high quality is in short supply. It also decreases the antigenic load transferred, thereby decreasing the risk of rejection. The graft is quadrisected to get four pie shaped smaller grafts. Surgery is however more difficult as it requires more time and patience by the surgeon to get it apposed as desired. By putting in a graft, albeit smaller, it allows rapid regaining of corneal clarity and thereby visual acuity and hence has advantages of DMEK. It also combines advantages of DSO by harnessing host peripheral endothelial cell migration. The host peripheral endothelial cell stimulation action of DMET may also be playing a role.

**Multiple Recipients from One Cornea**: Donor corneas are always in short supply, and the demand always far exceeds the availability. Customized component corneal transplantation involves the use of one donor cornea for multiple recipients. A DMEK or PDEK graft can be prepared from the posterior layers while the anterior layers of the donor cornea are used for lamellar keratoplasty. The stem cells may also be harvested for stem cell transplantation and the scleral rim for patch grafts. This is valuable in increasing the utilization of donor corneas and increasing utilization of high-quality tissues [46–48].

## 2.6 Techniques

**Air pump-assisted PDEK and E-PDEK or E-DMEK**: The air pump-assisted PDEK technique [49] was described by Soosan Jacob and uses pressurized air infusion for various steps of PDEK surgery. This is done with the help of an anterior chamber maintainer (ACM) which is connected to a source of pressurized air infusion (such as the fluid gas exchange system in vitrectomy machines) that is inserted into the anterior chamber to fill it with air. There are numerous advantages of using the pressurized air such as aiding descemetorhexis, arresting bleeding from synechiolysis or from the iris, promoting graft adhesion, unfolding graft edges, and helping in Host Descemetic scaffolding. It also helps maintain the depth of the AC intraoperatively and prevent graft damage from instrument touch.

The E-PDEK or E-DMEK technique [50] was also started by Soosan Jacob and is especially useful for determining graft orientation within the injector and inside the anterior chamber. It thus helps in confirming that the correct side of the graft is facing upwards.

**Host Descemetic Scaffolding**: Again, started by Soosan Jacob, this utilizes the peripheral rim of host Descemet's membrane to help scaffold the DMEK or PDEK graft in place. It thereby helps decrease the risk of graft detachment in high-risk cases. It may also be used in regular cases by beginner surgeons.

**Femtosecond EK**: Several studies in vitro and animal models have tried femtosecond laser for the lamellar cuts but the deep lamellar ablations are not as smooth as after Lasik flaps and the development of concentric rings in the dissection bed caused by compression of the cornea when applanated and pebbly contour to the dissection plane due to the loose fibrillar structure of the deep corneal stroma are further drawbacks which have led to disappointing results with the femtolaser for EK when compared to PK [51].

**Donor Insertion Techniques**: Insertion techniques like donor preparation techniques are continually evolving in order to decrease the endothelial cell loss and ensure ease of donor insertion. The various insertion techniques include [28]:

1. Forceps: Taco with 60/40 overfold, trifold, 40/60 underfold.
2. Glides: Busin, Sheets, Tan endoglide.
3. Inserters: Mechanical, closed chamber injector systems with a variety of mechanisms to fold retract and inject the donor tissue into the eye.

## 2.7 Objectives of an Ideal EK Procedure

Terry et al. [34] proposed certain objectives of an ideal EK procedure. These include smooth postoperative corneal surface with no significant change in astigmatism between pre and post op.

1. Healthy donor endothelium to resolve all corneal edema.
2. Highly predictable and stable refractive power.
3. Tectonically stable globe, free from injury and infection.
4. Optically clear cornea.
5. The procedure should be technically easy to perform.

First 4 objectives are readily achieved, and evolution of the technique may help in achieving an optically clear cornea with a technically easy surgical procedure.

EK represents a paradigm shift in corneal endothelial replacement with techniques continually evolving to provide faster and better visual recovery.

Lamellar keratoplasties have now replaced penetrating keratoplasties as the standard of care in corneal transplantation with ongoing research being directed to provide the best visual results to the patient.

**Financial Disclosure** The authors do not have any financial enclosure.

## References

1. Moffatt SL, Cartwright VA, Stumpf TH. Centennial review of corneal transplantation. Clin Exp Ophthalmol. 2005;33(6):642–57. https://doi.org/10.1111/j.1442-9071.2005.01134.x.
2. de Quengsy GP. Précis ou cours d'opérations sur la chirurgie des yeux. Paris: Didot; 1789.
3. Bigger SLL. An inquiry into the possibility of transplanting the cornea, with the view of relieving blindness (hitherto deemed incurable) caused by several diseases of that structure. Dublin J Med Sci. 1837;11(3):408–17.
4. Kissam R. Ceratoplastics in man. New York J Med. 1844;2:281–2.
5. Zirm E. Eine erfolgreiche totale Keratoplastik. Albr von Græfe's Arch für Ophthalmol. 1906;64(3):580–93.
6. Filatov VP. Transplantation of the cornea from preserved cadavers' eyes. Lancet. 1937;229(5937):1395–7.
7. Krumeich JH, Schoner P, Lubatschowski H, Gerten G, Kermani O. Excimer laser treatment in deep lamellar keratoplasty 100 micrometer over Descemet's membrane. Ophthalmologe. 2002;99(12):946–8. https://doi.org/10.1007/s00347-002-0670-5.
8. Hafezi F, Mrochen M, Fankhauser F 2nd, Seiler T. Anterior lamellar keratoplasty with a microkeratome: a method for managing complications after refractive surgery. J Refract Surg. 2003;19(1):52–7.
9. Price FW Jr. Air lamellar keratoplasty. Refract Corneal Surg. 1989;5:240–3.
10. Shimazaki J. The evolution of lamellar keratoplasty. Curr Opin Ophthalmol. 2000;11(4):217–23. https://doi.org/10.1097/00055735-200008000-00002.
11. Terry MA. The evolution of lamellar grafting techniques over 25 years. Cornea. 2000;19(5):611–6. https://doi.org/10.1097/00003226-200009000-00006.
12. Reinhart WJ, Musch DC, Jacobs DS, Lee WB, Kaufman SC, Shtein RM. Deep anterior lamellar keratoplasty as an alternative to penetrating keratoplasty: a report by the American Academy of Ophthalmology. Ophthalmology. 2011;118(1):209–18. https://doi.org/10.1016/j.ophtha.2010.11.002.
13. Forrester JV. Corneal transplantation. Imperial College Press; 2003.
14. Trevor-Roper PD. The history of corneal grafting. London: Butterworth; 1972.
15. Arenas E, Esquenazi S, Anwar M, Terry M. Lamellar corneal transplantation. Surv Ophthalmol. 2012;57(6):510–29. https://doi.org/10.1016/j.survophthal.2012.01.009.
16. Anwar M, Teichmann KD. Planned near-Descemet's dissection in deep lamellar keratoplasty, using air and fluid. In: Surgical techniques in anterior and posterior lamellar corneal surgery. New Delhi: Jaypee Brothers; 2006. p. 126–33.
17. Barraquer J. Queratomileusis para la correccion de la miopia. Arch Soc Am Oftalmol Optom. 1964;5:27–8.
18. Sugita J, Kondo J. Deep lamellar keratoplasty with complete removal of pathological stroma for vision improvement. Br J Ophthalmol. 1997;81(3):184. https://doi.org/10.1136/bjo.81.3.184.
19. Anwar M. Dissection technique in lamellar keratoplasty. Br J Ophthalmol. 1972;56(9):711–3.
20. Archila EA. Deep lamellar keratoplasty dissection of host tissue with intrastromal air injection. Cornea. 1984;3(3):217–8. http://www.ncbi.nlm.nih.gov/pubmed/6399886.
21. Manche EE, Holland GN, Maloney RK. Deep lamellar keratoplasty using viscoelastic dissection. Arch Ophthalmol. 1999;117(11):1561–5. https://doi.org/10.1001/archopht.117.11.1561.

22. Melles GR, Remeijer L, Geerards AJ, Beekhuis WH. A quick surgical technique for deep, anterior lamellar keratoplasty using visco-dissection. Cornea. 2000;19(4):427–32. https://doi.org/10.1097/00003226-200007000-00004.
23. Melles GR, Rietveld FJ, Beekhuis WH, Binder PS. A technique to visualize corneal incision and lamellar dissection depth during surgery. Cornea. 1999;18(1):80–6.
24. Anwar M. Technique in lamellar keratoplasty. Trans Ophthalmol Soc UK. 1974;94:163–71.
25. Suwan-Apichon O, Reyes JMG, Griffin NB, Barker J, Gore P, Chuck RS. Microkeratome versus femtosecond laser predissection of corneal grafts for anterior and posterior lamellar keratoplasty. Cornea. 2006;25(8):966–8. https://doi.org/10.1097/01.ico.0000226360.34301.29.
26. Azar DT. A new surgical technique of microkeratome-assisted deep lamellar keratoplasty with a hinged flap. Arch Ophthalmol. 2000;118(8):1112.
27. Tan DTH, Mehta JS. Future directions in lamellar corneal transplantation. Cornea. 2007;26(9 Suppl 1):S21–8. https://doi.org/10.1097/ICO.0b013e31812f685c.
28. Anshu A, Price MO, Tan DTH, Price FW. Endothelial keratoplasty: a revolution in evolution. Surv Ophthalmol. 2012;57(3):236–52. https://doi.org/10.1016/j.survophthal.2011.10.005.
29. Daneshgar F. Review of posterior lamellar keratoplasty techniques. J Transplant Technol Res. 2013;1:S2.
30. Tillett CW. Posterior lamellar keratoplasty. Am J Ophthalmol. 1956;41(3):530–3.
31. Ko W, Freuh B, Shield C, et al. Experimental posterior lamellar transplantation of the rabbit cornea (ARVO abstract). Invest Ophthalmol Vis Sci. 1993;34:1102.
32. Barraquer JI Jr. The technique for penetrating keratoplasty. In: Microsurgery of the cornea. Barcelona: Scriba; 1984. p. 289–94.
33. Melles GR, Eggink FA, Lander F, et al. A surgical technique for posterior lamellar keratoplasty. Cornea. 1998;17(6):618–26. https://doi.org/10.1097/00003226-199811000-00010.
34. Terry MA. Deep lamellar endothelial keratoplasty (DLEK): pursuing the ideal goals of endothelial replacement. Eye. 2003;17(8):982–8.
35. Melles GRJ, Wijdh RHJ, Nieuwendaal CP. A technique to excise the descemet membrane from a recipient cornea (descemetorhexis). Cornea. 2004;23(3):286–8. https://doi.org/10.1097/00003226-200404000-00011.
36. Price FW Jr, Price MO. Descemet's stripping with endothelial keratoplasty in 50 eyes: a refractive neutral corneal transplant. J Refract Surg. 2005;21(4):339–45.
37. Gorovoy MS. Descemet-stripping automated endothelial keratoplasty. Cornea. 2006;25(8):886–9. https://doi.org/10.1097/01.ico.0000214224.90743.01.
38. Melles GRJ, Lander F, Rietveld FJR. Transplantation of Descemet's membrane carrying viable endothelium through a small scleral incision. Cornea. 2002;21(4):415–8. https://doi.org/10.1097/00003226-200211000-00025.
39. McCauley MB, Price FW, Price MO. Descemet membrane automated endothelial keratoplasty. Hybrid technique combining DSAEK stability with DMEK visual results. J Cataract Refract Surg. 2009;35(10):1659–64. https://doi.org/10.1016/j.jcrs.2009.05.034.
40. Studeny P, Farkas A, Vokrojova M, Liskova P, Jirsova K. Descemet membrane endothelial keratoplasty with a stromal rim (DMEK-S). Br J Ophthalmol. 2010;94(7):909–14. https://doi.org/10.1136/bjo.2009.165134.
41. Dua HS, Faraj LA, Said DG, Gray T, Lowe J. Human corneal anatomy redefined: a novel pre-Descemet's layer (Dua's layer). Ophthalmology. 2013;120(9):1778–85.
42. Agarwal AAA, Dua HS, Narang P, et al. Pre-Descemet's endothelial keratoplasty (PDEK). Br J Ophthalmol. 2014;98(9):1181–5. https://doi.org/10.1136/bjophthalmol-2013-304639.
43. Lam FC, Bruinsma M, Melles GR. Descemet membrane endothelial transfer. Curr Opin Ophthalmol. 2014;25(4):353–7.
44. Iovieno A, Neri A, Soldani AM, Adani C, Fontana L. Descemetorhexis without graft placement for the treatment of Fuchs endothelial dystrophy: preliminary results and review of the literature. Cornea. 2017;36(6):637–41.
45. Zygoura V, Baydoun L, Ham L, Bourgonje VJ, van Dijk K, Lie JT, Dapena I, Oellerich S, Melles GR. Quarter-Descemet membrane endothelial keratoplasty (Quarter-DMEK) for Fuchs endothelial corneal dystrophy: 6 months clinical outcome. Br J Ophthalmol. 2018;102(10):1425–30.
46. Gadhvi KA, Coco G, Pagano L, Kaye SB, Ferrari S, Levis HJ, Parekh M, Romano V. Eye banking: one cornea for multiple recipients. Cornea. 2020;39(12):1599–603.
47. Siddharthan KS, Agrawal A, Reddy JK. Four in one: four recipients with a single donor tissue—a novel concept for eye transplantation surgery post-COVID-19. Indian J Ophthalmol. 2020;68(11):2471–4.
48. Vajpayee RB, Sharma N, Jhanji V, Titiyal JS, Tandon R. One donor cornea for 3 recipients: a new concept for corneal transplantation surgery. Arch Ophthalmol. 2007;125(4):552–4.

49. Jacob S. Use of pressurized air infusion for pre Descemet's endothelial keratoplasty (PDEK)—the air pump assisted PDEK technique. Open Ophthalmol J. 2018;12:175–80. https://doi.org/10.2174/1874364101812010175.
50. Jacob S, Agarwal A, Agarwal A, Narasimhan S, Kumar DA, Sivagnanam S. Endoilluminator-assisted transcorneal illumination for Descemet membrane endothelial keratoplasty: enhanced intraoperative visualization of the graft in corneal decompensation secondary to pseudophakic bullous keratopathy. J Cataract Refract Surg. 2014;40(8):1332–6. https://doi.org/10.1016/j.jcrs.2014.06.019. PMID: 25088633.
51. Cheng YYY, Schouten JSAG, Tahzib NG, et al. Efficacy and safety of femtosecond laser-assisted corneal endothelial keratoplasty: a randomized multicenter clinical trial. Transplantation. 2009;88(11):1294–302. https://doi.org/10.1097/TP.0b013e3181bc419c.

# 3 Evaluation of the Patient and Decision-Making: Posterior Lamellar Versus Penetrating Keratoplasty

Michael Tsatsos

Endothelial keratoplasty has revolutionized the treatment of corneal endothelial dysfunction as it leads to faster visual rehabilitation whilst maintaining the corneal architecture. Whilst DS(A)EK [Descement Stripping (Automated) Endothelial Keratoplasty] has seen massive improvements in technique modifications, DMEK (Descemet Membrane Endothelial Keratoplasty) and PDEK (Pre-Descemetic Endothelial Keratoplasty) are continuously being modified as they are being adopted by an ever growing number of surgeons.

## 3.1 Descemet Stripping [Automated] Endothelial Keratoplasty (DS[A]EK)

DS(A)EK can at least in theory replace PK (Penetrating Keratoplasty) in all eyes suffering from endothelial dysfunction or decompensation. DS(A)EK can be introduced using a variety of techniques and tools including the Endoserter (Fig. 3.1) or Busin Glide. Advances in DS(A)EK have rendered penetrating keratoplasty essential only in cases of dense stromal opacities with co-existing endothelial dysfunction [1].

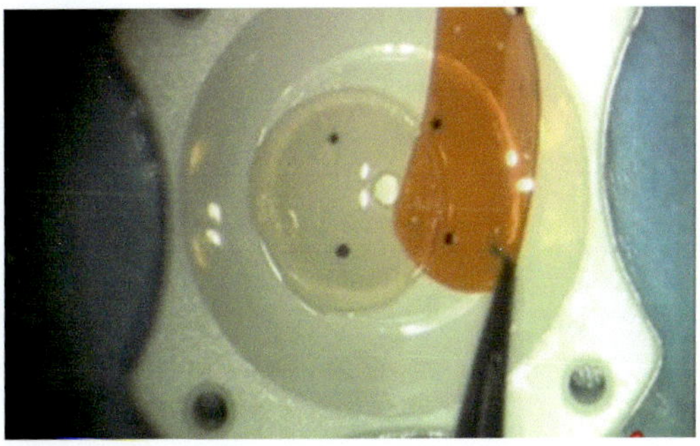

**Fig. 3.1** **DSAEK**: Loading of the DSEK lenticule on the Endoserter

M. Tsatsos (✉)
2nd Ophthalmology Department, Papageorgiou Hospital, Aristotle University of Thessaloniki, Thessaloniki, Greece

University Hospital Southampton, Southampton, UK


S. Jacob (ed.), *Mastering DMEK and PDEK*, https://doi.org/10.1007/978-981-97-3469-6_3

## 3.2 DMEK and PDEK

Descemet membrane endothelial keratoplasty (DMEK) offers an anatomical repair for endothelial pathology, replacing only endothelium and Descemet's membrane without any posterior stroma [2] (Fig. 3.2a–d). It is technically more challenging, requiring prolonged surgical time, associated with a steeper learning curve and possibly more potential complications [3, 4].

The description of the pre-Descemetic layer [4] and the subsequent development of the pre-Descemetic endothelial keratoplasty [5, 6] (PDEK) has led to a minimally additive procedure that shares the rapid visual rehabilitation of DMEK and the same time allowing easier and less laborious graft manipulation both outside and inside the eye (Fig. 3.3a, b, Table 3.1).

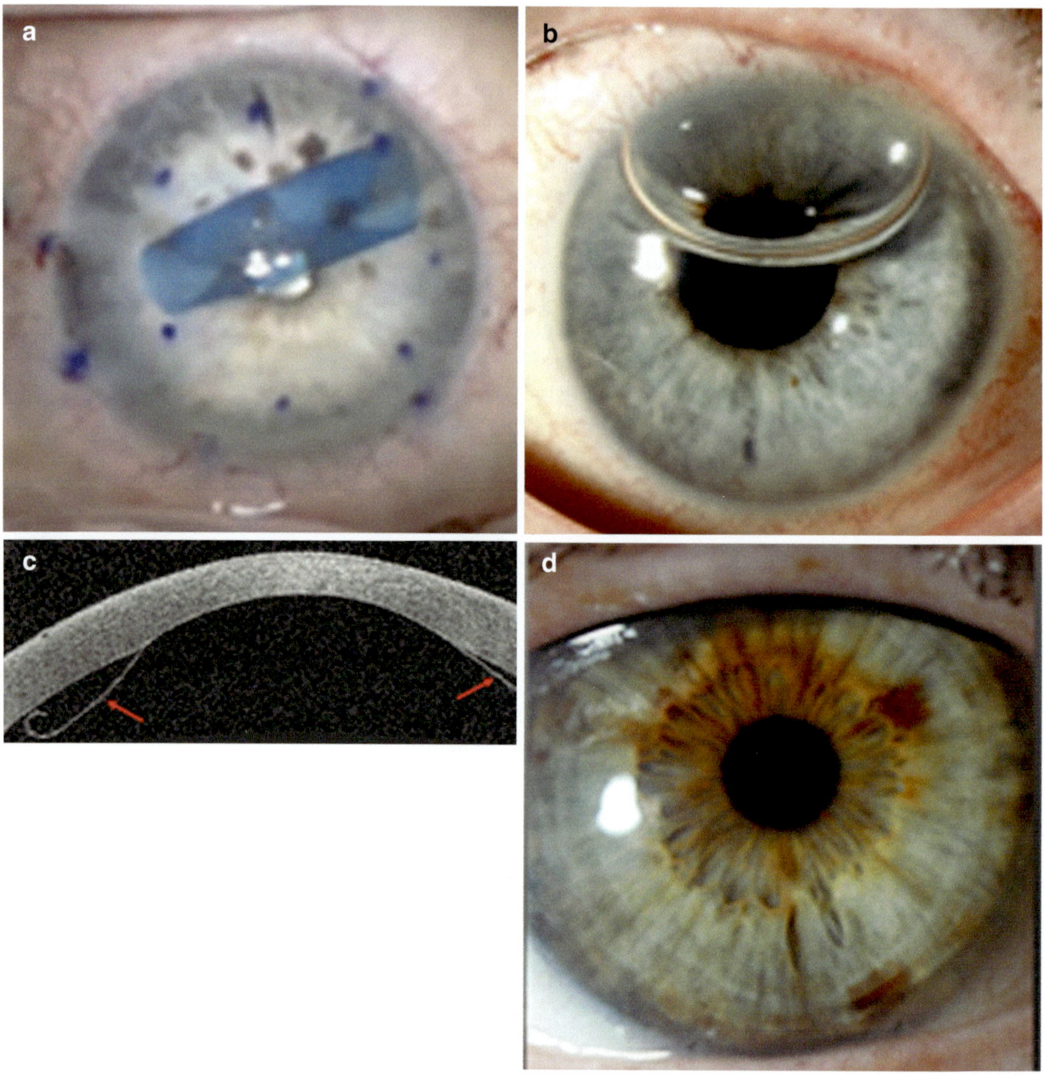

**Fig. 3.2** **DMEK**: (**a**) DMEK graft within anterior chamber. (**b**) First post-operative day appearance with clear cornea. (**c**) ASOCT in different patient showing a peripherally detached DMEK graft. The central DEMK graft remains well attached. (**d**) Clear cornea post DMEK

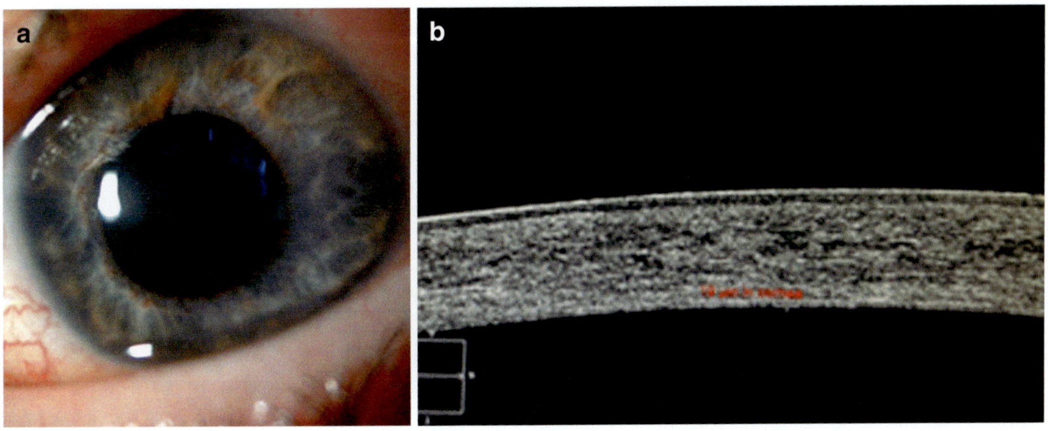


**Fig. 3.3** **PDEK**: (**a**) Clear graft seen after pre-Descemetic endothelial keratoplasty; (**b**) ASOCT image of the cornea 1 week after PDEK transplant

**Table 3.1** Differences between DMEK, PDEK, and DSAEK (Courtesy, Dr. Soosan Jacob)

| | DMEK | PDEK | DSAEK |
|---|---|---|---|
| Visual recovery | Fast | Fast | Slower |
| Visual outcome | Better | Better | Less |
| Induced refractive error | Less | Less | More |
| Rejection | Less | Less | More |
| Technical difficulty | More | Less | Less |
| Complex cases | Less easy | Easier | Easier |
| E-DMEK | Yes | Yes | Yes |
| Combined cases | Difficult | Easier | Easier |
| Vitrectomized monocameral eye | Difficult | Easier | Easier |
| Deep AC | Difficult | Easier | Easier |
| Donor age | Less than 40 years | More than 40 years | Any age |
| Donor thickness | 15 microns | 25–30 microns | 40–200 microns |
| Learning curve | Difficult | Less difficult | Easier |
| Graft handleability | Difficult | Easier | Easier |
| Graft loss while preparing | Possible | Possible | Less likely |

## 3.3 Host Evaluation

### 3.3.1 Patient Characteristics

Penetrating Keratoplasty (PK) has been the treatment of choice for a number of indications including endothelial dysfunction for almost a century since the description of the first successful PK in Olomouc (then Czechoslovakia) by Edward Zirm. Although when it comes to endothelial dysfunction it has been almost completely replaced by endothelial keratoplasty techniques, it still has an important role to play in cases of corneal pathology that involve more layers of the cornea, in specific situations where DMEK or PDEK could be very technically challenging (in most of these cases DSEK could be performed) or in areas where the surgical expertise for endothelial keratoplasty is lacking.

Although day-to-day referrals for endothelial dysfunction especially in busy tertiary referral centres include very complex cases sometimes with mixed pathology, it is important that novice surgeons embarking on endothelial membrane keratoplasty (DMEK and PDEK) begin with candidates that closely resemble the ideal host.

### 3.3.2 The Ideal Candidate and What Should Be Avoided During the Learning Curve

The ideal patient for a surgeon starting DMEK should be emmetropic or with a fairly early stage of Fuch's endothelial dystrophy with mild degree of corneal oedema allowing comfortable visualization of the cornea and the host corneal endothelium.

Pseudophakic patients are often preferred as the extra space in the AC would allow more space for manoeuvres and manipulations and also it would minimize the possibility of lens damage and cataract formation during graft insertion and manipulation. Low hyperopes should not be avoided especially if the surgeon has already got experience in DSEK/DSAEK or Ultrathin DS(A) EK surgery and Descemetorhexis manipulations in relatively shallow chambers. Extreme caution, however, has to be taken with hyperopic patients, especially when hyperopia is combined with high BMI (obesity) as these patients tend to have a positively high vitreous pressure which can lead to the expulsion of the DMEK graft out of the main corneal wound during graft insertion with an injector (Fig. 3.4). The surgeon should keep this in mind and intend to shallow the anterior chamber during graft injection into the AC to prevent the positive AC pressure from externalizing the DMEK graft when the graft injector is removed from the eye (Fig. 3.5). Mid to high myopes although do not form an absolute contraindication should probably be avoided by the novice membrane endothelial graft surgeon as graft opening may pose particularly challenging especially in tight (usually younger donor) DMEK rolls. The most problematic patients especially in the hands of surgeons that are still at the peak of their DMEK learning curve are vitrectomized patients and patients with very liquefied vitreous where there is little or no vitreous pressure making the anterior chamber very difficult to shallow and the DMEK graft very difficult to unroll. In these cases, the iris plane is not stable and tends to bow down with external manipulations making DMEK surgery very difficult even in the hands of expert surgeons. A number of techniques such as the double bubble technique [7] and air pump assisted PDEK [8] have been described to allow more experienced surgeons to perform DMEK even in these challenging cases (Fig. 3.6).

The difference between PDEK and DMEK lies not only in the behaviour of the graft and the tightness of the roll but also as mentioned above, in the ability to perform intraocular manoeuvres to unroll the PDEK graft without damaging it. This allows easier manipulation of the PDEK graft during unfolding in these challenging eyes extending the indications of PDEK even in cases where only DSEK could be considered as an alternative to the traditional penetrating keratoplasty.

Both PDEK and DMEK are indicated in Bullous keratopathy (BK), and they have largely replaced PK even in cases of severe BK where there is evidence of significant stromal scarring. The replacement of the host endothelium with a DSE(A)K, PDEK, or DMEK graft always leads to the improvement of the stromal opacity, therefore rendering the endothelial keratoplasty techniques the preferred choice in BK. The most challenging part of the PDEK or DMEK in these cases involves the visualization of the host Descemet's membrane as well as the visualization of the donor to allow graft unrolling and sticking to the host. Visualization is greatly enhanced after the removal of the host epithelium and the use of techniques such as Endoilluminator assisted Endothelial keratoplasty [9] (Fig. 3.7) or even the pretreatment of these patients with hypertonic NaCl 5% ointment (twice a day for 2–3 weeks pre-op) that reduces corneal oedema. These allow PDEK and DMEK to be performed even in cases of stromal opacities that were previously considered impossible and only suitable for penetrating keratoplasty.

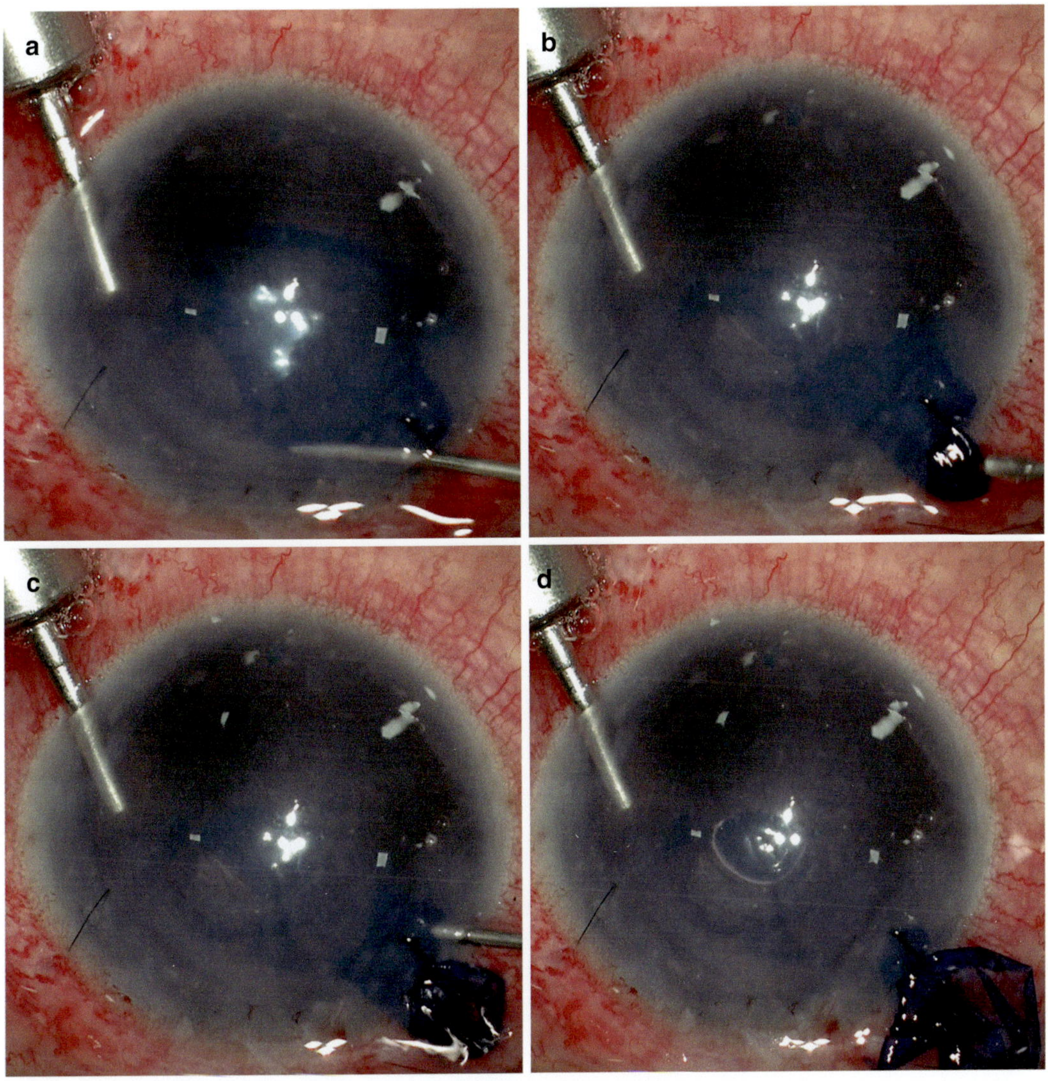


**Fig. 3.4** (**a–d**) Expulsion of the DMEK graft out of the main corneal wound during graft insertion with an injector. (Fig Courtesy Dr. Soosan Jacob, Dr. Agarwal's Eye Hospital, Chennai)

**Fig. 3.5** Avoiding the DMEK graft from being expelled out when the injector is removed. This is done by shallowing the AC as well as by applying gentle pressure over the wound in order to close it. (Fig Courtesy Dr. Soosan Jacob, Dr. Agarwal's Eye Hospital, Chennai)

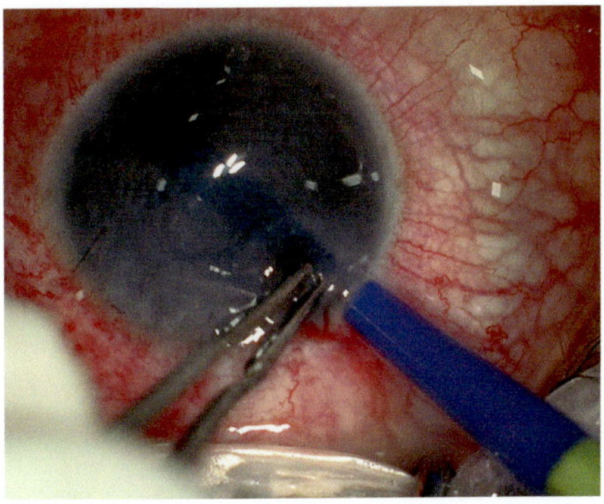

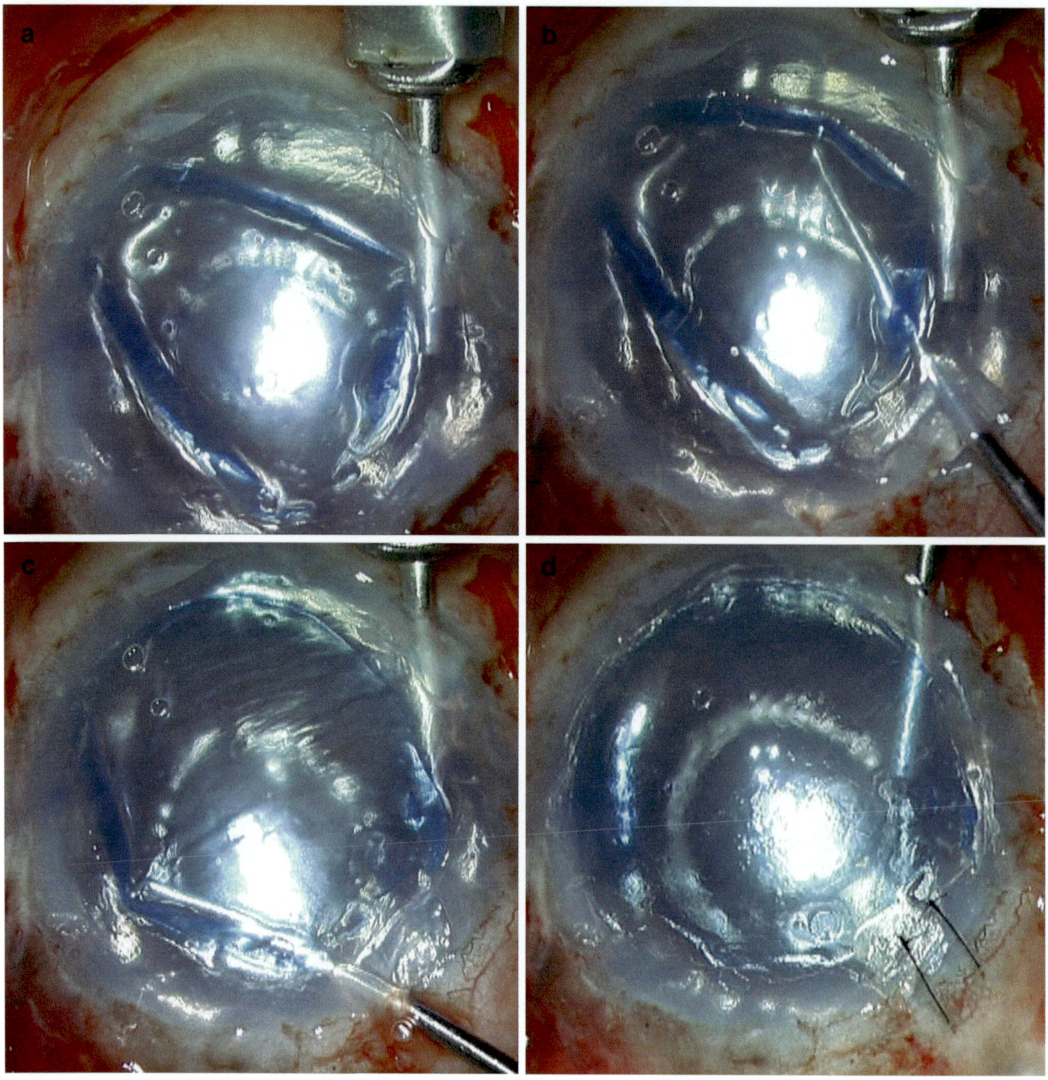


**Fig. 3.6** PDEK in glued IOL: the air pump assisted technique makes surgery easier even in vitrectomized eyes. The graft is floated up (**a**), and air is then used to hold it in place whilst any edge folds are removed and the graft is centred (**b–d**). (Fig Courtesy Dr. Soosan Jacob, Dr. Agarwal's Eye Hospital, Chennai)

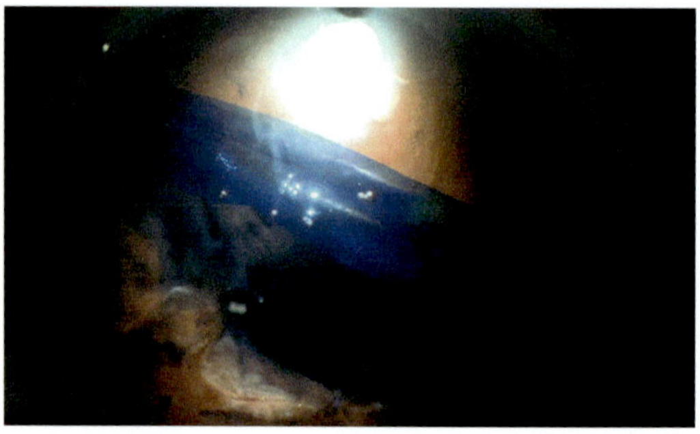

**Fig. 3.7** Endoilluminator assisted pre-Descemetic endothelial keratoplasty: the graft configuration can be visualized clearly with the oblique light of the endoilluminator. (Fig Courtesy Dr. Soosan Jacob, Dr. Agarwal's Eye Hospital, Chennai)

### 3.3.3 Trabeculectomy and Glaucoma Shunts

In eyes that had undergone trabeculectomy, air can escape through the area of the ostium/iridectomy, and the air or gas/air mixture bubble could escape through the trabeculectomy site. Although trabeculectomy should not be a contraindication for DMEK, it could possibly be avoided during the initial cases of a surgeon starting DMEK. Previous glaucoma shunt surgery should not be a contraindication for an experienced DMEK surgeon, and several techniques are used to make DMEK surgery as smooth as possible in eyes with previous shunts (Fig. 3.8) including filling the AC with air or air/gas mixture for longer, tying the tube of the glaucoma shunt, etc. However, the presence of the tube in the AC especially if placed over the iris reduces the space available for potential manipulations and could also lead to greater endothelial damage during graft opening or graft detachment and rebubbling as most manipulations take place on the iris plane.

### 3.3.4 Iris Defects and Aniridia

Large iris defects and aniridic patients either traumatic and iatrogenic or congenital (dominant or sporadic) where the absence of an intact iris plane can make the graft manipulations difficult should be avoided unless the surgeon is very experienced and familiar with a number of iris reconstruction techniques. Partial aniridia can ideally be repaired especially if iatrogenic or traumatic via techniques that aim to restore the iris anatomy with or without lens/cataract surgery [10]. In the case when the iris defect is anatomically repaired and the lens or IOL/iris plane is reconstructed, PDEK or DMEK can be performed by an experienced surgeon especially if modification techniques such as endothelial keratoplasty under continuous air infusion [8] are employed and a mixture of gas/air (SF6/Air = 15/85%) is injected intra and postoperatively to assist with graft attachment. The repair of the iris defect with the use of iris reconstruction IOL (such as the Ophtec 311 iris reconstruction IOL) makes surgery as lot less predictable as the compartmentalization of the eye remains incomplete and the maintenance of air or air/gas mixture in the AC in most cases proves very challenging. In complete congenital aniridia, most surgeons would accept that DMEK or PDEK surgery is not indicated (Fig. 3.9a). The slippage of the air mixed air/gas bubble through the iris defect (or the aniridic IOL/iris remnants plane in case or complete aniridia) could make the DMEK graft attachment to the host stroma extremely challenging. Therefore, most surgeons would opt for DSEK or PDEK surgery although in some occasions a keratoprosthesis might be preferred if ocular surface is also severely affected (aniridic keratopathy) (Fig. 3.9b–d). As Endothelial

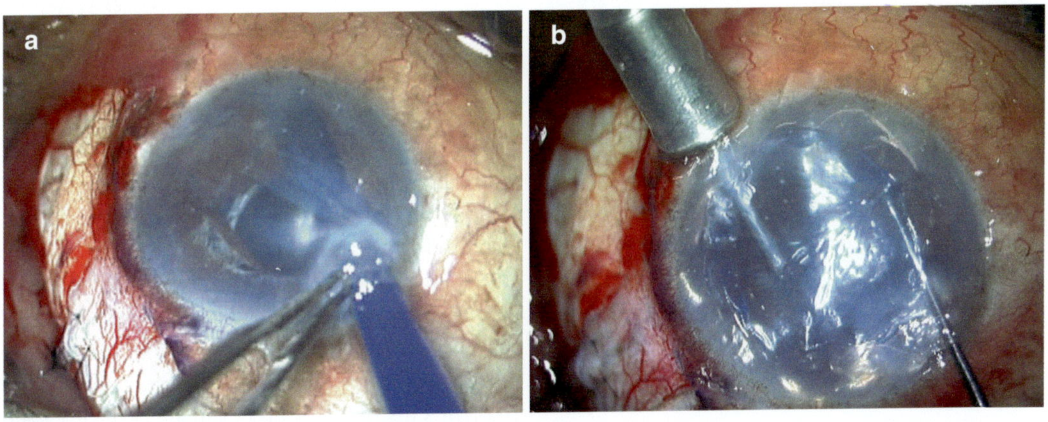

**Fig. 3.8** PDEK combined with Ahmed glaucoma valve: the AGV tube can be seen in the supero-temporal quadrant of the eye. It is placed behind the iris plane. (Fig Courtesy Dr. Soosan Jacob, Dr. Agarwal's Eye Hospital, Chennai)

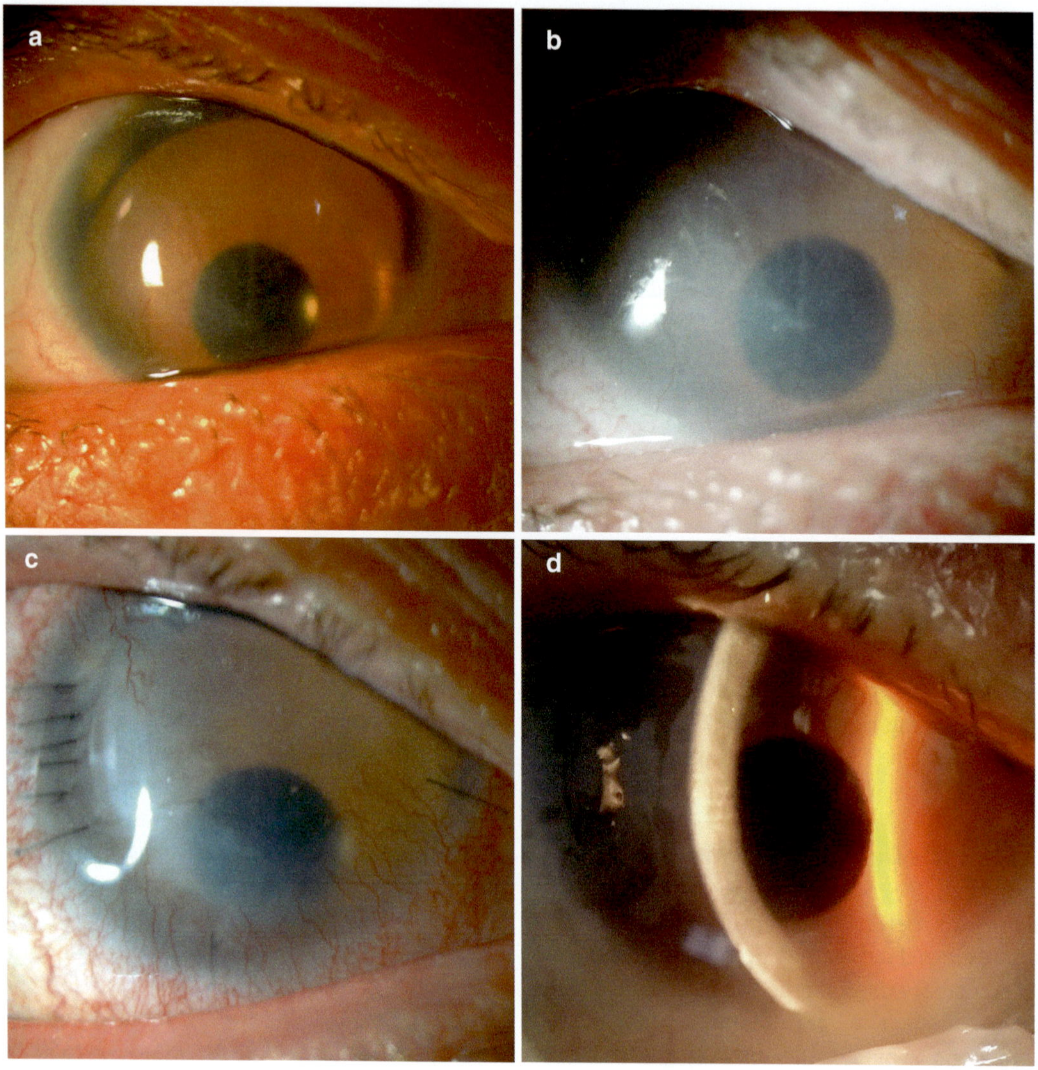


**Fig. 3.9** Aniridic keratopathy (**a**, **b**) treated with DSEK: aniridic keratopathy showing evidence of endothelial dysfunction, stromal oedema, and corneal neovascularization (**a**); close up photo of stromal oedema with DM folds (**b**); the graft is seen attached in 1 week after surgery (**c**); (**d**) 6 months post op DSEK showing greatly reduced corneal neovascularization

Keratoplasty procedures, instrumentation and expertise continue to advance, even Congenital Aphakia cases are operated with DMEK/PDEK.

### 3.3.5 Aphakia and Patients with AC-IOLs

Aphakia or the presence of an AC-IOL should not necessarily pose a complete contraindication against DMEK or PDEK although they form 2 separate entities with different risks associated with them. Aphakic patients can of course be first repaired with glued or sutured scleral fixation IOLs or even Iris clip IOL (clipped either antero or retro pupillary) after which DMEK or PDEK can be performed (Fig. 3.10). It is important of course to perform a complete assessment of the patient's history and fully evaluate clinically each patient with a case-by-case approach. Cases of traumatic aphakia require longer periods of rehabilitation after the initial injury as they are usually

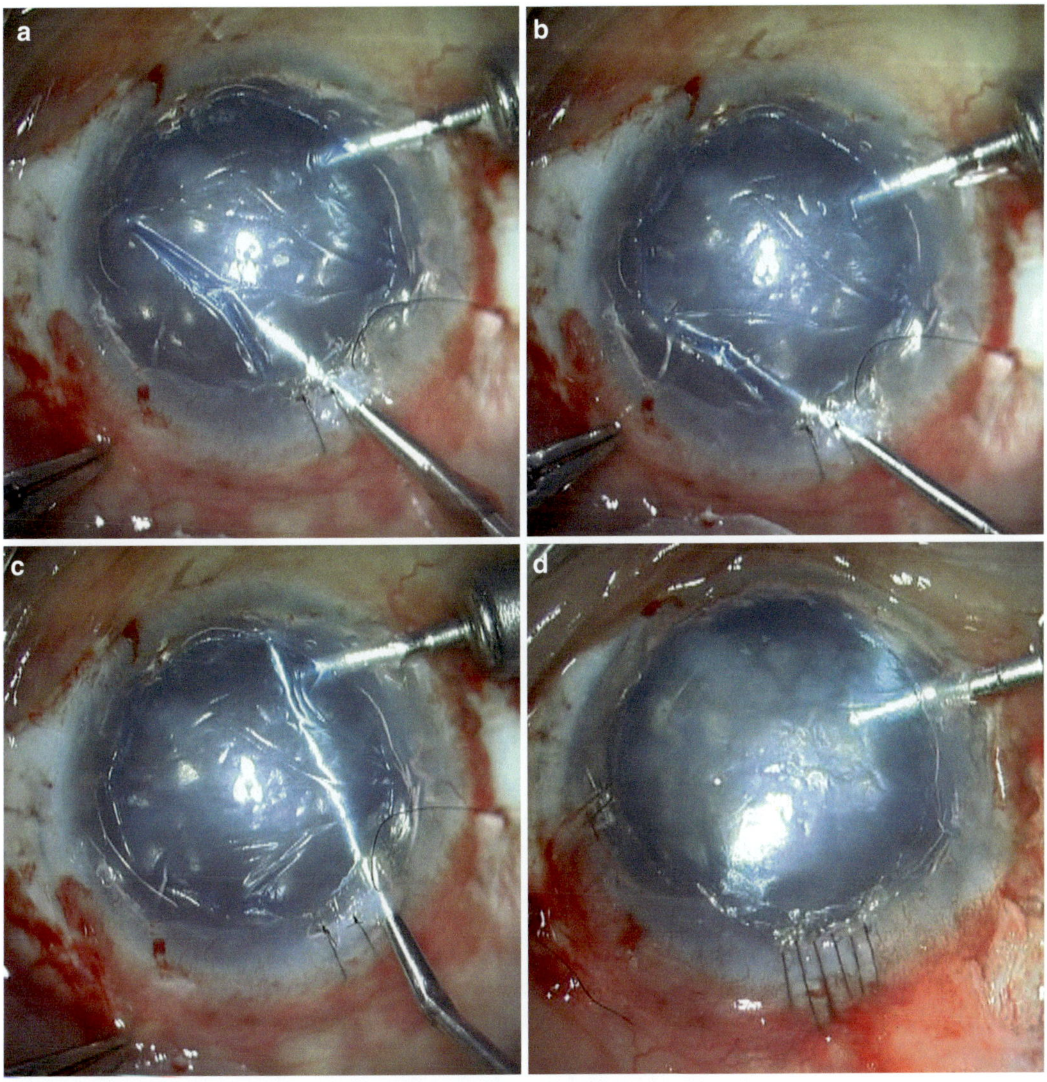


**Fig. 3.10** PDEK in glued IOL: the air pump assisted technique makes surgery easier even in vitrectomized eyes. The glued IOL has already been performed, haptics have been tucked in and flaps glued down. Next, the graft is floated up (**a**), and air is then used to hold it in place while any edge folds are removed and the graft is centred (**b**–**d**). (Fig Courtesy Dr. Soosan Jacob, Dr. Agarwal's Eye Hospital, Chennai)

associated with corneal, scleral or angle trauma and possible vitreous haemorrhage or retinal pathology. Aphakia resulting from complex cataract surgery complications such as Marfan's syndrome or previous retinal detachment surgery/vitrectomy or malignant/high myopia or severe pseudoexfoliation should be regarded as a temporary condition warranting intial treatment. This is especially important when the cornea is clear enough to allow manipulations needed in IOL fixation surgery. Combined IOL fixation and DSEK or DMEK/PDEK surgery should be considered only by experienced surgeons familiar with DMEK or PDEK in challenging eyes such as high myopia or vitrectomized eyes and only when there is clear evidence of corneal decompensation. It is not common to find a surgeon that would add another variable and difficult aspect to an already difficult surgery if there is even a slight chance of being able to avoid it.

In cases where the patient or surgeon decides to proceed without insertion of PC IOL or even iris clip or angle supported IOL, there is always the risk of the DMEK or PDEK graft ending up in the vitreous cavity. Therefore, a few manipulations have been introduced for the safer insertion of DMEK and PDEK grafts in aphakic patients [DMEK performed after insertion of an iris diaphragm]. These include apart from the relative hypotony that should be used when inserting the graft, the continuous low volume flow of air during graft insertion and manipulation, and the maintenance of a quite small pupil.

Patients with AC-IOLs pose different challenges. DMEK and PDEK can be performed in eyes with AC-IOL (either angle supported or iris clip) as long as the IOL is stable and not the sole cause of the corneal decompensation. In the later case, the AC-IOL should be removed and ideally replaced with a PC-IOL (Fig. 3.11).

In eyes with stable AC-IOLs, DMEK or PDEK can be performed and apart from the challenges associated with the presence of the IOL in the AC, the procedure appears to be largely successful in eyes with deep ACs. A well-accepted view that DSEK shows higher survival rates with AC depths greater than 3 mm can be transcended to DMEK or PDEK surgery as well. Endothelial keratoplasty can be cautiously performed in eyes with even shallower ACs as the width of conventional DSEK (approx. 150 microns) is replaced by a graft of 20–25 microns allowing more room for manipulation. Great caution should be taken as the AC IOL is less gentle than the iris or other ocular tissue to the donor's endothelium. Therefore, ideally few manoeuvres should be used during graft unfolding in the AC, and the patient should remain for a few minutes (10–30) in the flat position in the operating or recovery room to allow greater contact of the air/air/gas mixture bubble with the graft [11].

### 3.3.6 ICE Syndrome

As our experience with DSEK and ultrathin DSEK grafts continues to grow and a number of advances and modifications has led to smoother surgery and greater outcomes surgeons have begun to experiment with DSEK for a variety of indications that have been previously considered impossible. ICE syndrome and Peter's anomaly have been shown to have visual outcomes of questionable benefit after penetrating keratoplasty. DMEK and PDEK have been shown to be particularly challenging as graft manipulations can take considerable amount of time with negative impact on visual acuity. DSEK surgery with endothelial grafts of a smaller diameter (inside the iridocorneal attachments) has been shown to be more beneficial at least in short- to medium-term studies [12].

### 3.3.7 Failed PK

DMEK and PDEK have been reported to have great outcomes after repeat penetrating keratoplasty due to endothelial failure. DSEK has been reported in a number of studies and remains the preferred treatment option after PK endothelial failure for a large number of surgeons as it can easily be performed with or without a descemetorhexis. In case of DMEK and PDEK surgery, descemetorhexis should be performed inside the donor/host junction. The preferred location for the descemetorhexis is inside the graft/host junction as this allows the preservation of the weakest part of the cornea, the graft–host junction which remains intact. The presence of the descemetorhexis allows a stronger attachment of the new DMEK or PDEK graft with the corneal stromal of the first PK. Technically, a DMEK or PDEK is a lot easier without prior descemetorhexis but this greatly increases the rebubbling rate as the attachment of the DMEK on failed endothelium is not as strong as with corneal stroma. As mentioned above, ideally the host diseased Descemet's membrane is removed inside the graft/host junction; however, this is not always possible as the adhesion of even diseased Descemet's membrane can be very strong especially in neglected cases. These could benefit from DSE(A)K as lack of Descemetorhexis although not definitely necessary in PDEK or DMEK surgery is a lot more forgiving in the case of DS(A)EK (Fig. 3.12). All

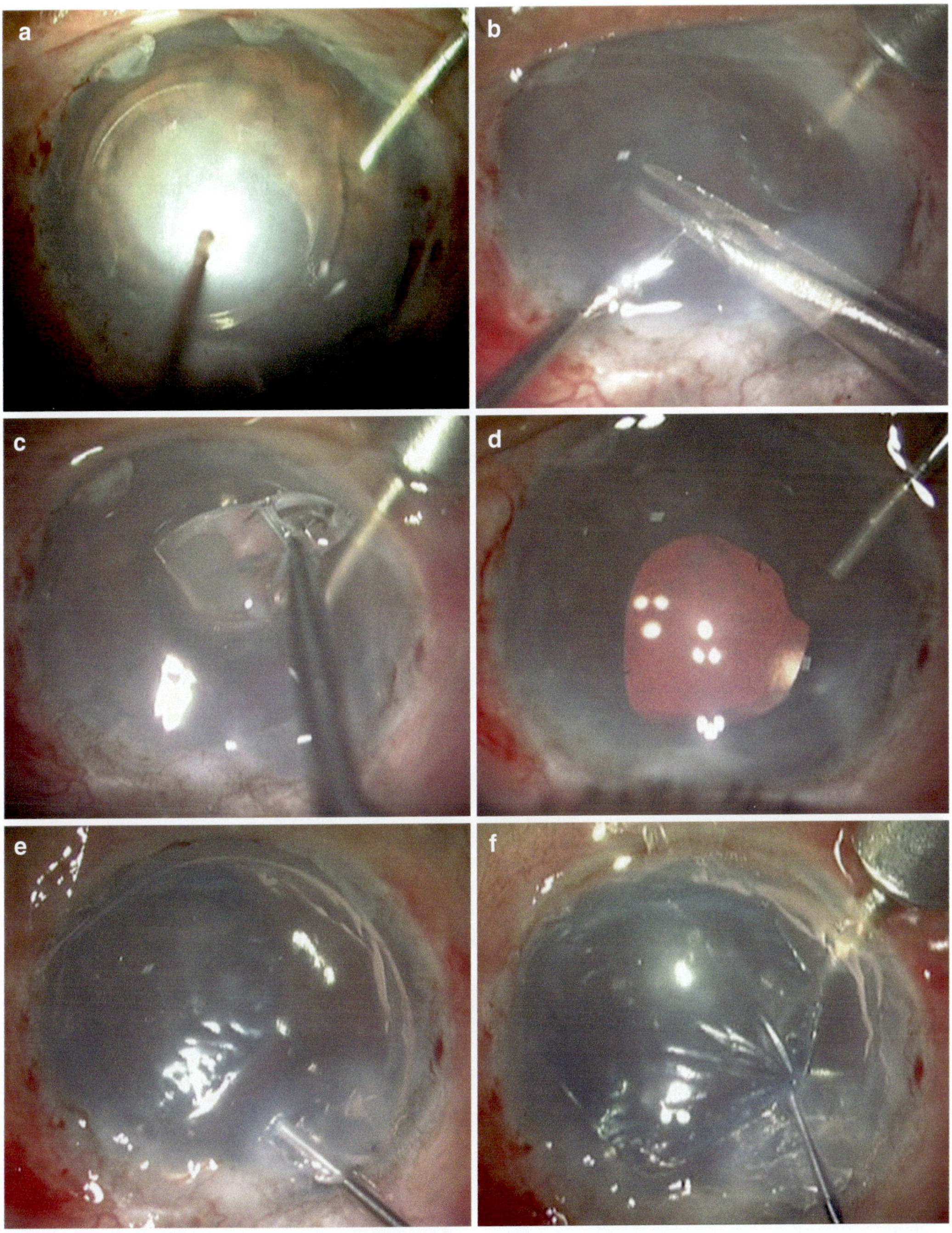


**Fig. 3.11** Pre-Descemetic endothelial keratoplasty performed after explantation of a PCIOL placed in AC (**a**); the PCIOL in AC is cut and explanted (**b**, **c**); a glued IOl is implanted (**d**); a PDEK graft is floated up and centred using the air pump assisted technique (**e**–**h**). (Fig Courtesy Dr. Soosan Jacob, Dr. Agarwal's Eye Hospital, Chennai)

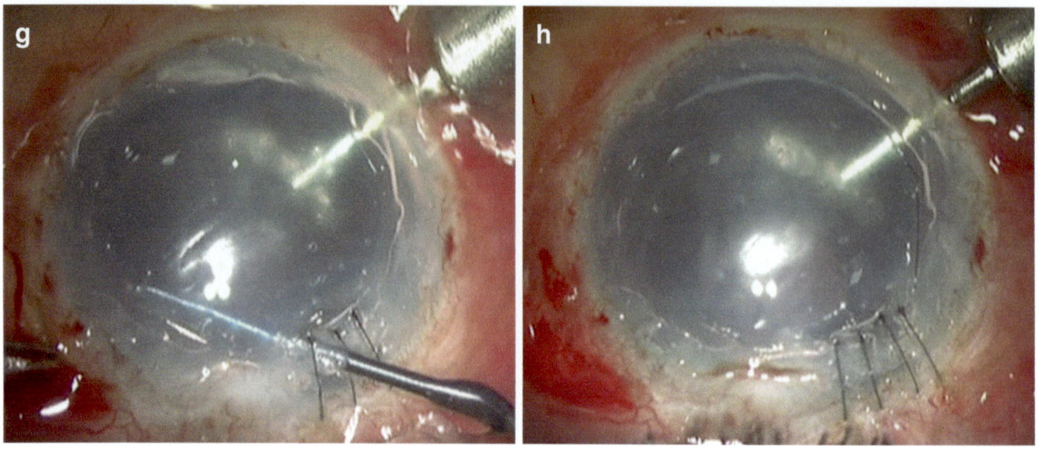


**Fig. 3.11** (continued)

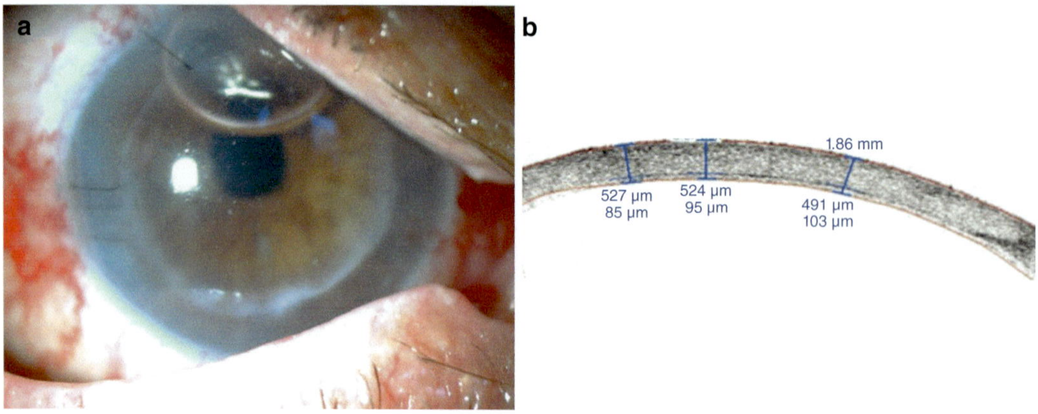


**Fig. 3.12** (**a**) DSAEK performed on a failed penetrating keratoplasty; (**b**) ASOCT of ultrathin DSEK on a PK with endothelial failure

the above should be performed if the graft/host junction is strong and intact and the patient is not suffering from high irregular astigmatism or worsening of the corneal ectasia at the graft/host junction as it is sometimes seen in keratoconus. In cases of very poor view of the AC even after the removal of the host epithelium, pretreatment with hypertonic ointment and use of the endoscope, repeat PK should be considered (Fig. 3.13). All the above indications would benefit from a repeat PK would be more beneficial as it would address anterior and posterior corneal pathology (Fig. 3.14).

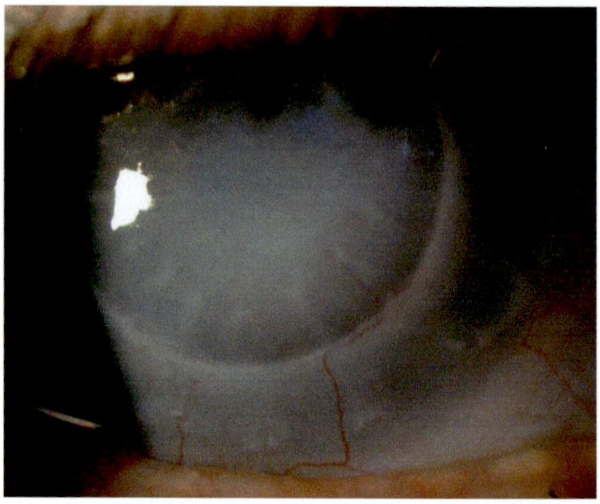

**Fig. 3.13** Failed PK with evidence of stromal opacification and interface host/donor junction neovascularization

### 3.3.8 Conjunctival Scarring/Short Fornices

Although mild cases of conjunctival scarring with some shortening of the fornices should not deter surgeons from performing DMEK or PDEK surgery, cases of severe conjunctival scarring with or without symblepharon with or without forniceal shortening are particularly challenging as the space for surgical manipulations is very limited. In any case of forniceal shortening, it is important to look for associated conditions and perform a detailed work-up with a full medical history and a thorough clinical examination as the root cause of scarring could be a number of conditions such as trauma (iatrogenic or accidental/non-accidental injury, chemical injury), trachoma, or ocular cicatricial pemphigoid.

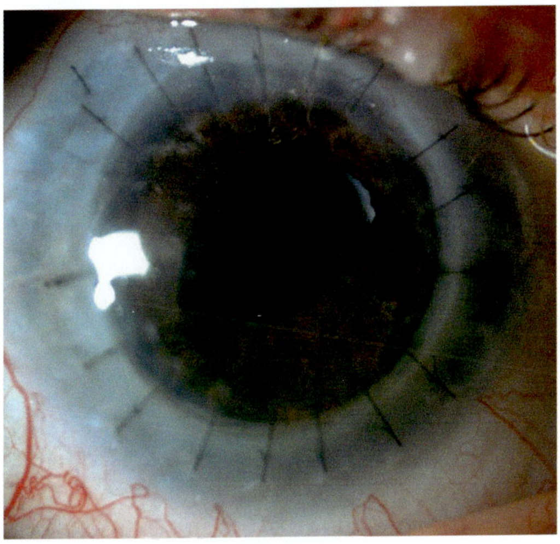

**Fig. 3.14** A repeat penetrating keratoplasty done for a failed penetrating graft

As the surgical manipulations and the post-surgical inflammation can lead to worsening of the ocular surface condition, it is imperative for the surgeon to use the technique that he or she is most comfortable and experienced with as in these eyes, the surgeon often has "one shot" at fixing the endothelial dysfunction before any significant inflammation and scarring impedes further surgery. It is also important to use a technique that needs little or no external (outside the eye) manipulations as this type of surgical manoeuvres are difficult in limited space.

Some surgeons would prefer PK over newer lamellar techniques but these would make sense only in cases of minimal or no ocular surface and adnexal involvement as in this case there would be very guarded prognosis for visual recovery and survival of the graft.

DS(A)EK and its modifications (ultrathin or nanothin) would be a good option that requires controlled manoeuvres. DMEK would be the most challenging option amongst Descemet membrane endothelial procedures as it most commonly requires extensive external manoeuvres and manipulations due to the tightness and frailty of the DMEK roll (Fig. 3.15a) compared to the more open and more rigid PDEK roll

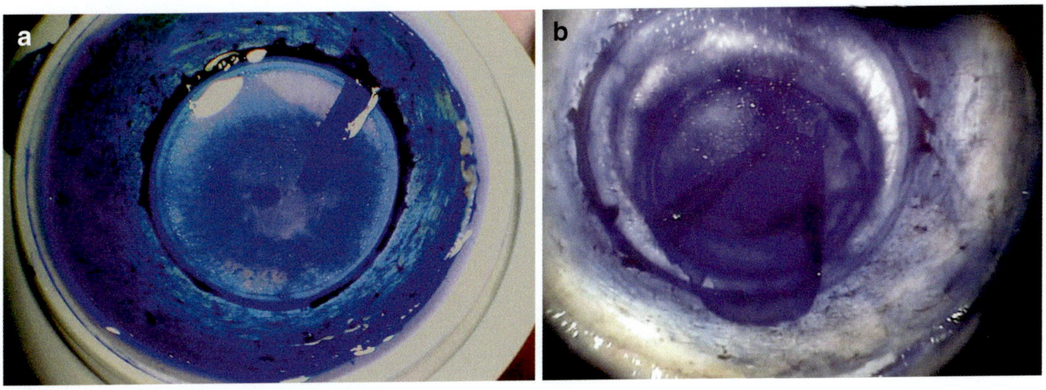


**Fig. 3.15** (**a**) DMEK roll. (**b**) PDEK roll

(Fig. 3.15b) that could most probably be positioned with inside of the eye manipulations alone, especially if PDEK is performed with air pump assisted method.

In summary, with improvements in instrumentation, DMEK surgery has started to grow in popularity due to the almost immediate improvement in visual acuity and minimal impact on post-operative refraction. PDEK enables the expansion of the surgical indications for membrane endothelial keratoplasty as it allows the use of younger donors (as young as 4 months old have been used, Figs. 3.16 and 3.17). PDEK also enables membrane endothelial keratoplasty to be performed in more complex cases as it can be manipulated to the right location and the right side via inside of the eye manoeuvres as well as outside of the eye. In cases of very complex eyes with very disturbed AC, DS(A)EK surgery can be performed as it is a lot more forgiving and easier to handle without serious compromise in visual acuity and the normal architecture and integrity of the host. Penetrating keratoplasty is reserved for cases where there is evidence of pathology in all the layers of the cornea or the visibility though the diseased cornea is so badly affected that intraocular surgery cannot be performed.

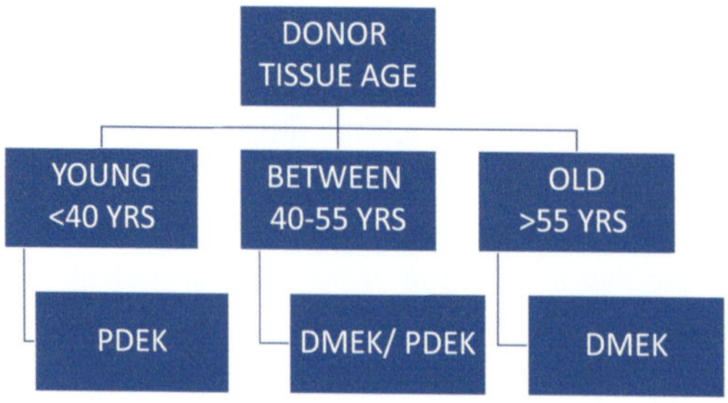


**Fig. 3.16** Tissue selection based on donor tissue age (Courtesy, Dr. Soosan Jacob). *DMEK* Descemet membrane endothelial keratoplasty, *PDEK* pre-Descemet's membrane endothelial keratoplasty

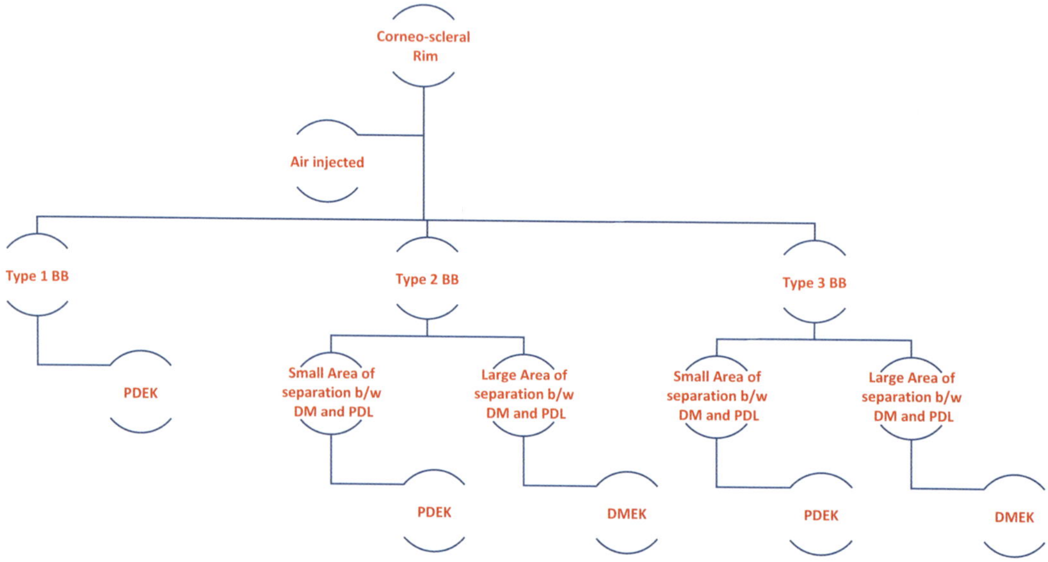


**Fig. 3.17** Complications while preparing graft (Courtesy, Dr. Soosan Jacob). *BB* big bubble, *DM* Descemet's membrane, *PDL* pre-Descemet's layer, *DMEK* Descemet membrane endothelial keratoplasty, *PDEK* pre-Descemet's membrane endothelial keratoplasty

## References


1. Tsatsos M, Athanasiadis I, Kopsachilis N, Krishnan R, Hossain P, Anderson D. Comparison of the Endosaver with noninjector techniques in Descemet's stripping endothelial keratoplasty. Indian J Ophthalmol. 2017;65(11):1133–7.
2. Melles GR, Ong TS, Ververs B, van der Wees J. Descemet membrane endothelial keratoplasty (DMEK). Cornea. 2006;25:987–90.
3. Terry MA. Endothelial keratoplasty: why aren't we all doing Descemet membrane endothelial keratoplasty. Cornea. 2012;31:469–71.
4. Price MO, Price FW Jr. Descemet's membrane endothelial keratoplasty surgery: update on the evidence and hurdles to acceptance. Curr Opin Ophthalmol. 2013;24(4):329–35.
5. Dua HS, Faraj LA, Said DG, Gray T, Lowe J. Human corneal anatomy redefined: a novel pre-Descemet's layer (Dua's layer). Ophthalmology. 2013;120(9):1778–85.
6. Agarwal A, Dua HS, Narang P, Kumar DA, Agarwal A, Jacob S, Agarwal A, Gupta A. Pre-Descemet's endothelial keratoplasty (PDEK). Br J Ophthalmol. 2014;98(9):1181–5.
7. Hayashi T, Kobayashi A. Double-bubble technique in Descemet membrane endothelial keratoplasty for vitrectomized eyes: a case series. Cornea. 2018;37(9):1185–8.
8. Jacob S. Use of pressurized air infusion for pre Descemet's endothelial keratoplasty (PDEK)—the air pump assisted PDEK technique. Open Ophthalmol J. 2018;12:175–18.
9. Jacob S, Agarwal A, Agarwal A, Narasimhan S, Kumar DA, Sivagnanam S. Endoilluminator-assisted transcorneal illumination for Descemet membrane endothelial keratoplasty: enhanced intraoperative visualization of the graft in corneal decompensation secondary to pseudophakic bullous keratopathy. J Cataract Refract Surg. 2014;40(8):1332–6.
10. Kumar DA, Agarwal A, Jacob S, Lamba M, Packialakshmi S, Meduri A. Combined surgical management of capsular and iris deficiency with glued intraocular lens technique. J Refract Surg. 2013;29(5):342–7.
11. Tsatsos M, Athanasiadis I, Ziakas N. To remove or not to remove (the AC-IOL)? This is the question. Int Ophthalmol. 2019;39(9):1917–8. https://doi.org/10.1007/s10792-018-1021-0. Epub 2018 Oct 22.
12. Fajgenbaum MA, Hollick EJ. Descemet stripping endothelial keratoplasty in iridocorneal endothelial syndrome: postoperative complications and long-term outcomes. Cornea. 2015;34(10):1252–8.

# 4 DMEK Graft Preparation

Monty Montoya

## 4.1 Introduction and Benefits

Descemet's Membrane Endothelial Keratoplasty (DMEK) has become the leading procedure in corneal transplants. Replacing the recipient's endothelium and Descemet's membrane using the DMEK method can lead to smaller incisions, faster recovery, and better overall vision for the patient [1–17]. Throughout this section, we will go over the stripping process, complications, and subsequent solutions during the peel, evaluation post-process and considerations in selecting a DMEK suitable cornea.

## 4.2 Process

Tools needed for stripping process include: Smooth bent forcep, toothed forceps, Sinskey hook, Teflon discs, trypan blue, corneal storage medium, WIC spears, 3 mm dermal punch, "S" stamp, and skin marker. Starting with the endothelial side up, using a bent forcep and toothed forcep to hold the sclera, strip out all the trabecular mesh work with the bent forcep around the entire cornea (e.g., Fig. 4.1).

With most of the meshwork removed, use a Sinskey hook to score the Descemet's membrane around the peripheral edge of the cornea, use trypan blue to visualize breaks in the Descemet's membrane (e.g., Fig. 4.2). Then use the Sinskey hook to find a break in the Descemet's membrane by sliding the hook between the Descemet's membrane and stroma to slightly lift the membrane trailing all the way around the cornea (e.g., Fig. 4.3).

Using the skin marker, mark a side on the sclera for an orientation mark. This will be a reference point for the location of the hinge (a small portion of the Descemet's membrane is left attached to the stroma in the periphery).

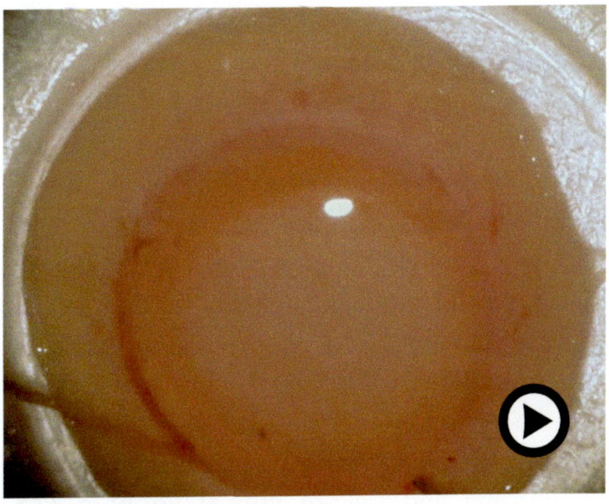

**Fig. 4.1** Removing the trabecular meshwork (https://doi.org/10.1007/000-dgr)

**Supplementary Information** The online version contains supplementary material available at https://doi.org/10.1007/978-981-97-3469-6_4. The videos can be accessed individually by clicking the DOI link in the accompanying figure caption or by scanning this link with the SN More Media App.

M. Montoya (✉)
CorneaGen, Seattle, WA, USA
e-mail: monty.montoya@corneagen.com


S. Jacob (ed.), *Mastering DMEK and PDEK*, https://doi.org/10.1007/978-981-97-3469-6_4

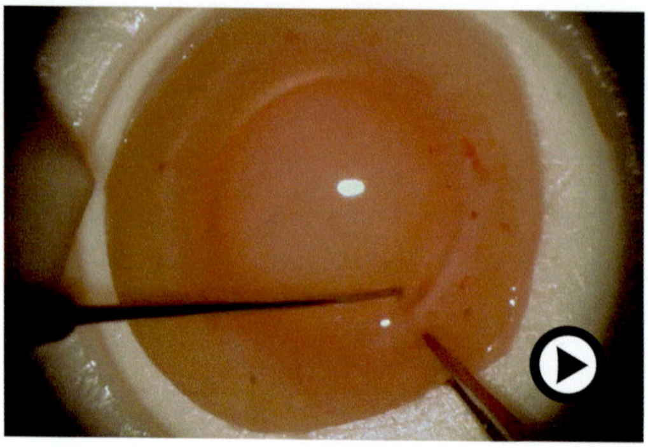

**Fig. 4.2** Using the Sinskey hook to score the Descemet's membrane (https://doi.org/10.1007/000-dgn)

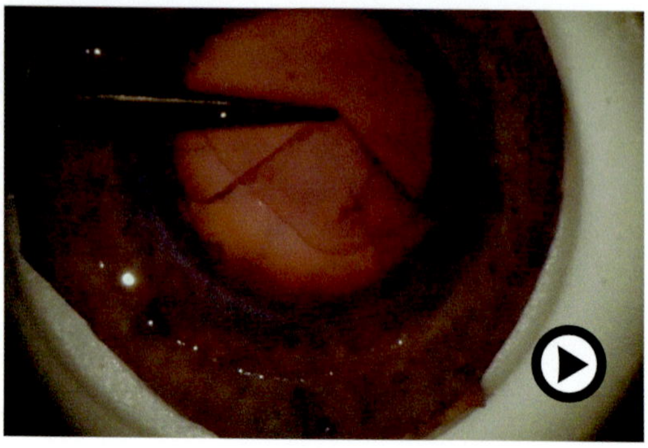

**Fig. 4.4** Peeling the Descemet's membrane (https://doi.org/10.1007/000-dgq)

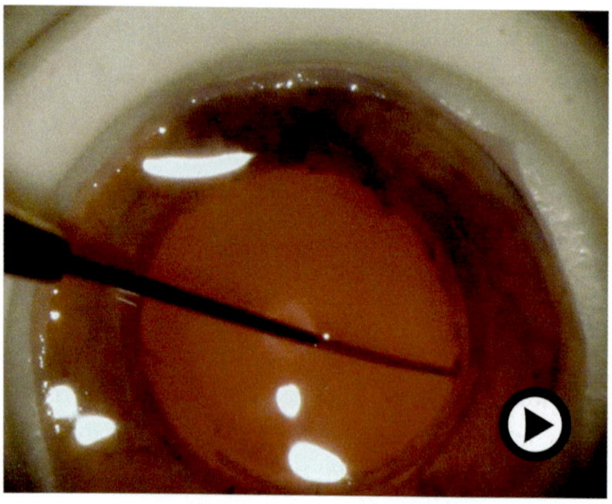

**Fig. 4.3** Using the Sinskey hook to lift and separate from the stroma (https://doi.org/10.1007/000-dgp)

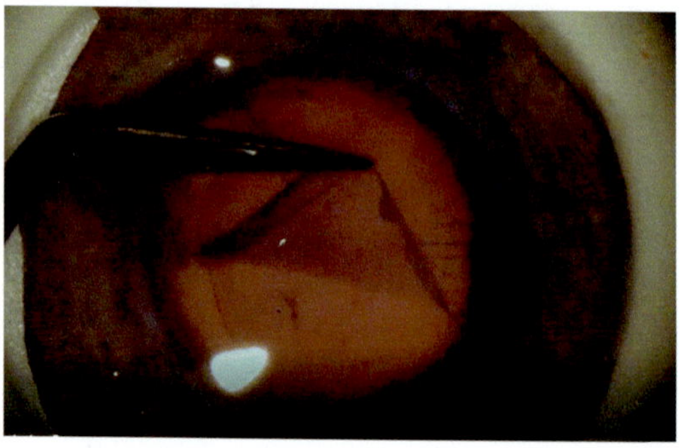

**Fig. 4.5** Peeling the Descemet's membrane

But, many find an orientation mark helpful to differentiate the anterior and posterior sides of the DMEK graft. This will describe the application of an "S" stamp on the anterior side of the Descemet's membrane. Once the orientation mark is made, start the peel on the opposite side. Fill the entire cornea with storage media, so the endothelial cells are submerged. Having it submerged helps with the Descemet's membrane separation and the fluidity of the graft when separating. Using the toothed forcep to hold the sclera, and the smooth bent forcep to grasp the Descemet's, slowly start peeling the Descemet's membrane away from the stroma and toward you at about a 135° angle, while keeping the graft submerged in media. If the graft seems to continuously tear on the periphery, release the graft to alleviate the tension, rotate the cornea 90°, and continue your peel, peeling the graft toward yourself and rotating until the graft is almost completely separated leaving about 10% of the Descemet's membrane attached for your hinge (e.g., Figs. 4.4 and 4.5).

At this point, the DMEK graft could be trephined and used for surgery. Once you have separated the Descemet's membrane, fold the graft toward your hinge and use a 3 mm dermal punch to create the window. Punch from stroma down to the epithelial layer to create the window and full-thickness plug (e.g., Figs. 4.6, 4.7 and 4.8).

Remove the 3-mm full thickness plug from the cornea and lay the Descemet's membrane graft back down to its original position and dry the graft to lay firmly back in place. Flip the cornea to the anterior portion and take a WIC spear to dry the Descemet's membrane through the stromal opening you have made (e.g., Fig. 4.9).

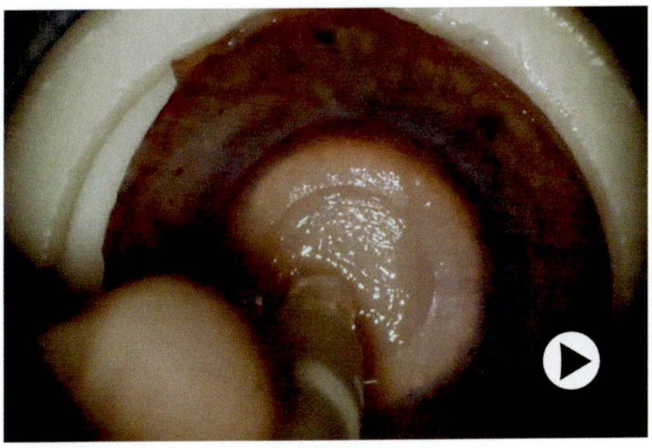

Fig. 4.6 Punching through the stromal layer (https://doi.org/10.1007/000-dgm)

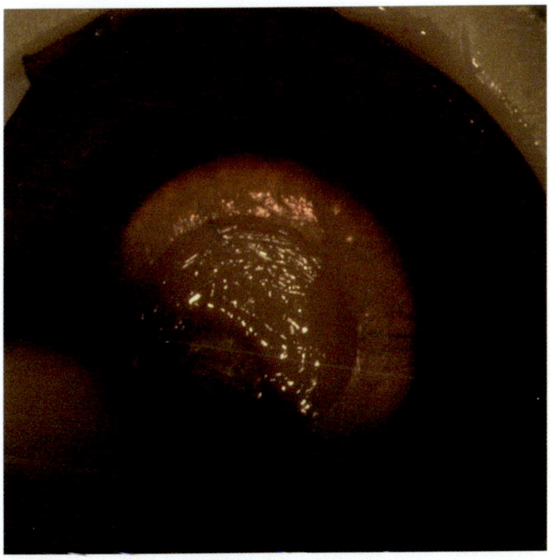

Fig. 4.7 Punch is made through the stroma with a 3 mm dermal punch

Once the graft is dry, take an inked s-stamp and stamp the anterior portion of the Descemet's membrane with the "S." With another dry WIC spear, wick up any excess ink from the s-stamp (e.g., Figs. 4.10 and 4.11).

Making sure to not have any excess liquid in the window you've created, replace the plug concave side down void of any bubbles underneath (e.g., Figs. 4.12 and 4.13). Having the endothelium portion side up, wick up any excess liquid from the peripheral of the graft to have the graft stay in place and to assess the plug (e.g., Fig. 4.14).

The graft can now be trephined to the desired graft diameter and used for transplant.

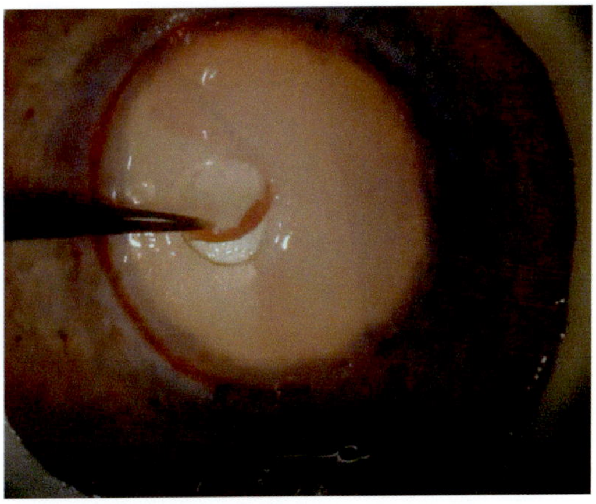

Fig. 4.8 Full thickness plug with hinge still attached

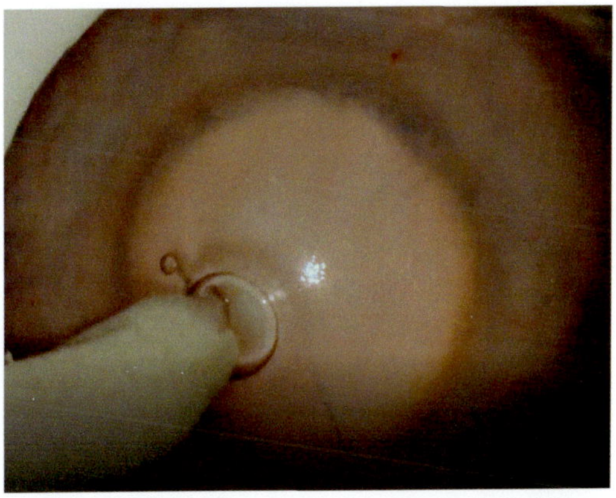

Fig. 4.9 Wicking up moisture before stamping the "S"

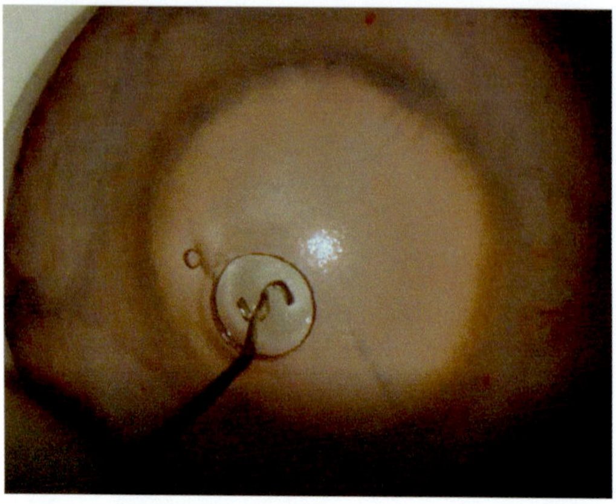

**Fig. 4.10** Stamping the "S"

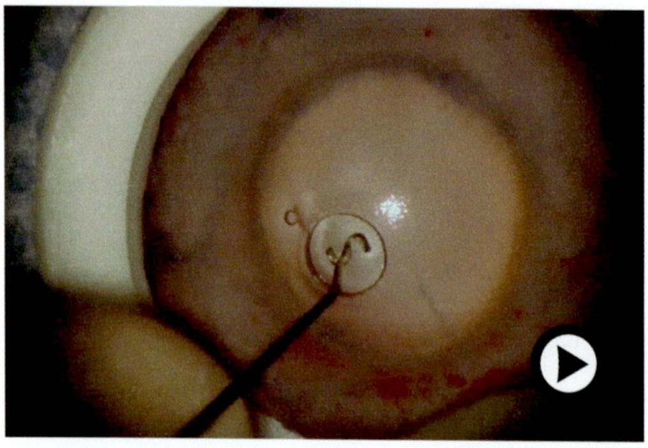

**Fig. 4.11** Drying the anterior side of Descemet's membrane to make the "s" (https://doi.org/10.1007/000-dgs)

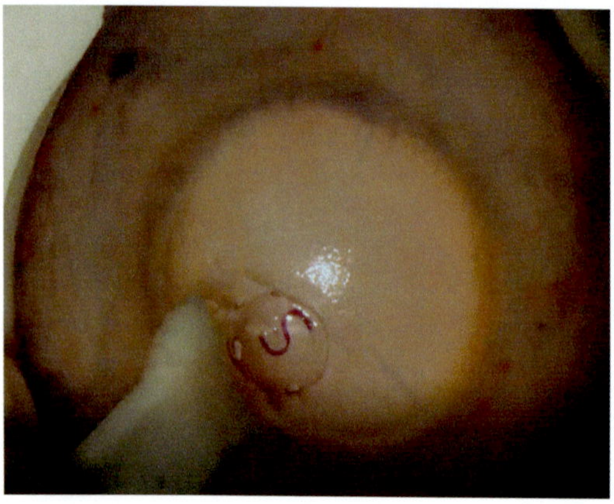

**Fig. 4.12** Replace the plug to original position. Use a wick to dry off excess fluid

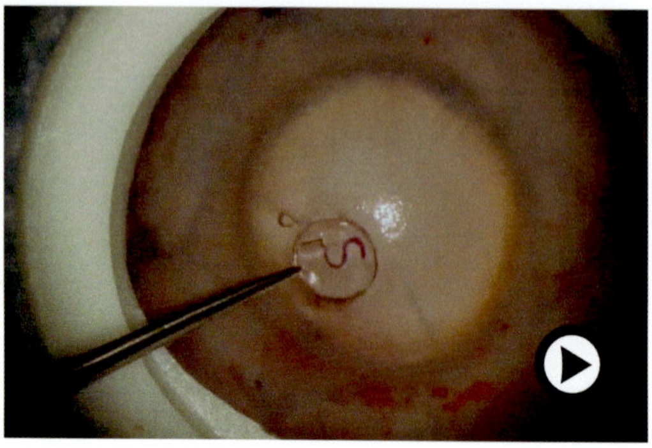

**Fig. 4.13** Replacing the plug to its original position (https://doi.org/10.1007/000-dgt)

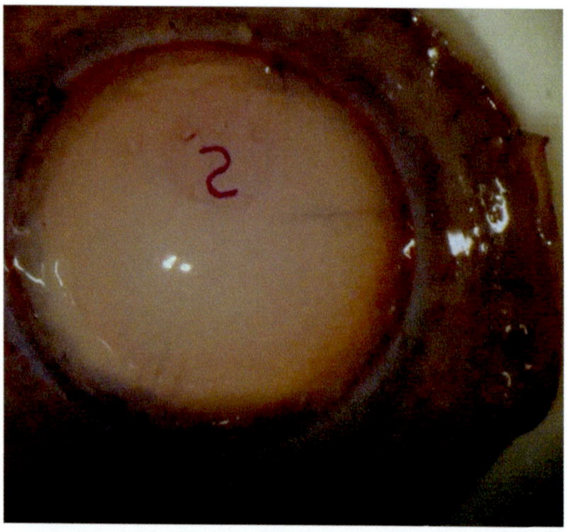

**Fig. 4.14** After replacing the plug, turn over to posterior side making sure there are no folds and graft is laid nicely back to original position. The graft is ready to be trephinated

## 4.3 Complications and How to Avoid Them

When peeling, a common complication to encounter is tears into the periphery of the cornea. In order to avoid extending the tear, each occurrence should be addressed as it arises. In order to prevent the tears from getting larger, a scalloped edge should be created. Creating this scalloped edge will prevent the tear from continuing into the center of the graft when proceeding to peel the rest of the Descemet's membrane.

When starting a peel, if there is a tear into the center, it is advisable to create a scalloped edge and keep that scallop as the hinge and continue to peel the rest of the Descemet's membrane opposite of the hinge.

To avoid complications while peeling the Descemet's membrane, play close attention to the horizon line while peeling. The line would ideally need to be straight and not create a "smile" so as to avoid tension in the graft (e.g., Fig. 4.15). A "smile" shape would be one where the Descemet's membrane is adhered tightly to the stroma resulting in the peripheral edges of the peel staying adhered at a higher point compared to the center point where the forceps are grasping the Descemet's membrane. If this line has a "smile" shape, there could be a tension point on the graft where a tear could arise. If you see a "smile" forming, it would be best to rotate the graph and start the peel again to the desired hinge.

When making the punch through the stroma, ensure that there is little to no residual fluid. Having a lot of fluid on the cornea when creating the window can cause the graft to float into the axis, accidentally punching the Descemet's membrane as you are punching through the stroma and damaging the graft.

It is important to consider the placement of the window. Preferably the window should be placed in the mid-periphery of the cornea. If the window is placed too peripheral and the size of the graft is not at least 9, there is risk of the graft sinking into the crevice of the window that was created, leaving the graft to be lifted and thus possibly having difficulty doing a full evaluation on the graft, creating a tear or causing damage to the endothelial layer.

Often times, when making the window, there can be a hinge left when punching through the stroma (e.g., Fig. 4.16). If a hinge is present while punching through the stroma, one can either use a stab knife or scissors to cut off the hinge. There are times when one can easily fold back the plug and the plug will stay in place, however if the stroma is too thick, the plug will want to go back to its original position. If the hinge is still in place, there is a chance that you will need to use your non-dominant hand to hold the plug-in place as you are drying and stamping the Descemet's membrane with the "S." Another option is to re-punch the window, however doing so would risk the chance of creating a bigger window, making it difficult for the plug to stay in place (e.g., Fig. 4.17).

There is a possibility that the plug does not stay in place if it is not properly adhered. Having bubbles underneath the plug can also make it

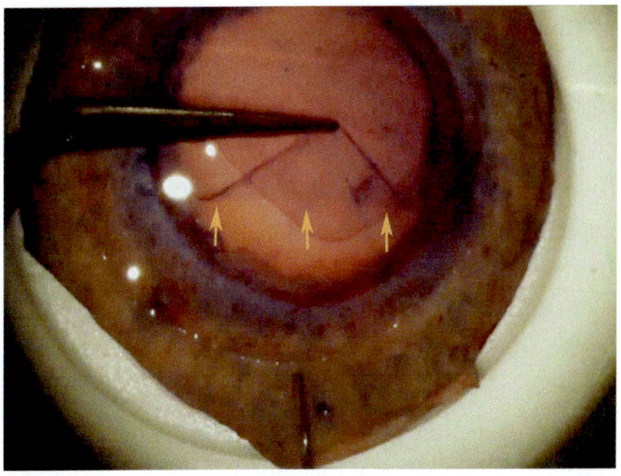

**Fig. 4.15** Ideal straight horizon line

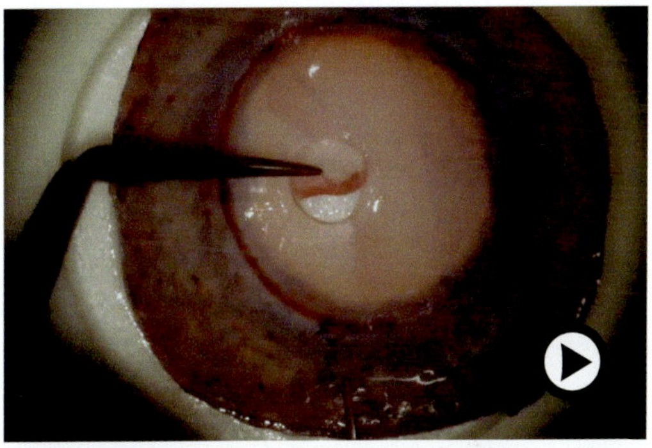

**Fig. 4.16** Hinge left when punching through the stroma (https://doi.org/10.1007/000-dgv)

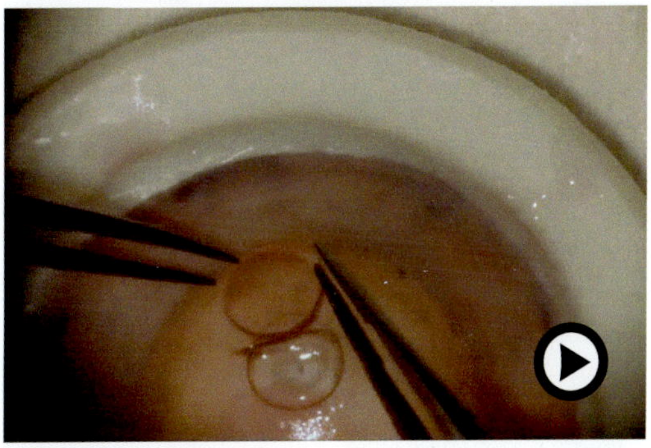

**Fig. 4.17** Hinge when making the window (https://doi.org/10.1007/000-dgw)

difficult for the plug to stay in place during transport and may lift the graft making it difficult to perform a post-evaluation. The amount of liquid, coupled with the movement from transport, can force the plug to come out of place and force the graft to lift. If the graft seems to be lifted, grab from where the hinge is marked and let the flow of liquid and gravity lay the graft back down to its original state (e.g., Figs. 4.18 and 4.19).

In some cases, the window created can be too big and the plug may not fit back into its original position. Making sure the plug is in the correct orientation is beneficial during transport, if the plug is in the wrong orientation it could come out of the window and fall out, no longer protecting the Descemet's membrane graft. It is still possible to trephinate the graft without the plug-in place; however, if the graft is not laid down and free of folds, there is a chance for the graft to sink into the window, making the graft uneven. Another common problem is having multiple tears created around the periphery of the cornea. If the tears do not come too far into the center of the graft, it is still possible to transplant the graft as long as the graft size is to the desired trephinated size designated by the surgeon.

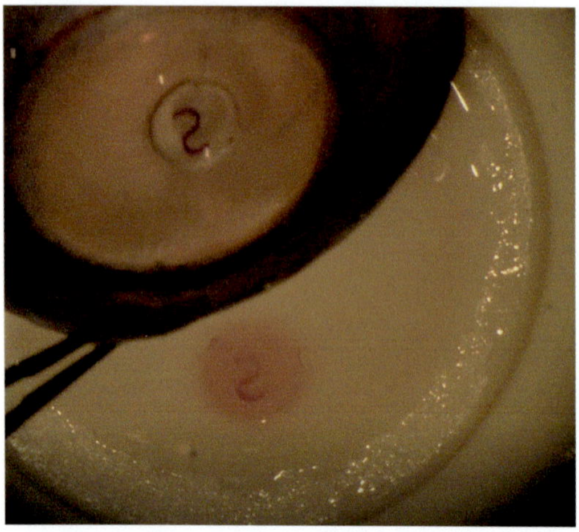

**Fig. 4.18** Example of plug easily coming out. Still transplantable without the plug

## 4.4 Slit Lamp and Evaluation

The evaluation is the final step to our DMEK process. After the Descemet's is peeled, a full evaluation is done to make sure the integrity of the cornea is intact and is still transplantable. A full evaluation consists of capturing a specular image and analysis of the corneal endothelium to make sure the endothelial cells are healthy for transplant as well as a slit lamp evaluation to evaluate the overall integrity of the Descemet's layer (i.e., no major defects were made during the process, endothelial cells are present throughout the whole cornea, no tears or horseshoe tears, and a measurement of the overall graft for the surgeon). Defects are noted for the surgeon and is still transplantable if it is within an acceptable range of the surgeon's graft. The evaluation also consists of making sure the "S" stamp is suitable for the surgery and is placed well within the desired size of the trephination punch (e.g., Figs. 4.20 and 4.21).

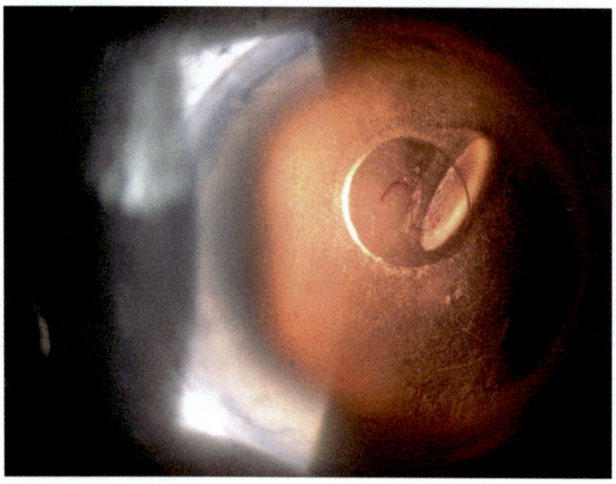

**Fig. 4.19** Slit lamp view of plug not adhered. Slit lamp view of inverted plug

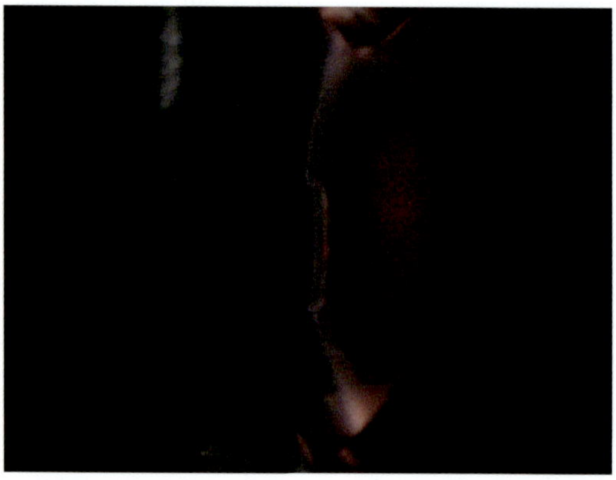

**Fig. 4.20** Retroillumination on slit lamp

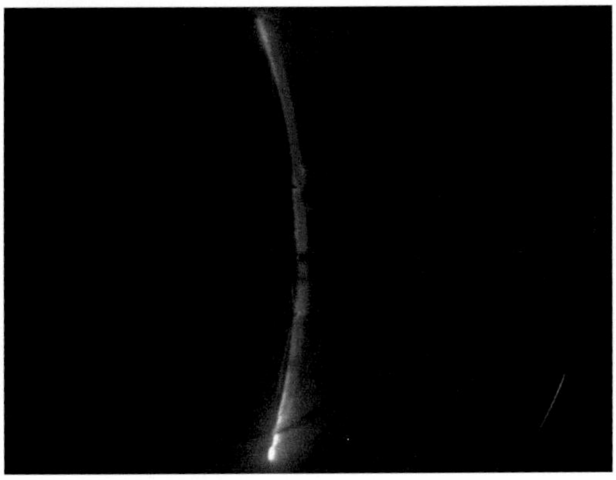

**Fig. 4.21** Narrow slit on the slit lamp

## 4.5 Choosing Placement of Corneas

DMEK suitable corneas consist of a variety of factors that play a part in having a successful procedure [18]. Typically, the age criteria of DMEK suitable corneas range from 40 to 75 years of age. Younger donors are typically more fragile and more pliable, making it a little unpredictable on the flow of the cornea. Younger donors also have a tighter scroll making it complicated when unscrolling in the patient's eye. Older donors ranging from 60 to 75 are ideal when transplanting into the recipient and are generally a little thicker opposed to younger grafts.

Whether or not the donor had diabetes also plays into successful graft preparation. CorneaGen has categorized the severity of diabetes from level 1 to 5. Based on the severity of diabetes, a DM score is designated to the donor tissue: 1—being more likely to be successful vs level 5—being more difficult. Generally, donors who possess a diabetes score of DM5 have proven to be more adhered to the stroma or frail during the peeling process, creating more tears, and has a higher chance of not being successful.

## References


1. Melles GRJ, Lander F, Rietveld FJR. Transplantation of Descemet's membrane carrying viable endothelium through a small scleral incision. Cornea. 2002;21(4):415–8. https://doi.org/10.1097/00003226-200211000-00025.
2. Melles GR, Ong TS, Ververs B, van der Wees J. Descemet membrane endothelial keratoplasty (DMEK). Cornea. 2006;25:987–90.
3. Baydoun L, Ham L, Borderie V, et al. Endothelial survival after Descemet membrane endothelial keratoplasty. Effect of surgical indication and graft adherence status. JAMA Ophthalmol. 2015;133:1277–85.
4. Brockmann T, Brockmann C, Maier AB, Schroeter J, Bertelmann E, Torun N. Primary Descemet's membrane endothelial keratoplasty for Fuchs endothelial dystrophy versus bullous keratopathy: histopathology and clinical results. Curr Eye Res. 2018;43:1221–7.
5. Oellerich S, Baydoun L, Peraza-Nieves J, et al. Multicenter study of 6-month clinical outcomes after Descemet membrane endothelial keratoplasty. Cornea. 2017;36:1467–76.
6. Schlötzer-Schrehardt U, Bachmann BO, et al. Reproducibility of graft preparations in Descemet's membrane endothelial keratoplasty. Ophthalmology. 2013;120:1769–77.
7. Greiner MA, Rixen JJ, Wagoner MD, et al. Diabetes mellitus increases risk of unsuccessful graft preparation in Descemet membrane endothelial keratoplasty: a multicenter study. Cornea. 2014;33:1129–33.
8. Yoeruek E, Bartz-Schmidt KU. Novel surgical instruments facilitating Descemet membrane dissection. Cornea. 2013;32:523–6.
9. Kruse FE, Laaser K, Cursiefen C, et al. A stepwise approach to donor preparation and insertion increases safety and outcome of Descemet membrane endothelial keratoplasty. Cornea. 2011;30:580–7.
10. Muraine M, Gueudry J, He Z, et al. Novel technique for the preparation of corneal grafts for Descemet membrane endothelial keratoplasty. Am J Ophthalmol. 2013;156:851–9.
11. McKee HD, Jhanji V. Femtosecond laser-assisted graft preparation for Descemet membrane endothelial keratoplasty. Cornea. 2018;37:1342–4.
12. Matsuzawa A, Hayashi T, Oyakawa I, et al. Use of four asymmetric marks to orient the donor graft during Descemet's membrane endothelial keratoplasty. BMJ Open Ophthalmol. 2017;1(1):e000080.
13. Parekh M, Baruzzo M, Favaro E, et al. Standardizing Descemet membrane endothelial keratoplasty graft preparation method in the eye bank-experience of 527 Descemet membrane endothelial keratoplasty tissues. Cornea. 2017;36:1458–66.
14. Veldman PB, Dye PK, Holiman JD, et al. Stamping an S on DMEK donor tissue to prevent upside-down grafts: laboratory validation and detailed preparation technique description. Cornea. 2015;34:1175–8.
15. Bhogal M, Maurino V, Allan BD. Use of a single peripheral triangular mark to ensure correct graft orientation in Descemet membrane endothelial keratoplasty. J Cataract Refract Surg. 2015;41:2022–4.
16. Majmudar PA, Johnson L. Enhancing DMEK success by identifying optimal levels of trypan blue

dye application to donor corneal tissue. Cornea. 2017;36:217–21.
17. Hayashi T, Yuda K, Oyakawa I, Kato N. Use of brilliant blue G in Descemet's membrane endothelial keratoplasty. Biomed Res Int. 2017;2017:9720389.
18. Heinzelmann S, Huther S, Bohringer D, et al. Influence of donor characteristics on Descemet membrane endothelial keratoplasty. Cornea. 2014;33:644–8.

# Processing of Donor Tissue for PDEK

# 5

Eric Abdullayev

In 2013, Harminder Dua MD (UK) was the first to describe a pre-Descemet's layer (PDL) of collagen, present between the corneal stroma and DM [1], and Dr. Amar Agarwal MD (India) applied this knowledge to produce a new EK variant: pre-Descemet membrane endothelial keratoplasty (PDEK) [2]. PDEK has a number of advantages over previous EK methods. For one, PDEK donor graft is thicker (than DMEK) and is of about 25–30 microns. In addition, it permits the use of younger tissue (dramatically increasing the potential donor pool) and it also yields tissue that typically has a far greater endothelial cell density than typical DMEK grafts. The result should be a faster resolution of post-procedural corneal edema and improved graft longevity relative to DMEK-prepared grafts (Figs. 5.1 and 5.2).

**Supplementary Information** The online version contains supplementary material available at https://doi.org/10.1007/978-981-97-3469-6_5. The videos can be accessed individually by clicking the DOI link in the accompanying figure caption or by scanning this link with the SN More Media App.

E. Abdullayev (✉)
Lions World Vision Institute, Tampa, FL, USA
e-mail: eabdullayev@lionseyeinstitute.org



S. Jacob (ed.), *Mastering DMEK and PDEK*, https://doi.org/10.1007/978-981-97-3469-6_5

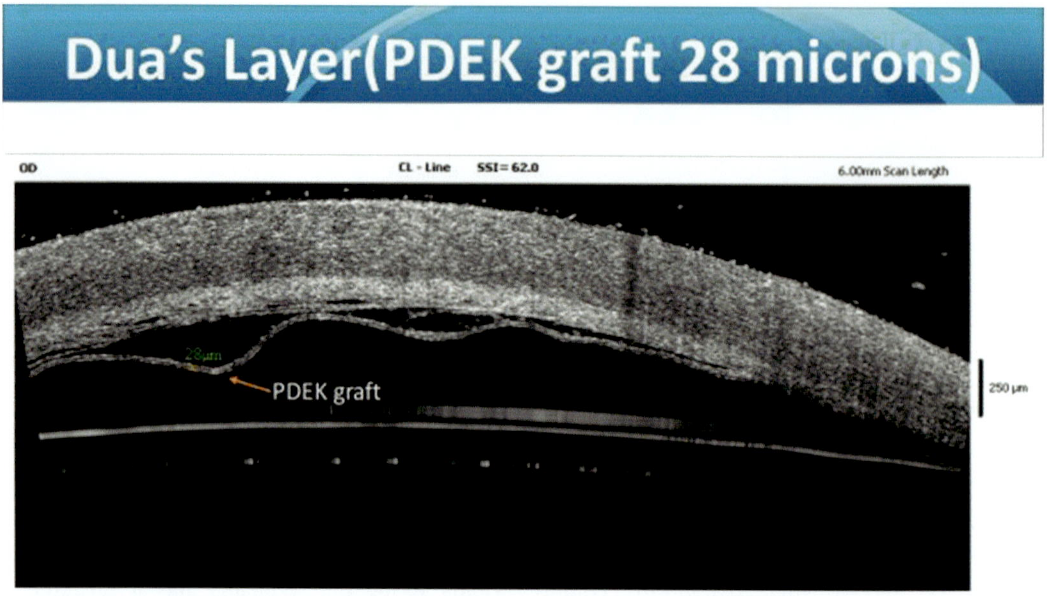


**Fig. 5.1** OCT of 28 microns thick PDEK graft. (Image provided by Eric Abdullayev MD, MBA, CEBT)

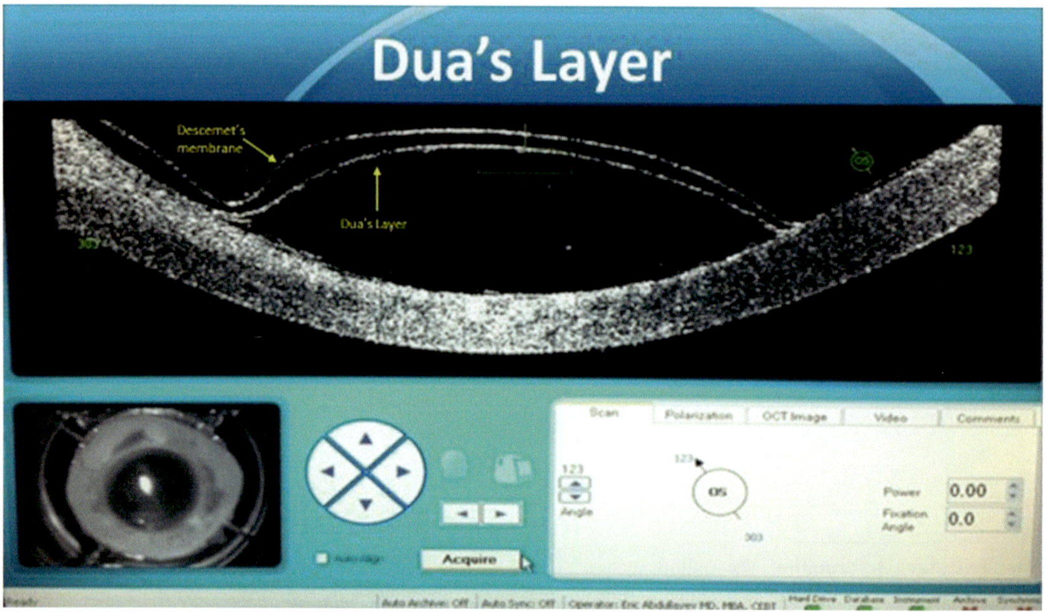


**Fig. 5.2** OCT image of Dua's layer separated from Descemet's membrane. (Image provided by Eric Abdullayev MD, MBA, CEBT)

## 5.1 Donor Tissue Selection

1. Slit lamp, specular, and backlight examination must be performed prior to preparing cornea
2. Donor age—any
3. Epithelium may have defects
4. Donor rim size at least 1.0 mm
5. Intact Descemet's membrane
6. No evidence of prior corneal surgery that compromises the graft such as penetrating stromal wounds (i.e., IOL/cataract scars)
7. Mild or few folds in Descemet's membrane
8. Few central diffused or several peripheral endothelial stress lines
9. Endothelial cell density at least 3000 cells per square millimeter mild or no cell loss. No guttata
10. No ocular or intraocular inflammation or evidence of ocular infection
11. No corneal diseases that might compromise the graft:
    - Ectasia
    - Ulceration
    - Marginal degeneration
    - Endothelial dystrophy
12. The following are acceptable:
    - Epithelial dystrophies
    - Anterior and posterior stromal edema or scars
13. Mild or no polymegathism or pleomorphism
14. Tissue processed for DMEK may be performed at any time up to 10 days post mortem. Anything more will be the responsibility of the transplanting surgeon
15. After tissue has been processed, the cornea shall be re-evaluated using cells staining, slit lamp, backlight, and specular microscopy. Approval/rejection will then be made if tissue is suitable for transplant

## 5.2 Techniques

Donor graft preparation is the most important part of the PDEK procedure. Formation of a type 1 bubble is essential and involves the separation of the pre-Descemet's layer with the Descemet's membrane endothelium complex from the residual stroma. This is unlike a Descemet's membrane endothelial keratoplasty procedure, which involves the formation of a type 2 bubble with the passage of air in between the pre-Descemet's layer and the Descemet's membrane-endothelial complex and leads to the harvesting of only the Descemet's membrane-endothelial layer, leaving the pre-Descemet's layer attached behind in the donor graft. Dr. Amar Agarwal MD (India) prepares PDEK graft with injecting air. Eric Abdullayev MD, MBA, CEBT (Lions Eye Institute for Transplant and Research, Tampa USA) at ASCRS 2018 in Washington, DC introduced a no-touch hydro separation BLISTER method with instant staining for the PDEK graft preparation [3]. In contrast with Dr. Agarwal's method where air is used to separate pre-Descemet's membrane, BLISTER method is separation of the pre-Descemet's membrane with fluid (cornea storage media Optisol GS). Because fluid is not compressible, injection of the small amount of Optisol GS under the Dua's layer basically instantly separates it from the stroma without much stroma infiltration (bumpy deformity) which always takes place when air used for separation. That is why when PDEK graft prepared with BLISTER method it is possible to perform post-processing specular microscopy to confirm viability of endothelial cells: (Fig. 5.3).

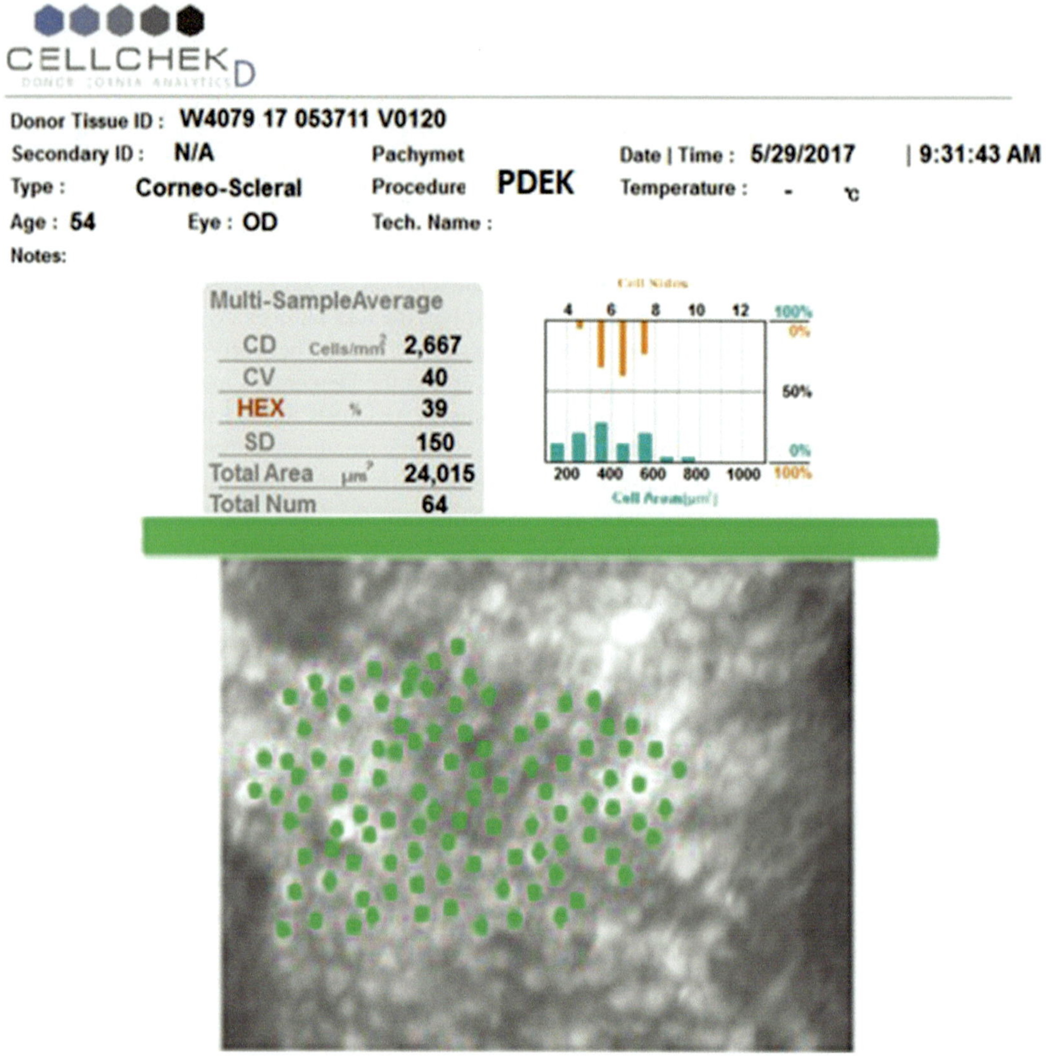


**Fig. 5.3** Endothelial cell count

## 5.3 Preparation of PDEK Graft with Air Injection

The steps include:

**A**: A 30-gauge needle connected to a syringe with air enters the cornea from the edge of the sclera. The donor cornea is kept endothelial side up.

**B**: The needle is gradually passed to the center of the cornea, taking care not to perforate the endothelial side. Once it reaches the center of the cornea, air is injected into the corneal layers.

**C**: A type 1 big bubble is formed. The air is now between the pre-Descemet's layer and stroma. Note the big bubble does not reach the periphery of the cornea because there are firm adhesions between the pre-Descemet's and stroma in the periphery. If a bubble is created to the edge of the cornea, it is a type 2 big bubble. This means the air has formed between the Descemet's membrane and the pre-Descemet's layer. If a type 2 big bubble forms, one cannot do PDEK and will have to do DMEK.

**D**: Trypan blue is injected into the type 1 big bubble as the bubble has been perforated. This helps to stain the tissue and also helps the surgeon get a clear view of the lenticule.

**E**: A trephine is taken, matching the size of the type 1 big bubble and trephination done.

**F**: Any area that has not been clearly cut is cut with Vannas scissor, and the entire lenticule is lifted. This graft now contains endothelium, Descemet's membrane, and pre-Descemet's layer (Fig. 5.4). (Image courtesy Jacob S)

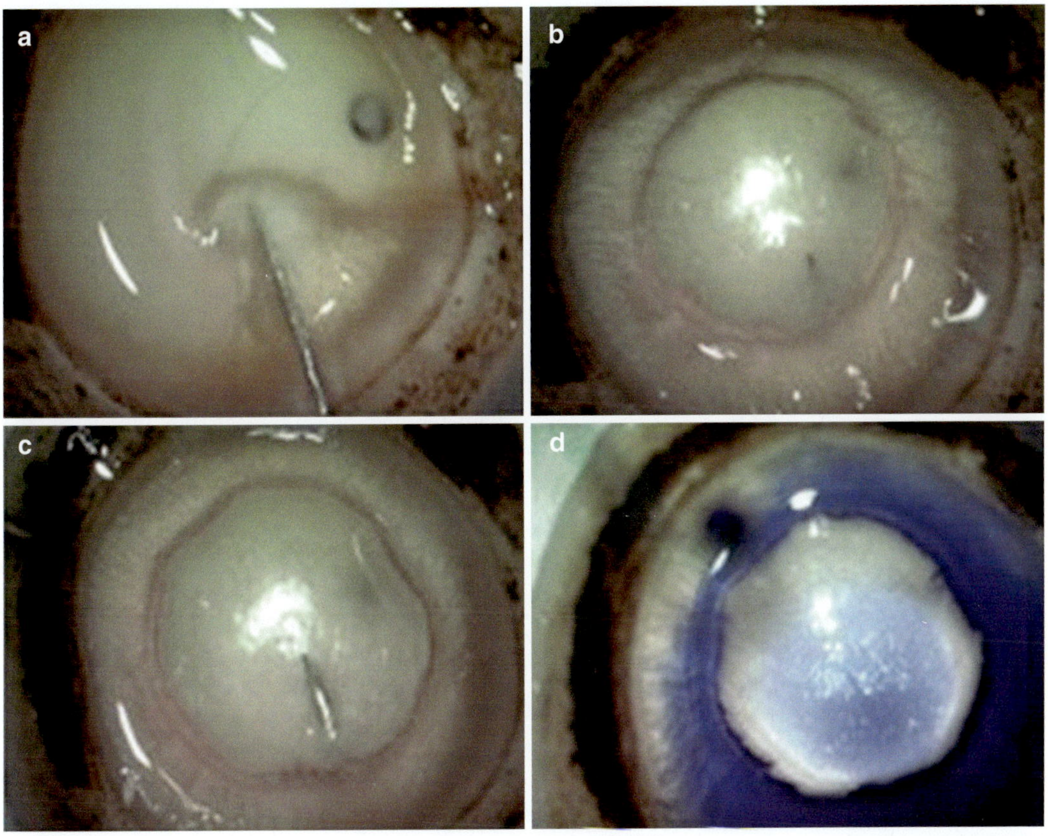


**Fig. 5.4** Preparation of PDEK graft with air injection. (**a**) 30-gauge needle connected to a syringe with air enters the cornea from the edge of the sclera. The donor cornea is kept endothelial side up. (**b**) The needle is gradually passed to the center of the cornea, taking care not to perforate the endothelial side. Once it reaches the center of the cornea, air is injected into the corneal layers. (**c**) A type 1 big bubble is formed. The air is now between the pre-Descemet's layer and stroma. Note the big bubble does not reach the periphery of the cornea because there are firm adhesions between the pre-Descemet's and stroma in the periphery. If a bubble is created to the edge of the cornea, it is a type 2 big bubble. This means the air has formed between the Descemet's membrane and the pre-Descemet's layer. If a type 2 big bubble forms, one cannot do PDEK and will have to do DMEK. (**d**) Trypan blue is injected into the type 1 big bubble as the bubble has been perforated. This helps to stain the tissue and also helps the surgeon get a clear view of the lenticule. (**e**) A trephine is taken, matching the size of the type 1 big bubble and trephination done. (**f**) Any area that has not been clearly cut is cut with Vannas scissor, and the entire lenticule is lifted

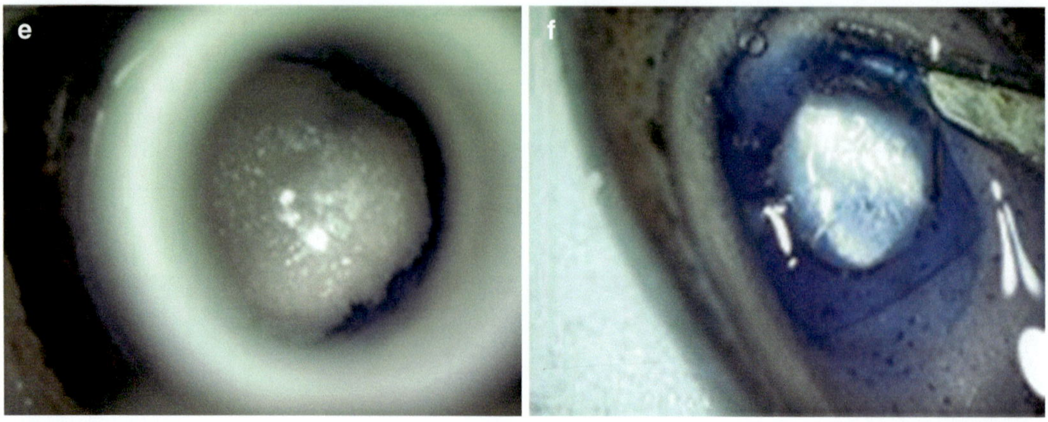


**Fig. 5.4** (continued)

## 5.4 Preparation of PDEK Graft with BLISTER Method (Hydroseparation)

Four step procedure (Fig. 5.5):

A. 30G needle, attached to 1 cc syringe with Optisol GS, inserted horizontally as possible into the sclera and Optisol GS injected into the stroma
B. Continue to move needle and inject Optisol GS into the stroma with soft pressure with needle. When needle appr. 3.0–3.5 mm from the limbus stroma “BLISTER” created and PreDM detachment initiated.
C. The “Blister” continues (Trypan blue can be used) to expand and separates PreDM until it reaches the 7.5–8.0 mm slightly unevenly.
D. Optisol (or Trypan blue) drained out of prepared “BLISTER” by several needle punctures at the edge of the graft.

Separation of pre-Descement’s membrane for PDEK is more difficult than separation of Descemet’s membrane due to Dua’s layer anatomy (Fig. 5.6). It is only an average of 7.5–8 mm diameter and doesn’t reach the limbus as the Descemet’s membrane does. This 7.5-8mm dome-shaped bubble however translates to a slightly larger graft size (by about 0.5mm) in the recipient’s eye as the dome-shaped configuration changes into a flatter configuration on floating up against the host stroma.

That is why separation of the Dua’s layer with BLISTER method should start exactly from the center portion of the cornea by positioning the needle in the posterior stroma as close to Dua’s layer as possible. If those steps are done properly, it will always be possible to obtain pre-Descemet’s membrane with the BLISTER method.

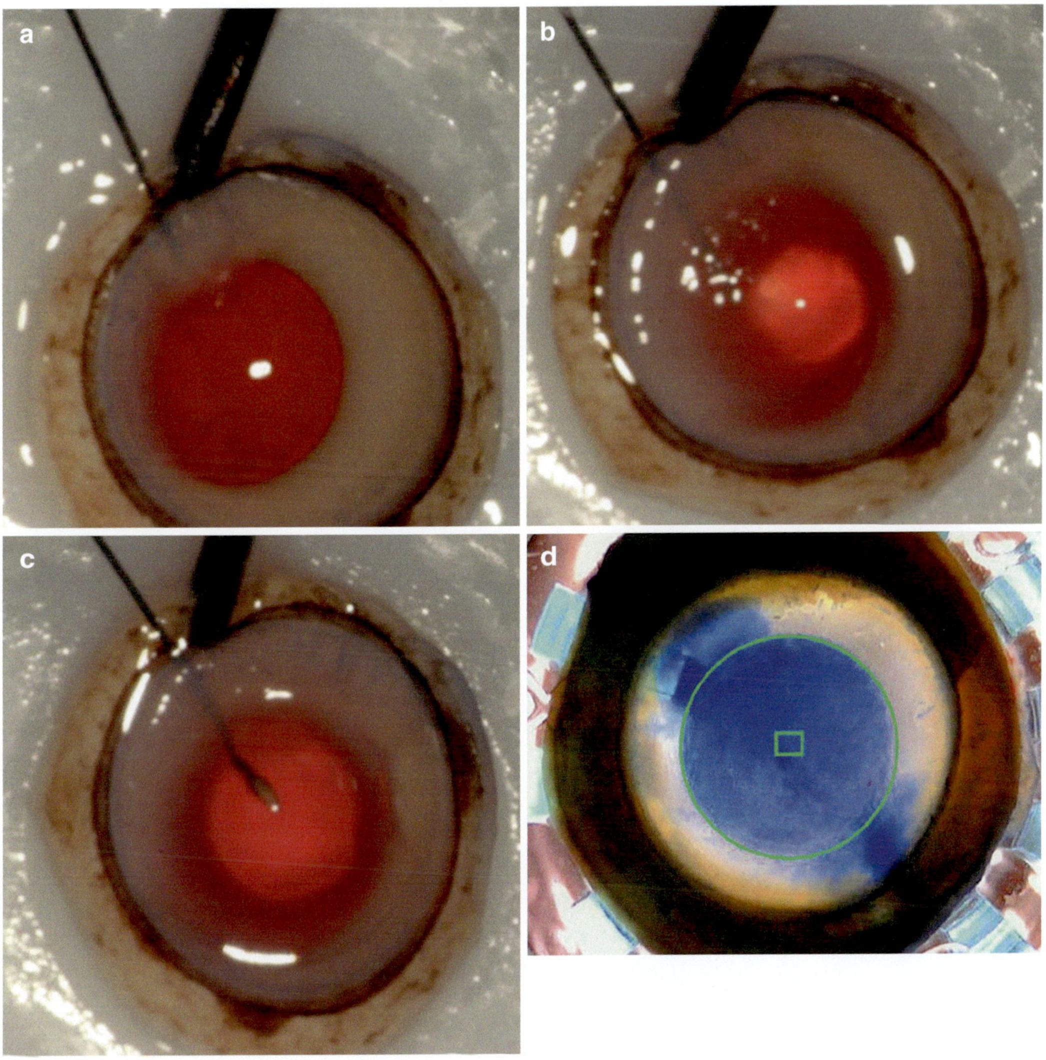


**Fig. 5.5** Preparation of PDEK graft with BLISTER method (hydro separation). (**a**) 30G needle, attached to 1 cc syringe with Optisol GS, inserted horizontally as possible into the sclera and Optisol GS injected into the stroma. (**b**) Continue to move needle and inject Optisol GS into the stroma with soft pressure with needle. When needle appr. 3.0–3.5 mm from the limbus stroma "BLISTER" created and PreDM detachment initiated. (**c**) The "Blister" continues (Trypan blue can be used) to expand and separates PreDM until it reaches the 7.5–8.0 mm slightly unevenly. (**d**) Optisol (or Trypan blue) drained out of prepared "BLISTER" by several needle punctures at the edge of the graft

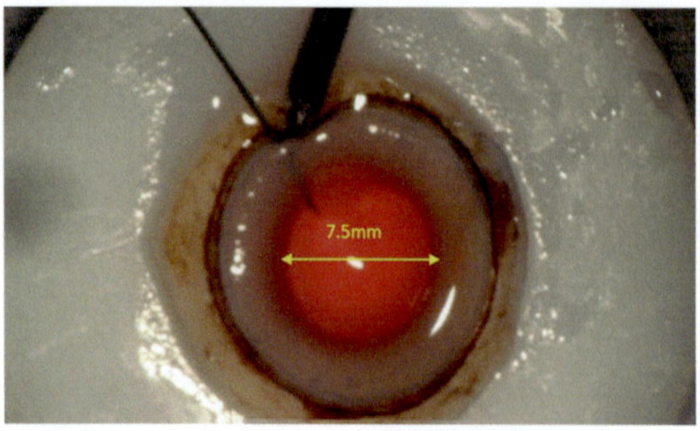


**Fig. 5.6** Pre-Descemet's membrane dimension

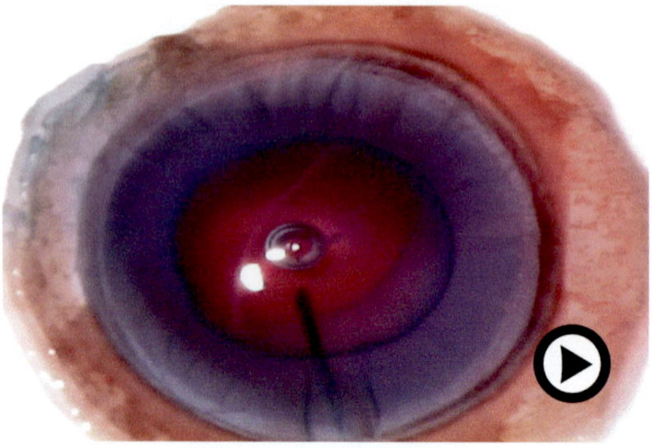

PDEK graft preparation by hydroseparation (https://doi.org/10.1007/000-dgy)

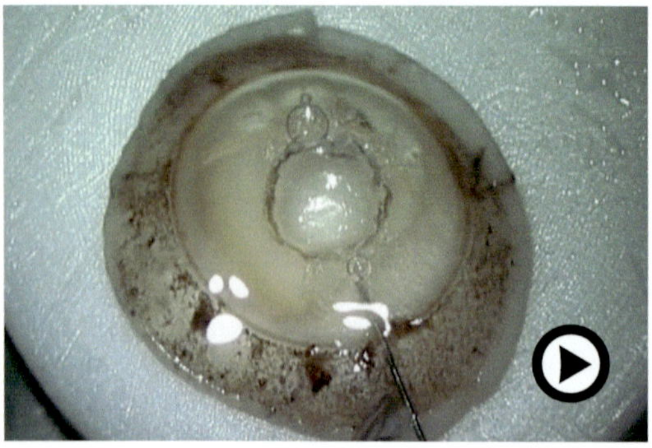

PDEK graft preparation with air (https://doi.org/10.1007/000-dgx)

## References

1. Dua HS, et al. Human corneal anatomy redefined: a novel pre-Descemet layer (Dua's layer). Ophthalmology. 2013;120:1778–85.
2. Agarwal A, Dua HS, Narang P, Kumar DA, Agarwal A, Jacob S, Agarwal A, Gupta A. Pre-Descemet's endothelial keratoplasty (PDEK). Br J Ophthalmol. 2014;98:1181–5. https://doi.org/10.1136/bjophthalmol-2013-304639.
3. Abdullayev E. New method for preparation of injector-preloaded and transplant-ready pre-Descemet endothelial keratoplasty (PDEK) grafts. In: 2018 ASCRS symposium and congress, scientific paper session, 2018, Washington, DC, USA.

# DMEK: Surgical Technique

# 6

Björn Bachmann, Mario Matthaei, Claus Cursiefen, and Takahiko Hayashi

## 6.1 Introduction

Descemet membrane endothelial keratoplasty (DMEK) has become a standard surgery for endothelial decompensation in Fuchs endothelial corneal dystrophy (FECD) [1]. The indications have been gradually expanded to other situations such as pseudophakic bullous keratopathy [2, 3] or endothelial dysfunction in more complex situations, namely after vitrectomy [4–7], after glaucoma surgery (filtrating surgery or shunt tube surgery) [8], eyes of aphakia or with iris defect [6], or eyes after penetrating keratoplasty (PKP) [9–11]. Almost all patients with blurred vision or glare/photophobia caused by corneal endothelial dysfunction or by corneal guttae in FECD are suitable for DMEK (Fig. 6.1) [12, 13]. An intact iris diaphragm is important for the unfolding process and prevents graft loss into the vitreous. Surgeons who are new to the technique of DMEK should start with such patients and make sure that the anterior chamber (AC) has a normal depth [6, 7, 14]. As there is a certain learning curve to master DMEK, an average of 25 cases are necessary until repeatable results in normal eyes are achieved by otherwise experienced intraocular surgeons [15, 16]. The learning curve might be flattened under the instructions of experienced surgeons (who have experiences of over 100 cases).

Special care should be taken on eyes with deep AC (e.g., vitrectomized eyes, high myopic eyes) or shallow AC (small eyes, phakic eyes). These and other more challenging situations like eyes after glaucoma surgeries (Fig. 6.2), aphakia, or eyes with large iris defects (Fig. 6.3) are suitable for DMEK but should be avoided by beginners. Surgeons taking the step toward more complex situations can influence intracameral unfolding of the DMEK roll already by choosing a graft with correct donor age. In principle, both old (above the age of 55 years) and young donors are suitable for transplantation in DMEK [17]. It is well known that DMs from young donors form tighter rolls and are therefore more suitable for eyes with shallow anterior chambers. On the contrary, DMs from older donors show less rolling and therefore allow easier unfolding in patients with deep anterior chamber. The handling of tight DM rolls in a very deep anterior chamber is dem-

**Supplementary Information** The online version contains supplementary material available at https://doi.org/10.1007/978-981-97-3469-6_6. The videos can be accessed individually by clicking the DOI link in the accompanying figure caption or by scanning this link with the SN More Media App.

B. Bachmann (✉) · M. Matthaei · C. Cursiefen
Department of Ophthalmology, University of Cologne, Cologne, Germany
e-mail: bjoern.bachmann@uk-koeln.de; claus.cursiefen@uk-koeln.de

T. Hayashi
Department of Ophthalmology, University of Cologne, Cologne, Germany

Department of Ophthalmology, Yokohama Minami Kyosai Hospital, Kanagawa, Japan


S. Jacob (ed.), *Mastering DMEK and PDEK*, https://doi.org/10.1007/978-981-97-3469-6_6

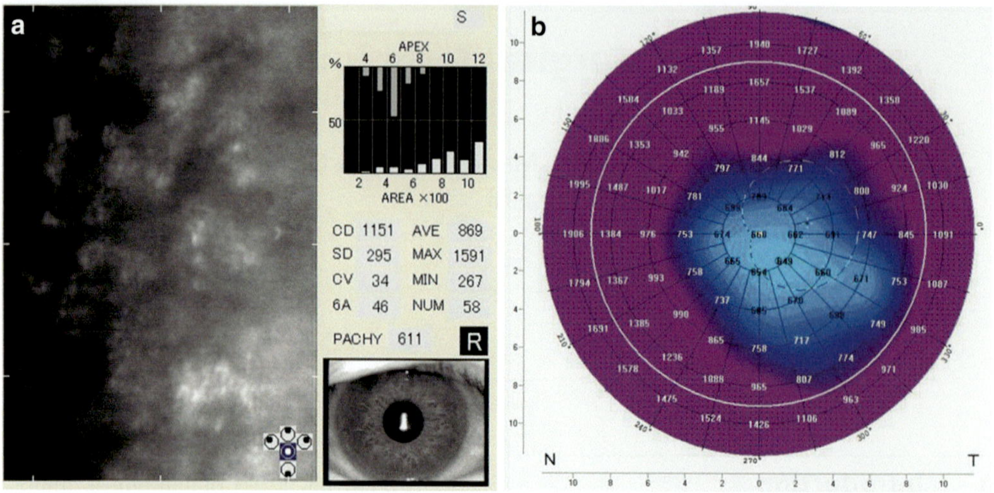


**Fig. 6.1** Corneal guttae. (**a**) Endothelial cells in a patient with Fuchs endothelial corneal dystrophy (FECD). Even if pictures by a specular microscope can be achieved, the true number of endothelial cells cannot be calculated. Cell distribution and the occurrence of guttae have a high variability across the posterior corneal surface. Even patients with no or mediocre corneal edema (**b**) can suffer from blurred vision and reduced contrast sensitivity caused by dense guttae

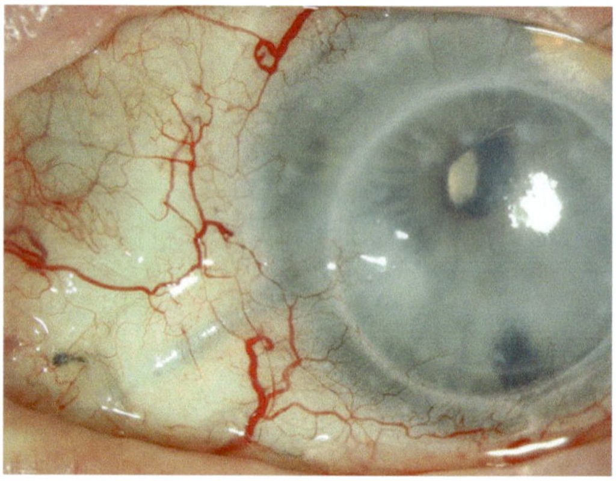

**Fig. 6.2** Eyes after glaucoma surgeries. A certain number of patients will develop corneal endothelial decompensation after the implantation of a glaucoma drainage device. Long tubes can have contact to the posterior corneal surface and need to be shortened before insertion of a DMEK graft

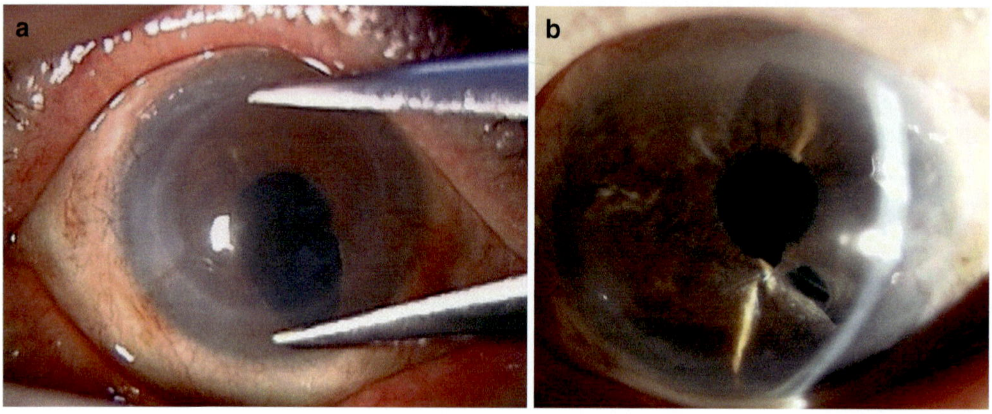


**Fig. 6.3** DMEK in eyes with iris defects. In eyes with large iris defects in the presence of corneal endothelial decompensation (**a**) iris reconstruction by sutures (**b**) or by the implantation of artificial iris devices can be combined with DMEK. An intact lens-iris-diaphragm eases the process of graft unfolding and prevents the loss of the DMEK roll into the vitreous cavity

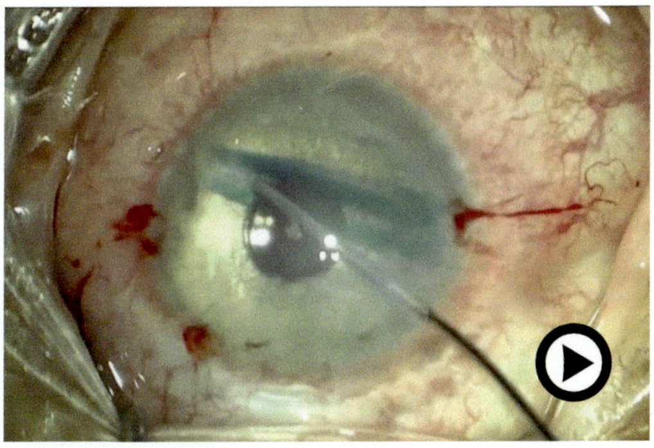

**Fig. 6.4** Tight DMEK roll (https://doi.org/10.1007/000-dh5)

onstrated in Fig. 6.4. Finally, the graft was unfolded while pressed against the corneal stroma by a small air bubble.

## 6.2 Graft Preparation

There is a growing number of eye banks providing prestripped or even preloaded DMEK grafts [18, 19]. The use of prestripped grafts shifts the risk for preparation failures into the eye bank. However, once the technique of graft preparation has been adapted, the rate of graft loss due to difficulties during preparation can be below 1% [19]. The time for graft preparation by trained surgeons depends on donor characteristics and ranges between 5 and 20 min. Most eye banks will charge an extra fee for graft preparation. Therefore, many surgeons trained well in the technique currently perform graft preparations by themselves. Graft preparation also offers the opportunity to become familiar with the individual graft characteristics, and it helps to avoid additional stress to the endothelial cells caused by transportation of prestripped tissue [20, 21].

For graft preparation, surgeons should keep in mind the following points:

1. DMs from young donors are thinner. So far there is no evidence that these thinner DMs are more prone to tearing during stripping. However, DMs from younger donors form a tight scroll and are more difficult to unfold in deeper ACs [22]. When comparing the final visual acuity, rebubbling rate and the loss of endothelial cells caused by DMEK, there seems to be no significant difference between old and young donors [17, 23].
2. Donor corneas from pseudophakic eyes have scars around the entrance wound of the paracentesis and the main incision. DM will tear around these scars during stripping. Still these corneas are usable for DMEK but graft preparation might take longer and in some cases will result in smaller grafts when the entrance wounds are located toward the corneal center [24].
3. Donor corneas from patients with diabetes mellitus have been shown to result in graft preparation failures as high as 15.3% [25].

Surgeons learning the technique of graft preparation should use tissue from phakic donors aged over 55 years without a history of diabetes mellitus.

Different techniques for the separation of Descemet's membrane (DM) from the corneal stroma exist [26–35]. The original method was introduced by Melles et al. in which the DM is lifted and separated from the outer side of trabecular meshwork [1]. Alternatively DM can be separate by predescemetal injection of either air or fluid [29, 31, 33].

Kruse et al. described a technique resulting in high success rates which is easy to adapt to corneas from pseudophakic donors [27]. Here we describe a modified technique (Fig. 6.5). It is important during all preparation steps to keep the endothelium wet.

1. A narrow strip of the outer most DM is removed in a continuous circular shape close to the trabecular meshwork (Fig. 6.6).
2. To highlight the resulting edge of DM, 0.06% trypan blue (TB) is used to stain DM. A couple of drops for 5–10 s are sufficient. Excess dye can be absorbed by the use of a surgical sponge. After the first staining step, the graft should be carefully checked for typical staining patterns indicating endothelial scars after cataract surgery.
3. Using a blunt golf shaped blade, the resulting edge of DM is lifted and checked for tears (Fig. 6.6). Irregular notches need to be trimmed to avoid tear enlargement when stripping DM.

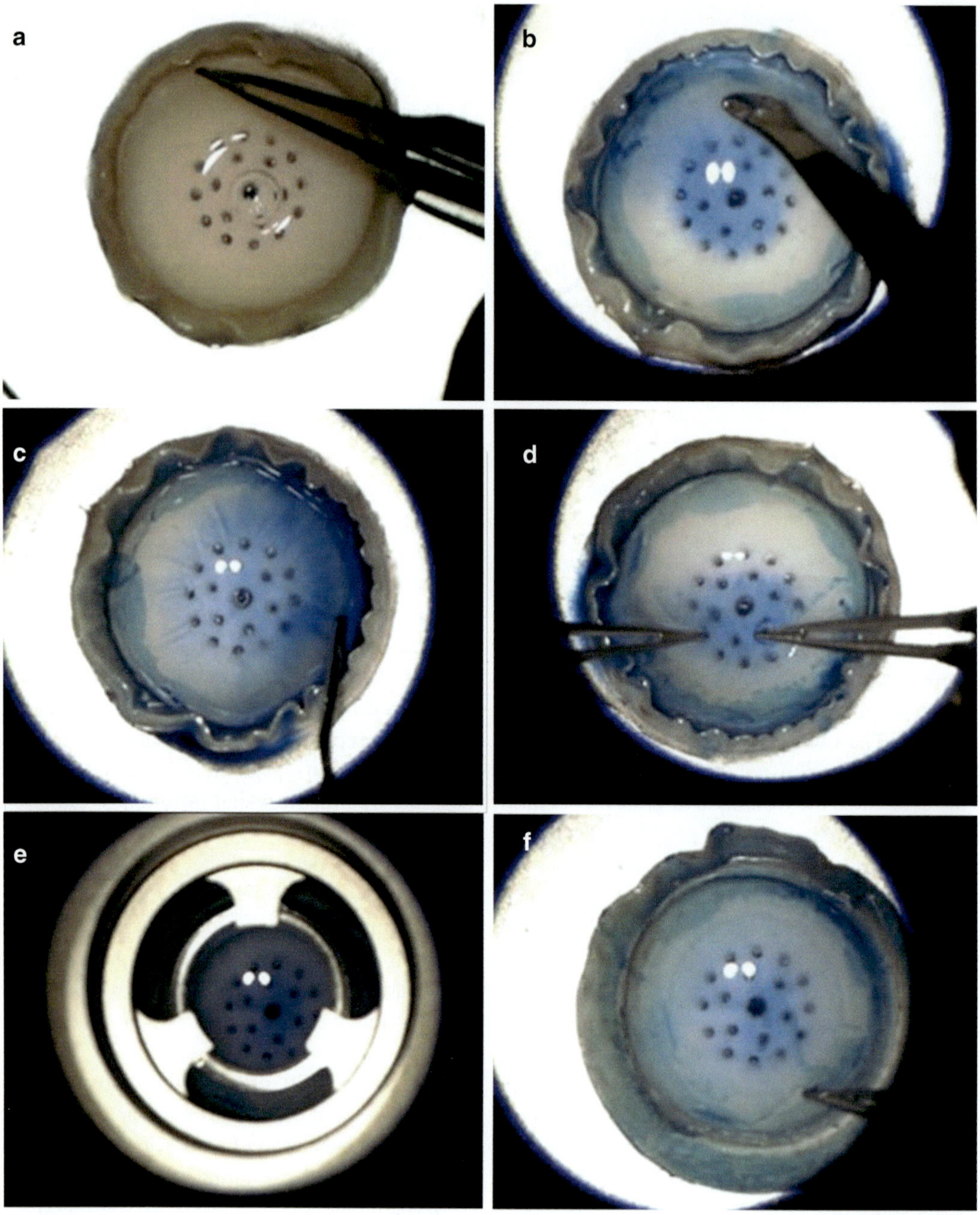


**Fig. 6.5** Graft preparation: stripping technique. Using a blade or forceps, the peripheral endothelium is cut in a continuous manner (**a**). To check the cutting edge, trypan blue is dripped on the outer surface (**b**). Using a golf blade, the peripheral edge is lifted (**c**). If there is an irregular notch, the rim should be removed to make the shape round. This procedure is very important to prevent tearing of DM when pulling centrally. Gentle stripping can be performed with one or two forceps. (**d**) Bimanual stripping results in a more even distribution of the traction forces over DM [28]. After stripping DM can be trephined (**e**). After punching, the peripheral excess tissue is removed (**f**). Using a 1.0-mm derma-punch, three markings are created asymmetrically allowing the identification of the graft orientation after insertion (**g**, **h**)

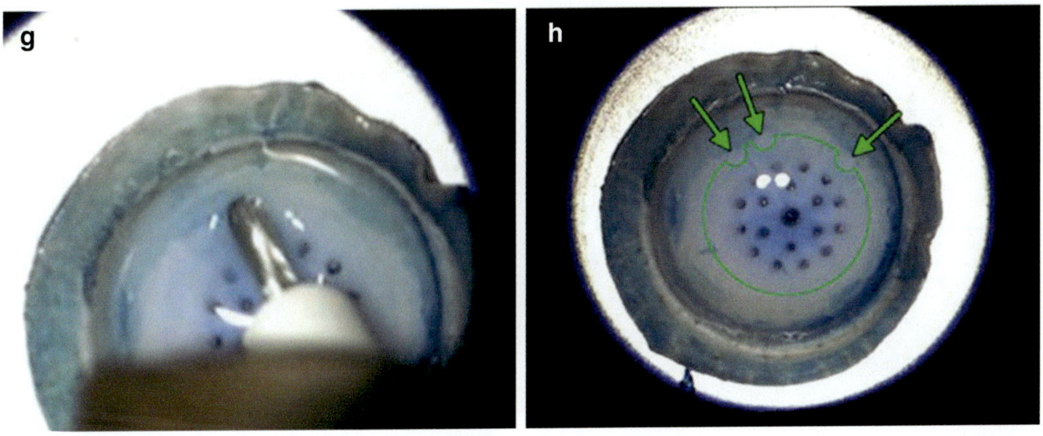


**Fig. 6.5** (continued)

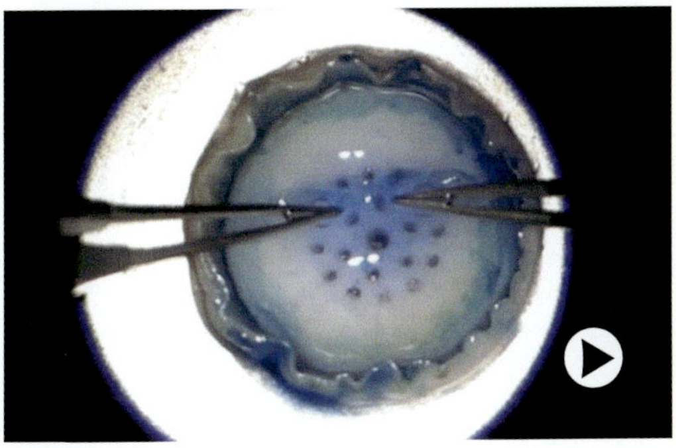

**Fig. 6.6** DMEK graft preparation (https://doi.org/10.1007/000-dh0)

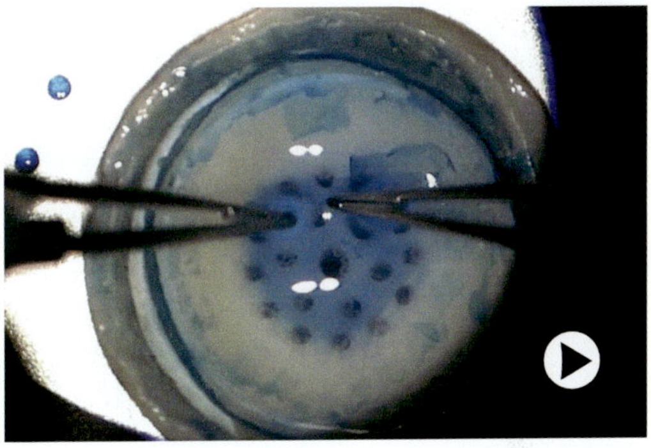

**Fig. 6.7** DMEK graft tear (https://doi.org/10.1007/000-dh1)

4. After lifting the complete circumference of the DM edge stripping can be started using either one or two forceps (Figs. 6.5 and 6.6). While pulling DM special care has to be taken to look for signs indicating tear formation. While stripping DM dye clouds that suddenly appear behind the line of detached DM indicate small tears through which the dye passes from the anterior to the posterior side of DM ("cloud of dirt," Fig. 6.7).
5. Most surgeons are using trephined grafts for implantation. The trephine diameter for "normal" cases usually ranges between 8.0 and 9.5 mm. Smaller diameters can be chosen for smaller, hyperopic eyes or for very focal DMEKs as in acute hydrops in keratoconus. For graft diameters of 5 mm or below, the procedure was termed "Mini-DMEK" [36]. To identify the correct graft orientation during surgery, different techniques have been described such as 3-point-marking [37], 4-point-marking [38], triangle marking [39], S stamp [40], or F stamp [41], etc. In stamping techniques, the marker dye is stamped from the stromal side on Descemet's membrane. Orientation marks are placed at the edge of the graft by using a 1.0-mm punch. Orientation marks at the graft's edge allow to monitor the correct graft orientation not only during surgery but also during the postoperative course (Fig. 6.5) [37].
6. Before loading the graft into the injector (Figs. 6.8, 6.9 and 6.10), proper staining is necessary for sufficient visualization during intracameral unfolding. DM can be stained much better than the endothelial cells. Moreover, trypan blue, the most common used dye for graft staining in DMEK, has some toxic effect on endothelial cells at high

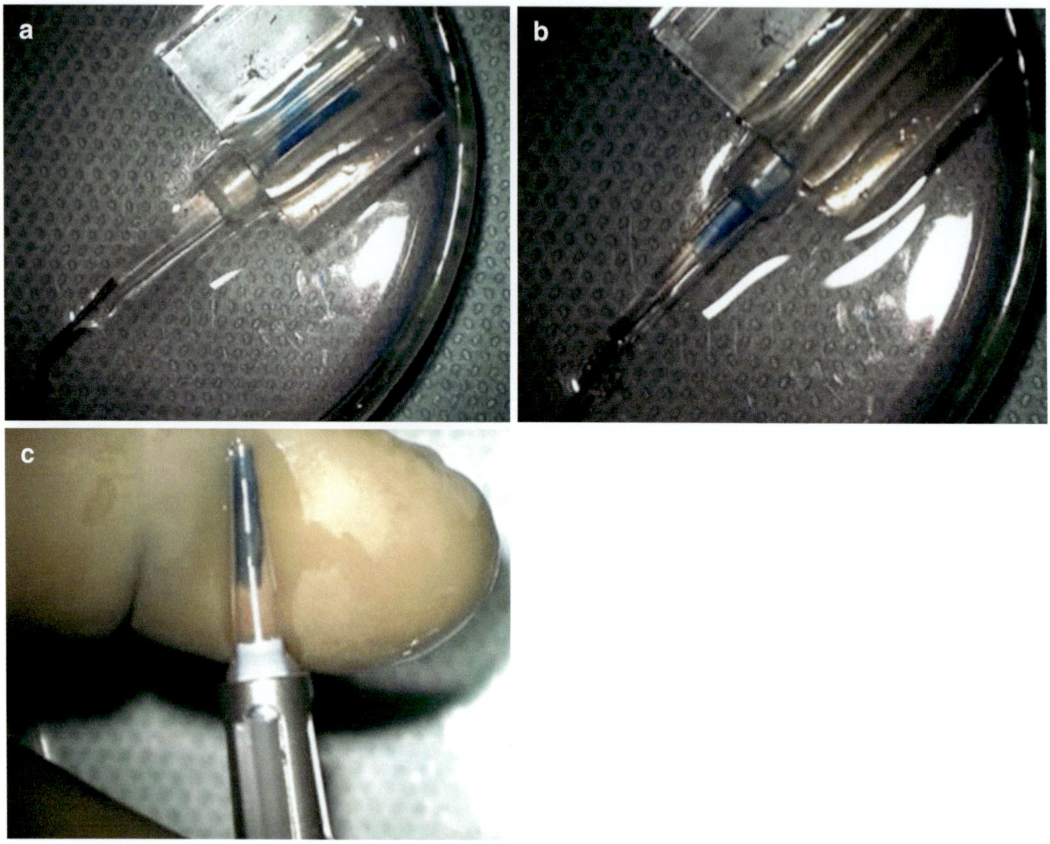


**Fig. 6.8** Graft loading into an IOL injector. The graft can be moved into the cartridge by suction from a canula (**a**, **b**). The plunger should be moved forward until there is only little distance between the graft and the tip opening. Here the graft can be turned easily by a small canula until the graft opening is correctly orientated (**c**)

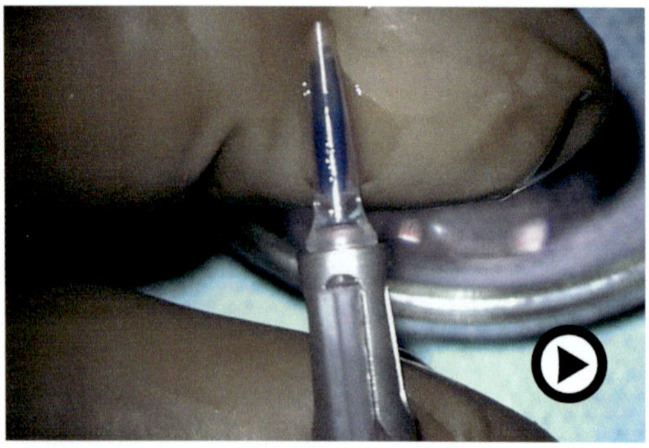

**Fig. 6.9** Loading graft into IOL injector (https://doi.org/10.1007/000-dh2)

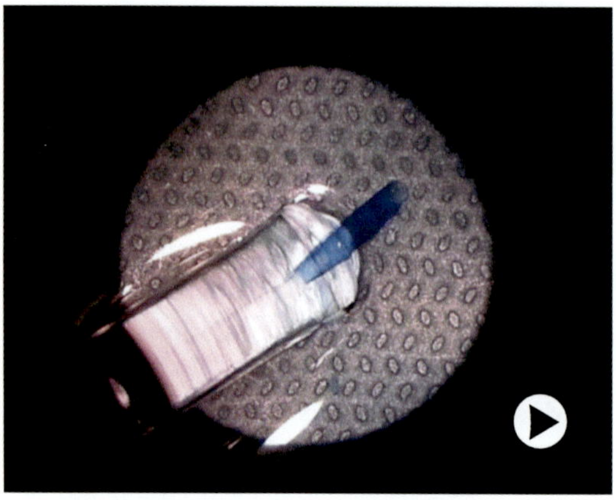

**Fig. 6.10** Loading graft into glass injector (https://doi.org/10.1007/000-dh3)

concentration at longer exposure times [42]. Therefore, the dye should be applied at the stromal side of DM rather than on top of the endothelial cells. Alternative dyes are Brilliant Blue G (BBG) [43, 44] and patent blue [45, 46] which exhibit less staining intensity compared to trypan blue. Different injector systems for graft implantation are available such as commercially available glass injectors [1, 18, 47] or DIY injectors [48]. A very eco-

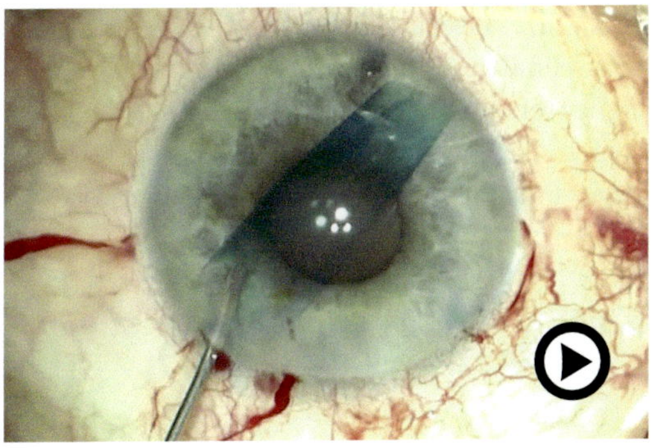

**Fig. 6.11** Opening the scrolls (https://doi.org/10.1007/000-dh4)

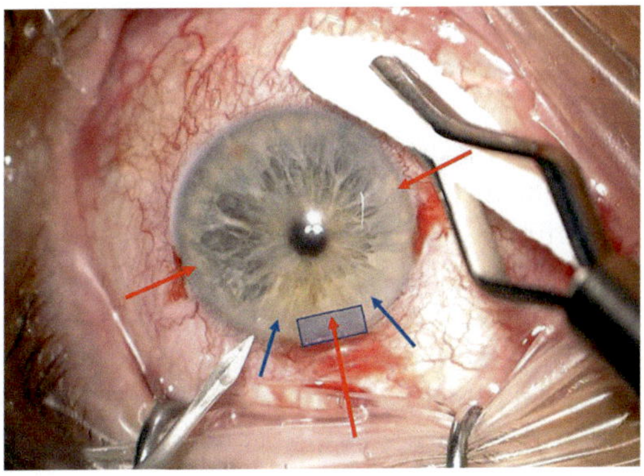

**Fig. 6.12** Incisions. Two paracenteses (commonly at 3 and 9 o'clock position) and one main incision (at 12 o'clock) are necessary. Two additional paracenteses can be added according to the surgeon's preference at 1 and 11 o'clock

nomic and effective injector solution is the use of intraocular lens injectors also suitable for DMEK graft insertion [27, 49, 50]. Most systems currently in use are based on either flushing the graft into the anterior chamber by a fluid jet (glass injector systems) or on pushing the graft into the anterior chamber with a plunger (IOL injector systems) [51]. Pushing systems (e.g., IOL injectors) allow the graft to be reoriented during the insertion process by simply rotating the shooter device (Fig. 6.11). A third approach is the use of long and thin forceps to grasp the graft from the shooter opening and to pull it into the anterior chamber (pull-through technique). Both the pull-through technique and the pushing technique give very good control over the graft orientation during graft insertion [51]. For the pull-through technique, the graft is manually folded into the "tri-fold" formation. In contrast to the spontaneous roll formation of the DMEK graft where the endothelial cells are located on the outer side in the tri-fold formation, the endothelial cells are located at the inner side of the roll [52–54].

## 6.3 Surgery

### 6.3.1 Anesthesia

General anesthesia is less stressful for both the surgeon and the patient. In general, vitreous pressure is lower compared to local anesthesia which makes unfolding of the graft easier. However, more experienced surgeons will be able to perform DMEK surgery also under local anesthesia. All types of topical anesthesia such as sub-Tenon block, retrobulbar block, or even anesthetic eye drops combined with intracameral injection of lidocaine are suitable. The patient's ability to move the eye during local anesthesia with eye drops can be used to direct the graft in the anterior chamber through targeted eye movements.

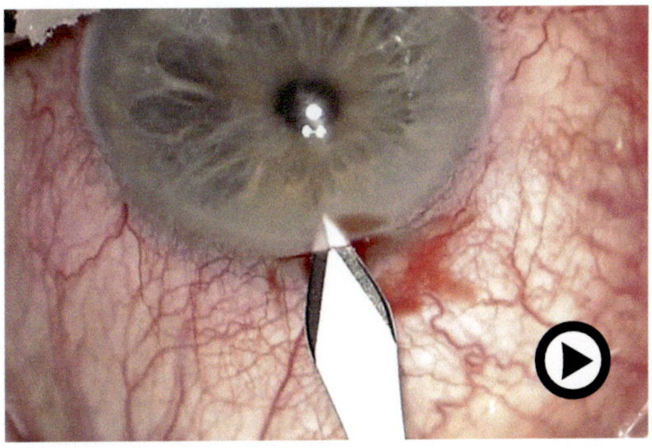

**Fig. 6.13** Incisions for DMEK (https://doi.org/10.1007/000-dgz)

### 6.3.2 Entrance Wounds

A main tunnel and at least two or even more paracentesis are recommended (Fig. 6.12). The width of the wound needs to be adapted to the injector system used. In our technique, a 2.5 mm-corneal incision is created at 12 o'clock (Fig. 6.13).

### 6.3.3 Descemetorhexis (Figs. 6.14 and 6.15)

Descemetorhexis can be easily performed under air at a high contrast. We recommend continuous air perfusion, e.g., via an infusion canula. During this procedure, the ocular surface should be clean of ophthalmic viscosurgical device (OVD) as this will cause the formation of many air bubbles on the entire ocular surface that interferes with the visualization of the recipient's DM. The size of the descemetorhexis should be adapted to the donor size. Overlapping areas more often lead to postoperative graft detachment [55, 56]. Even if higher rebubbling rates result in similar final outcomes, a descemetorhexis diameter 0.5 mm larger than the graft size is recommended [57].

### 6.3.4 Surgical Peripheral Iridectomy (PI) (Figs. 6.16 and 6.17)

For the prevention of a pupillary block [58], a peripheral iridectomy (PI) at the 6 o'clock posi-

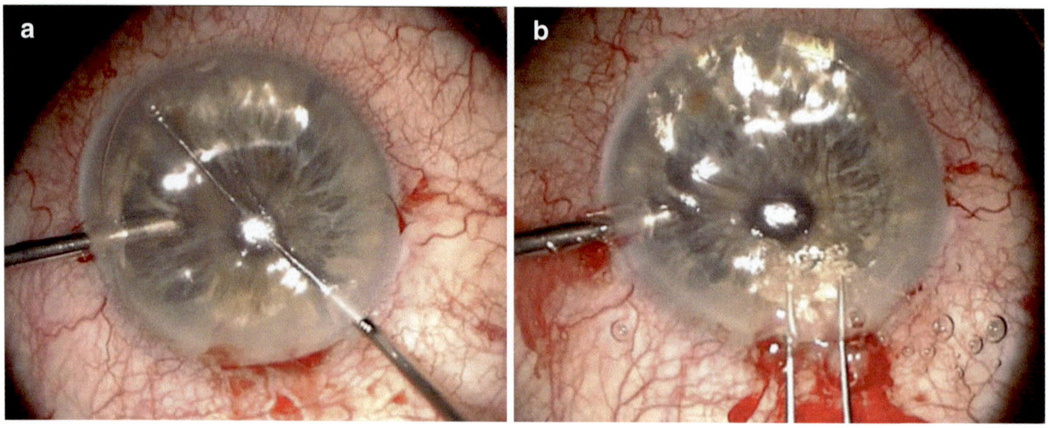


**Fig. 6.14** Descemetorhexis. Descemetorhexis can be performed under water as well as under air. Air gives better visualization and contrast of DM while removing. Current phaco machines often allow for continuous air insufflation which helps to maintain the anterior chamber filled with air during intracameral manipulation with instruments

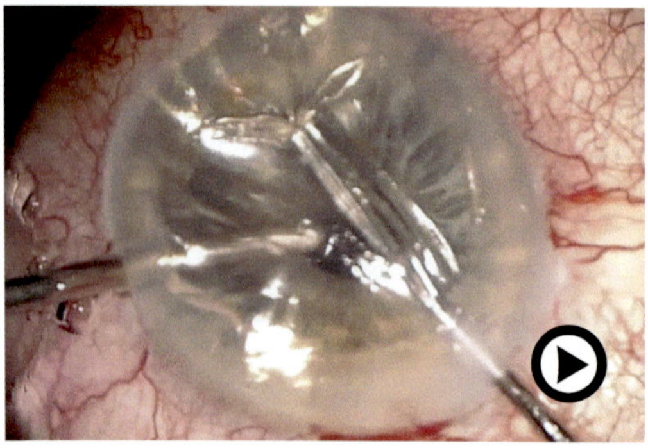

**Fig. 6.15** Descemetorhexis (https://doi.org/10.1007/000-dh6)

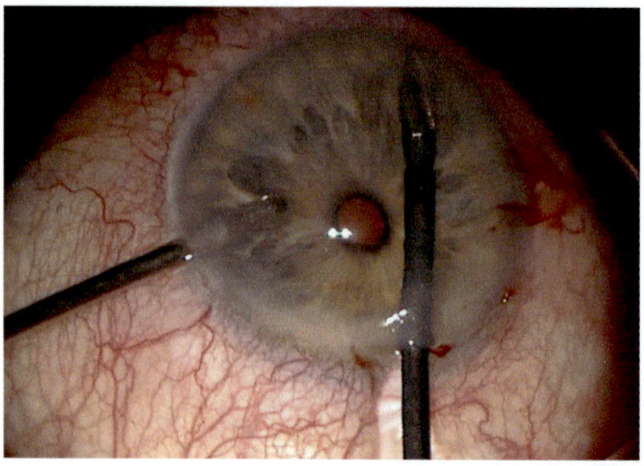

**Fig. 6.16** Peripheral iridotomy. A peripheral iridotomy (PI) is necessary for the prevention of a postoperative pupillary block caused by an intracameral air bubble. A laser iridotomy at least 1 day before DMEK reduces the risk of bleeding caused by a primary intraoperative iridectomy. Just by blunt spreading with scissors, this iridotomy can be easily enlarged during surgery

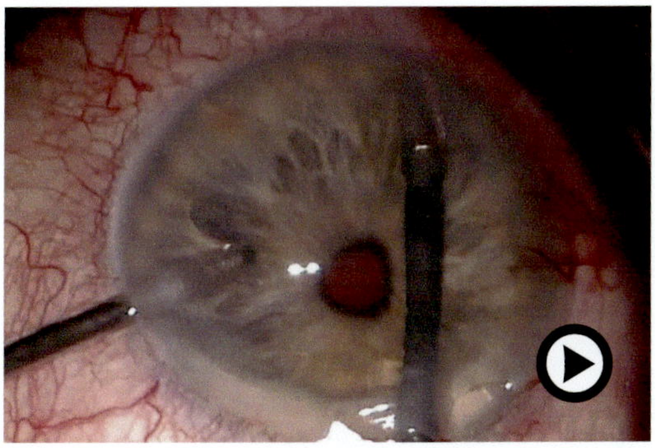

**Fig. 6.17** Peripheral iridectomy (https://doi.org/10.1007/000-dh7)

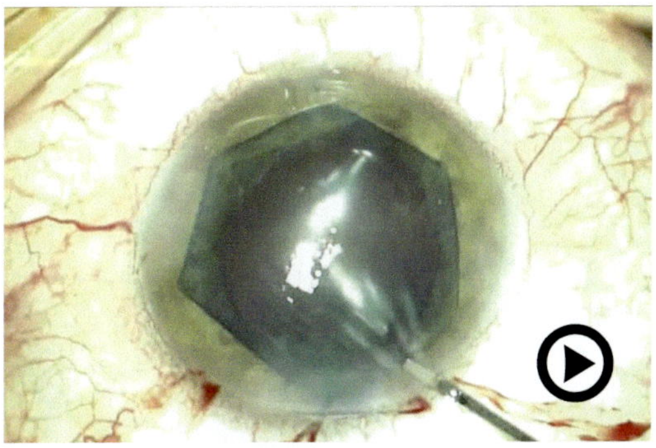

**Fig. 6.18** Opening the loose scrolls (https://doi.org/10.1007/000-dh8)

tion is necessary. The PI can be created with an intraocular scissor or a vitreous cutter using the preexisting paracentesis. However, a freshly introduced iridectomy can cause massive bleeding during surgery which prolongs the surgery and can lead to complications during the following surgical steps [59]. Blood clotting and fibrin formation inhibit unfolding of the DMEK graft [52]. To prevent bleeding, a laser iridotomy should be placed at least the day before surgery. In case of intraoperative bleeding from iris vessels, the intraocular pressure (IOP) should be kept high. A retinal coagulator can be used for iris vessel coagulation.

### 6.3.5 Graft Insertion (Figs. 6.11 and 6.18)

Graft insertion is one of the most crucial parts of DMEK. The technique for graft insertion depends on the injector system used. Anterior chamber (AC) depth is maintained either by an irrigation handpiece or by an AC maintainer when an IOL injector system is used for graft insertion. Here the irrigation has to be stopped when around 2/3 of the graft has passed the tip of the injector [27]. Insertion by flushing systems is usually performed without irrigating the anterior chamber.

IOL injector systems allow control of graft orientation before (Figs. 6.19 and 6.20) and during insertion (Fig. 6.11). Keeping the correct orientation during insertion of the graft is helpful for atraumatic unfolding.

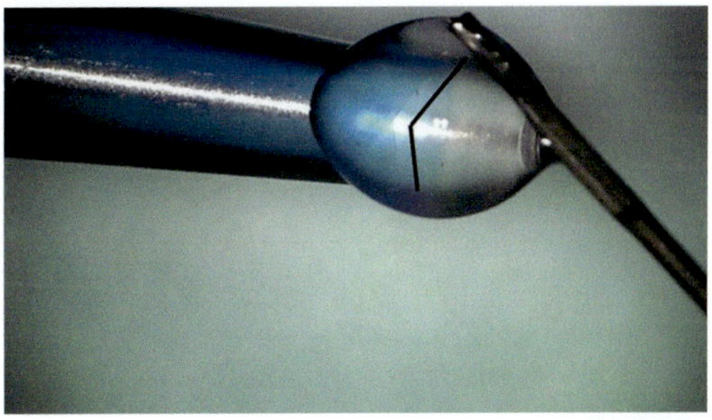

**Fig. 6.19** Orientation of the graft directly before implantation. Correct orientation can be confirmed by a V-shaped overlap zone of the graft (see black line). This overlap zone must be aligned upwards when inserting

### 6.3.6 Graft Unfolding (Figs. 6.11 and 6.18)

After insertion, the first step is to identify correct orientation. Wrong graft orientation is among the main causes for primary graft failure [60, 61]. In cases of severe corneal edema, epithelial debridement should be performed to improve visualization. Different methods have been described for intraoperative identification of the graft orientation. Besides the above described marking techniques [37–39], slit-beam illumination, insertion of a spatula or cannula into the roll (Moutsouris' sign) [62, 63] and the use of intraoperative OCT help to visualize graft orientation (Fig. 6.21) [64–66].

Once correct orientation has been confirmed continuous, corneal tapping with a canula on each side of the graft will unfold the roll. During the unfolding process, the anterior chamber depth

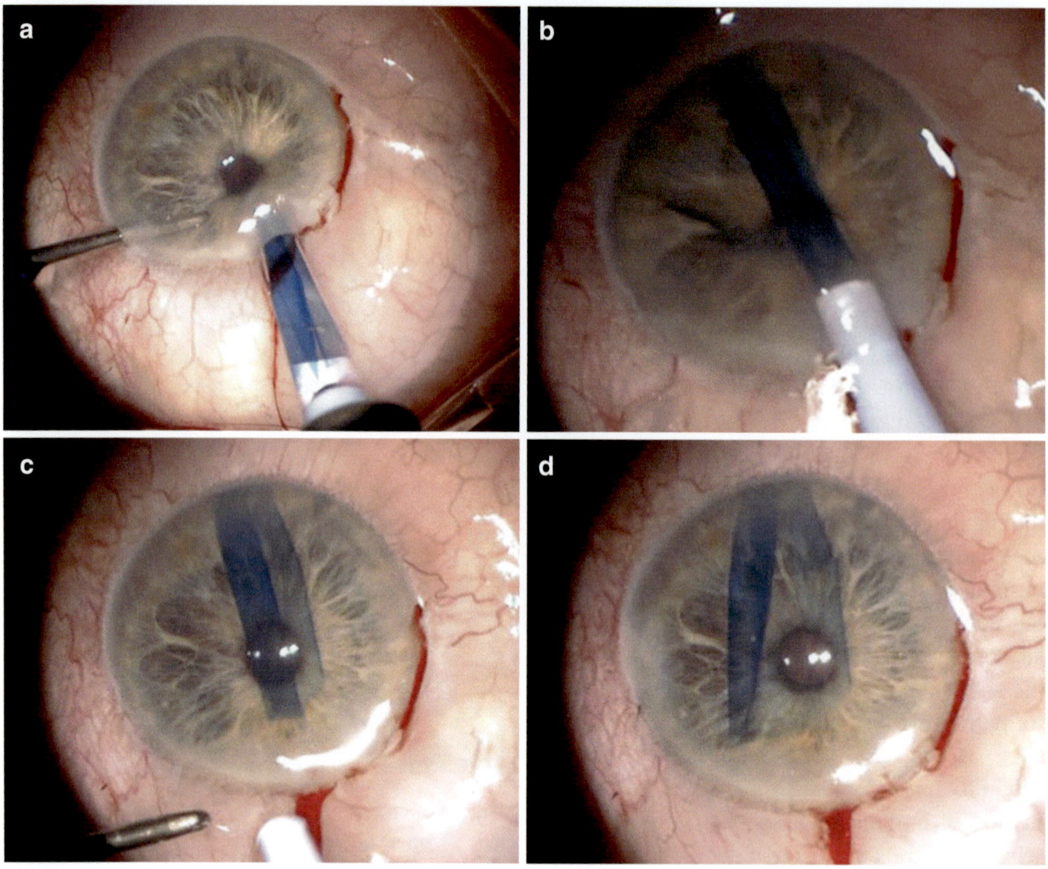


**Fig. 6.20** Graft insertion. The injector tip is introduced through the main incision. When an IOL shooter is used for graft insertion, the AC depth can be adjusted using an AC maintainer or an irrigation hand piece (**a**). During slow insertion by moving the plunger forward orientation of the graft can be readjusted by turning the shooter. The irrigation should be stopped once around halve of the graft has passed the tip opening (**b**) while the plunger is continuously moved forward until the graft has completely entered the anterior chamber (**c**). If the graft is placed in correct orientation (**d**) unfolding can be easily achieved by tipping onto the cornea at both ends of the graft

needs to be adjusted: If the roll tilts, or if there is a risk of taco formation with roll opening to the side, the anterior chamber should be deepened by gentle BSS injection to allow the graft to reorient itself. If unfolding progresses shallowing the anterior chamber by release of fluid via a paracentesis helps to keep the graft unfolded (Fig. 6.18) [67]. Alternatively an air bubble can be placed inside the DMEK roll to unfold the graft (Fig. 6.11) [68]. However, in most cases, simple tapping without the use of intracameral instruments and without the use of an air bubble is sufficient to unfold the graft.

In case of upside-down graft orientation, the AC should be deepened allowing the graft to form a roll again. Once the roll has reformed, it can be easily turned by tapping the cornea or by gentle BSS bursts.

It is difficult to unfold the graft in eyes after vitrectomy, because the AC cannot be flattened to keep the graft unfolded. In such situations, even if unfolding succeeds, the graft is likely to reform a roll immediately. Certain techniques have been described to overcome the problem of the deep AC in high myopic or vitrectomized eyes such as the double-bubble technique (Fig. 6.22) [69], the temporary diaphragm technique [70], C-press technique [71], or holding technique [72].

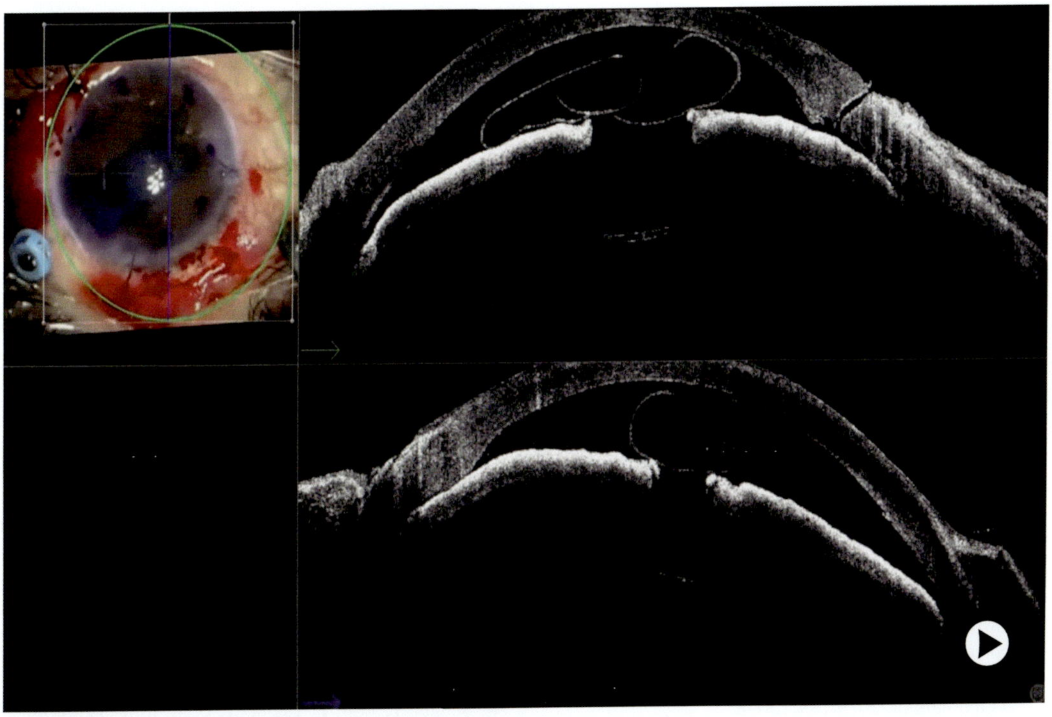

**Fig. 6.21** Intraoperative OCT assisted DMEK (https://doi.org/10.1007/000-dh9)

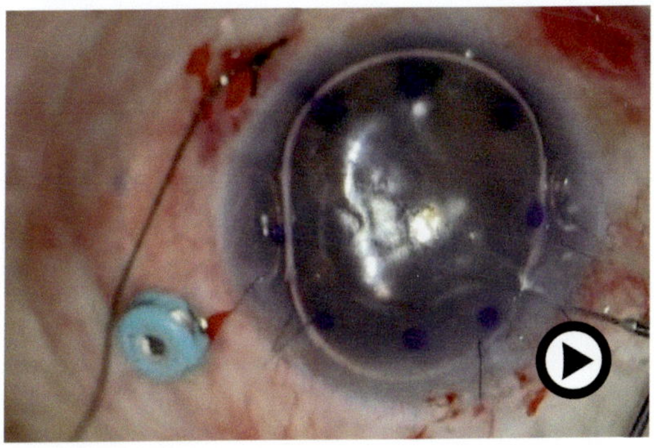

**Fig. 6.22** Graft opening—double bubble (https://doi.org/10.1007/000-dha)

### 6.3.7 Graft Attachment

After unfolding, the graft is attached to the posterior stromal surface by an air bubble which is placed underneath the graft. It must be ensured that the graft is well centered before the application of the first air bubble. Even if the graft is attached by a small air bubble, very strong tapping of the cornea or the use of specialized forceps is needed to move the graft. After complete unfolding and attachment of the graft, either room air or SF6 in concentrations up to 20% can be used for the final AC tamponade. Compared to room air SF6 in a concentration of 20% persists 4–5 days longer and has been shown to reduce the rebubbling rate significantly [73, 74]. If a sufficient PI has been placed, the AC can be filled almost completely. However, it should be ensured that there is no posterior movement of the lens-iris diaphragm. Postoperatively, parts of the gas can be easily released via one of the horizontal paracentesis at the slit-lamp with a blunt probe, e.g., an angled tear duct probe, in case of a pupillary block. This procedure should also be performed in patients where continuous IOP measurements within the first 24 h after surgery cannot be performed.

## References

1. Melles GR, Ong TS, Ververs B, van der Wees J. Descemet membrane endothelial keratoplasty (DMEK). Cornea. 2006;25:987–90.
2. Baydoun L, Ham L, Borderie V, et al. Endothelial survival after Descemet membrane endothelial kera-

toplasty. Effect of surgical indication and graft adherence status. JAMA Ophthalmol. 2015;133:1277–85.
3. Brockmann T, Brockmann C, Maier AB, Schroeter J, Bertelmann E, Torun N. Primary Descemet's membrane endothelial keratoplasty for Fuchs endothelial dystrophy versus bullous keratopathy: histopathology and clinical results. Curr Eye Res. 2018;43:1221–7.
4. Liarakos VS, Ham L, Dapena I, et al. Endothelial keratoplasty for bullous keratopathy in eyes with an anterior chamber intraocular lens. J Cataract Refract Surg. 2013;39:1835–45.
5. Yoeruek E, Rubino G, Bayyoud T, et al. Descemet membrane endothelial keratoplasty in vitrectomized eyes: clinical results. Cornea. 2015;34:1–5.
6. Weller JM, Tourtas T, Kruse FE. Feasibility and outcome of descemet membrane endothelial keratoplasty in complex anterior segment and vitreous disease. Cornea. 2015;34:1351–7.
7. Sorkin N, Einan-Lifshitz A, Ashkenazy Z, et al. Enhancing Descemet membrane endothelial keratoplasty in postvitrectomy eyes with the use of pars plana infusion. Cornea. 2017;36:280–3.
8. Birbal RS, Tong CM, Dapena I, et al. Clinical outcomes of Descemet membrane endothelial keratoplasty in eyes with a glaucoma drainage device. Am J Ophthalmol. 2019;199:150–8.
9. Pasari A, Price MO, Feng MT, Price FW Jr. Descemet membrane endothelial keratoplasty for failed penetrating keratoplasty: visual outcomes and graft survival. Cornea. 2019;38:151–6.
10. Einan-Lifshitz A, Belkin A, Sorkin N, et al. Descemet membrane endothelial keratoplasty after penetrating keratoplasty: features for success. Cornea. 2018;37:1093–7.
11. Pierné K, Panthier C, Courtin R, et al. Descemet membrane endothelial keratoplasty after failed penetrating keratoplasty. Cornea. 2019;38:280–4.
12. Arnalich-Montiel F, Mingo-Botín D, De Arriba-Palomero P. Preoperative risk assessment for progression to DMEK following cataract surgery in Fuchs endothelial corneal dystrophy. Am J Ophthalmol. 2019;208:76–86. https://doi.org/10.1016/j.ajo.2019.07.012. [Epub ahead of print].
13. Schaub F, Gerber F, Adler W, et al. Corneal densitometry as a predictive diagnostic tool for visual acuity results after Descemet membrane endothelial keratoplasty. Am J Ophthalmol. 2019;198:124–9.
14. MikeStraiko. http://www.ascrs.org/sites/default/files/000556_25730132_Straiko_DMEK_tips.pdf.
15. Oellerich S, Baydoun L, Peraza-Nieves J, et al. Multicenter study of 6-month clinical outcomes after Descemet membrane endothelial keratoplasty. Cornea. 2017;36:1467–76.
16. Debellemanière G, Guilbert E, Courtin R, et al. Impact of surgical learning curve in Descemet membrane endothelial keratoplasty on visual acuity gain. Cornea. 2017;36:1–6.
17. Schaub F, Enders P, Zachewicz J, et al. Impact of donor age on Descemet membrane endothelial keratoplasty outcome: evaluation of donors aged 17–55 years. Am J Ophthalmol. 2016;170:119–27.
18. Terry MA, Straiko MD, Veldman PB, Talajic JC, VanZyl C, Sales CS, Mayko ZM. Standardized DMEK technique: reducing complications using prestripped tissue, novel glass injector, and sulfur hexafluoride (SF6) gas. Cornea. 2015;34:845–52.
19. Schlötzer-Schrehardt U, Bachmann BO, et al. Reproducibility of graft preparations in Descemet's membrane endothelial keratoplasty. Ophthalmology. 2013;120:1769–77.
20. Abdin A, Daas L, Pattmöller M, et al. Negative impact of dextran in organ culture media for pre-stripped tissue preservation on DMEK (Descemet membrane endothelial keratoplasty) outcome. Graefes Arch Clin Exp Ophthalmol. 2018;256:2135–42.
21. Menzel-Severing J, Walter P, Plum WJ, et al. Assessment of corneal endothelium during continued organ culture of pre-stripped human donor tissue for DMEK surgery. Curr Eye Res. 2018;43:1439–44.
22. Heinzelmann S, Huther S, Bohringer D, et al. Influence of donor characteristics on Descemet membrane endothelial keratoplasty. Cornea. 2014;33:644–8.
23. Sáles CS, Terry MA, Veldman PB, et al. Relationship between tissue unscrolling time and endothelial cell loss. Cornea. 2016;35:471–6.
24. Schaub F, Pohl L, Enders P, et al. Impact of corneal donor lens status on 2-year course and outcome of Descemet membrane endothelial keratoplasty (DMEK). Graefes Arch Clin Exp Ophthalmol. 2017;255:2407–14.
25. Greiner MA, Rixen JJ, Wagoner MD, et al. Diabetes mellitus increases risk of unsuccessful graft preparation in Descemet membrane endothelial keratoplasty: a multicenter study. Cornea. 2014;33:1129–33.
26. Melles GRJ, Rietveld FJR. Transplantation of Descemet's membrane carrying viable endothelium through a small scleral incision. Cornea. 2002;21:415–8.
27. Kruse FE, Laaser K, Cursiefen C, et al. A stepwise approach to donor preparation and insertion increases safety and outcome of Descemet membrane endothelial keratoplasty. Cornea. 2011;30:580–7.
28. Yoeruek E, Bartz-Schmidt KU. Novel surgical instruments facilitating Descemet membrane dissection. Cornea. 2013;32:523–6.
29. Anwar M, Teichmann KD. Big-bubble technique to bare Descemet's membrane in anterior lamellar keratoplasty. J Cataract Refract Surg. 2002;28:398–403.
30. Sikder S, Ward D, Jun AS. A surgical technique for donor tissue harvesting for Descemet membrane endothelial keratoplasty. Cornea. 2011;30:91–4.
31. Busin M, Scorcia V, Patel AK, et al. Pneumatic dissection and storage of donor endothelial tissue for Descemet's membrane endothelial keratoplasty: a novel technique. Ophthalmology. 2010;117:1517–20.
32. Studeny P, Farkas A, Vokrojova M, et al. Descemet membrane endothelial keratoplasty with a stromal rim (DMEK-S). Br J Ophthalmol. 2010;94:909–14.

33. Agarwal A, Dua HS, Narang P, et al. Pre-Descemet's endothelial keratoplasty (PDEK). Br J Ophthalmol. 2014;98:1181–5.
34. Muraine M, Gueudry J, He Z, et al. Novel technique for the preparation of corneal grafts for Descemet membrane endothelial keratoplasty. Am J Ophthalmol. 2013;156:851–9.
35. McKee HD, Jhanji V. Femtosecond laser-assisted graft preparation for Descemet membrane endothelial keratoplasty. Cornea. 2018;37:1342–4.
36. Bachmann B, Händel A, Siebelmann S, Matthaei M, Cursiefen C. Mini-Descemet membrane endothelial keratoplasty for the early treatment of acute corneal hydrops in keratoconus. Cornea. 2019;38:1043–8.
37. Bachmann BO, Laaser K, Cursiefen C, Kruse FE. A method to confirm correct orientation of Descemet membrane during Descemet membrane endothelial keratoplasty. Am J Ophthalmol. 2010;149:922–5.
38. Matsuzawa A, Hayashi T, Oyakawa I, et al. Use of four asymmetric marks to orient the donor graft during Descemet's membrane endothelial keratoplasty. BMJ Open Ophthalmol. 2017;1(1):e000080. https://doi.org/10.1136/bmjophth-2017-000080. eCollection 2017.
39. Parekh M, Baruzzo M, Favaro E, et al. Standardizing Descemet membrane endothelial keratoplasty graft preparation method in the eye bank-experience of 527 Descemet membrane endothelial keratoplasty tissues. Cornea. 2017;36:1458–66.
40. Veldman PB, Dye PK, Holiman JD, et al. Stamping an S on DMEK donor tissue to prevent upside-down grafts: laboratory validation and detailed preparation technique description. Cornea. 2015;34:1175–8.
41. Bhogal M, Maurino V, Allan BD. Use of a single peripheral triangular mark to ensure correct graft orientation in Descemet membrane endothelial keratoplasty. J Cataract Refract Surg. 2015;41:2022–4.
42. Majmudar PA, Johnson L. Enhancing DMEK success by identifying optimal levels of trypan blue dye application to donor corneal tissue. Cornea. 2017;36:217–21.
43. Hayashi T, Yuda K, Oyakawa I, Kato N. Use of brilliant blue G in Descemet's membrane endothelial keratoplasty. Biomed Res Int. 2017;2017:9720389. https://doi.org/10.1155/2017/9720389. Epub 2017 Jun 6.
44. Siebelmann S, Matthaei M, Hörster R, et al. Lutein and brilliant blue-based dye for donor preparation and transplantation in Descemet membrane endothelial keratoplasty. Cornea. 2017;36:440–4.
45. Chen SY, Tran KD, Wehrer S, et al. Patent blue V as an alternative stain for DMEK grafts: safety, stain retention, and feasibility. Cornea. 2019;38:1322–7.
46. Ho WT, Chang JS, Chen TC, et al. Evaluation of patent blue as the vital dye in an animal model of Descemet membrane endothelial keratoplasty. Cornea. 2019;38:360–3.
47. Yoeruek E, Bartz-Schmidt KU, Hofmann J. Impact of the radius of the injector system on the cell viability in Descemet membrane endothelial keratoplasty: an ex-vivo experimental study. Acta Ophthalmol. 2016;94:e1–5. https://doi.org/10.1111/aos.12787.
48. Kim EC, Bonfadini G, Todd L, et al. Simple, inexpensive, and effective injector for Descemet membrane endothelial keratoplasty. Cornea. 2014;33:649–52.
49. Güell JL, Morral M, Gris O, Elies D, Manero F. Bimanual technique for insertion and positioning of endothelium-Descemet membrane graft in Descemet membrane endothelial keratoplasty. Cornea. 2013;32:1521–6.
50. Price MO, Giebel AW, Fairchild KM, Price FW Jr. Descemet's membrane endothelial keratoplasty: prospective multicenter study of visual and refractive outcomes and endothelial survival. Ophthalmology. 2009;116:2361–8.
51. Siebelmann S, Janetzko M, König P, et al. Flushing versus pushing technique for graft implantation in Descemet membrane endothelial keratoplasty (DMEK). Cornea. 2019.; [Epub ahead of print].;39:605.
52. Ang M, Mehta JS, Newman SD, et al. Descemet membrane endothelial keratoplasty: preliminary results of a donor insertion pull-through technique using a donor mat device. Am J Ophthalmol. 2016;171:27–34. https://doi.org/10.1016/j.ajo.2016.08.023. Epub 2016 Aug 24.
53. Romano V, Ruzza A, Kaye S, Parekh M. Pull-through technique for delivery of a larger diameter DMEK graft using endothelium-in method. Can J Ophthalmol. 2017;52(5):e155–6. https://doi.org/10.1016/j.jcjo.2017.03.006. Epub 2017 Apr 20.
54. Busin M, Leon P, D'Angelo S, et al. Clinical outcomes of preloaded Descemet membrane endothelial keratoplasty grafts with endothelium tri-folded inwards. Am J Ophthalmol. 2018;193:106–13.
55. Tourtas T, Schlomberg J, Wessel JM, et al. Graft adhesion in Descemet membrane endothelial keratoplasty dependent on size of removal of host's Descemet membrane. JAMA Ophthalmol. 2014;132:155–61.
56. Röck T, Bramkamp M, Bartz-Schmidt KU, et al. Causes that influence the detachment rate after Descemet membrane endothelial keratoplasty. Graefes Arch Clin Exp Ophthalmol. 2015;253:2217–22.
57. Schrinttenlocher S, Bachman B, Cursienfen C. Impact of donor tissue diameter on postoperative central endothelial cell density in Descemet membrane endothelial keratoplasty. Acta Ophthalmol. 2019;97(4):e618–22.
58. Gonzalez A, Price FW Jr, Price MO, Feng MT. Prevention and management of pupil block after Descemet membrane endothelial keratoplasty. Cornea. 2016;35:1391–5.
59. Crews JW, Price MO, Lautert J, et al. Intraoperative hyphema in Descemet membrane endothelial keratoplasty alone or combined with phacoemulsification. J Cataract Refract Surg. 2018;44:198–201.
60. Veldman PB, Dye PK, Holiman JD, et al. The S-stamp in Descemet membrane endothelial keratoplasty safely eliminates upside-down graft implantation. Ophthalmology. 2016;123:161–4.

61. Ham L, van der Wees J, Melles GR. Causes of primary donor failure in Descemet membrane endothelial keratoplasty. Am J Ophthalmol. 2008;145:639–44.
62. Kevin JS, Straiko MD, Greiner MA. https://pdfs.semanticscholar.org/c487/beeb8f388021e6b7d921c600fa3b70083dbf.pdf. Accessed 5 Mar 2020.
63. Dapena I, Moutsouris K, Droutsas K, et al. Standardized "no-touch" technique for Descemet membrane endothelial keratoplasty. Arch Ophthalmol. 2011;129:88–94.
64. Steven P, Le Blanc C, Velten K, et al. Optimizing Descemet membrane endothelial keratoplasty using intraoperative optical coherence tomography. JAMA Ophthalmol. 2013;131:1135–42.
65. Saad A, Guilbert E, Grise-Dulac A, Sabatier P, Gatinel D. Intraoperative OCT-assisted DMEK: 14 consecutive cases. Cornea. 2015;34:802–7.
66. Patel AS, Goshe JM, Srivastava SK, Ehlers JP. Intraoperative optical coherence tomography-assisted Descemet membrane endothelial keratoplasty in the DISCOVER study: first 100 cases. Am J Ophthalmol. 2019;210:167–73. https://doi.org/10.1016/j.ajo.2019.09.018. [Epub ahead of print].
67. Yoeruek E, Bayyoud T, Hofmann J, Bartz-Schmidt KU. Novel maneuver facilitating Descemet membrane unfolding in the anterior chamber. Cornea. 2013;32:370–3.
68. Price MO, Lisek M, Kelley M, Feng MT, Price FW Jr. Endothelium-in versus endothelium-out insertion with Descemet membrane endothelial keratoplasty. Cornea. 2018;37:1098–101.
69. Hayashi T, Kobayashi A. Double-bubble technique in Descemet membrane endothelial keratoplasty for vitrectomized eyes: a case series. Cornea. 2018;37:1185–8.
70. Saad A, Awwad ST, El Salloukh NA, et al. C-press technique to facilitate Descemet membrane endothelial keratoplasty surgery in vitrectomized patients: a case series. Cornea. 2019;38:1198–201.
71. Yoeruek E, Bartz-Schmidt KU. Novel technique for improving graft unfolding in vitrectomized eyes using a temporary diaphragm in Descemet membrane endothelial keratoplasty. Cornea. 2018;37:1334–6.
72. Kobayashi A, Yokogawa H, Mori N, Masaki T, Sugiyama K. Development of a donor tissue holding technique for Descemet's membrane endothelial keratoplasty using a 25-gauge graft manipulator. Case Rep Ophthalmol. 2018;9:431–8. https://doi.org/10.1159/000493571.
73. Güell JL, Morral M, Gris O, et al. Comparison of sulfur hexafluoride 20% versus air tamponade in Descemet membrane endothelial keratoplasty. Ophthalmology. 2015;122:1757–64.
74. Schaub F, Enders P, Snijders K, et al. One-year outcome after Descemet membrane endothelial keratoplasty (DMEK) comparing sulfur hexafluoride (SF6) 20% versus 100% air for anterior chamber tamponade. Br J Ophthalmol. 2017;101:902–8.

# 7 Air Pump Assisted PDEK

Soosan Jacob

## 7.1 Introduction

Pre-Descemet's endothelial keratoplasty (PDEK) differs from Descemet's membrane endothelial keratoplasty (DMEK) in having an additional layer—the pre-Descemet's layer (PDL) or the Dua's layer in the graft. To understand this better, it is important to understand the difference between the type 1 bubble and the type 2 big bubbles. When air is injected into a donor corneoscleral rim, it may form one of three different types of grafts—type 1, type 2, and type 3 (Fig. 7.1a–c) [1]. The type 1 big bubble is formed when air dissects into the plane between the PDL and the overlying stroma, thus giving a big bubble composed of three layers—PDL, Descemet's membrane (DM), and the endothelium. This type 1 big bubble is harvested to obtain the PDEK graft. The PDL layer is tough and resilient in nature as compared to a DMEK graft and does not tear easily. It provides a splinting property to the graft, making graft management easier. The type 2 big bubble is obtained when air instead dissects into a plane between the PDL and the DM, thus giving a big bubble composed of two layers—the DM and the endothelium. This type 2 bubble is harvested to obtain the DMEK bubble. Type 3 bubble formation refers to when both type 1 and type 2 are obtained in the same graft, and this is a mixed bubble formation. When the type 2 component is still small, the graft can still be utilized as a PDEK graft. However if type 2 formation is significant, it can be further expanded to obtain a DMEK graft which can then be used (Fig. 7.1c).

A PDEK graft has advantages of being stronger and more resistant to tear. It provides the ability for younger grafts to be used, thereby giving a larger quantum of endothelial cell transfer [2]. These properties are utilized for performing safe and effective surgery by the air pump assisted technique which has been described by the author [3, 4].

**Supplementary Information** The online version contains supplementary material available at https://doi.org/10.1007/978-981-97-3469-6_7. The videos can be accessed individually by clicking the DOI link in the accompanying figure caption or by scanning this link with the SN More Media App.

S. Jacob (✉)
Dr. Agarwal's Refractive and Cornea Foundation, Chennai, India

Dr. Agarwal's Eye Hospital and Eye Research Centre, Chennai, India



S. Jacob (ed.), *Mastering DMEK and PDEK*, https://doi.org/10.1007/978-981-97-3469-6_7

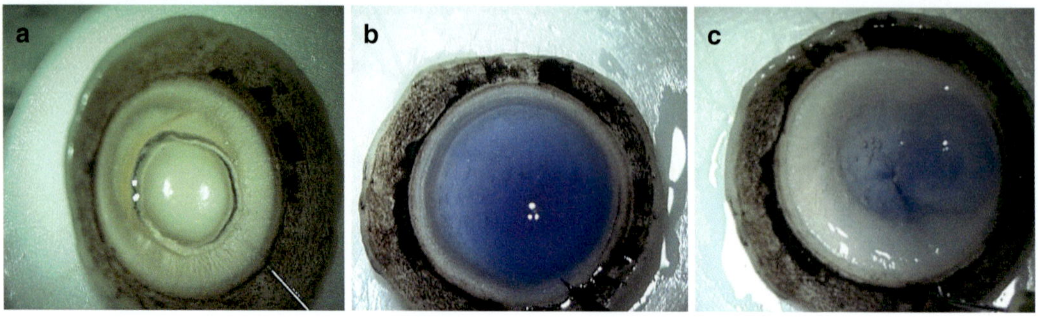


**Fig. 7.1** Big bubble types: (**a**) Type 1 (PDEK graft); (**b**) Type 2 (DMEK graft); (**c**) Type 3 (mixed graft)

## 7.2 Technique

Pressurized air infusion from either the fluid air exchange system of a vitrectomy machine or the pressurized system from newer phaco machines is used (Fig. 7.2). Surgery starts out with creating a side port in the inferotemporal quadrant for inserting an anterior chamber maintainer (ACM). This is made tangential to the limbus in such a way that when the ACM is inserted, it is directed toward the angle and not the pupil. The ACM is also not directed toward any iridectomy to prevent air from entering the posterior chamber through it. A main port is partially created in the upper right quadrant (for right handed surgeons). Air infusion is then started through the anterior chamber maintainer, and a descemetorhexis of the desired diameter is performed using a reverse Sinskey hook. This is made easy by the continuous air infusion which maintains a well formed AC and also allows good visualization of the tearing edge of the Descemet's membrane and thereby allows greater control over size and shape of the rhexis. The tearing edge can be folded over similar to performing a capsulorhexis and can be pulled inwards from all edges.

Under air, a small, inferior peripheral iridectomy (PI) is then created using a vitrector. The continuous air infusion maintains a well-formed anterior chamber (AC) for this as well and prevents bleeding from the PI into the AC. The PI may be performed prior to the descemetorhexis to give time for any bleeding to stop before removing air (Fig. 7.3a–d).

### 7.2.1 Bubble Test

Next what I refer to as the "Bubble test" is performed. This consists of removing the ACM and injecting an air bubble into the AC and seeing how well it stays in the AC without migrating posteriorly. A good tamponade at this stage confirms that a good post-operative tamponade will be obtained in the post-operative period also, thus increasing the risk of graft detachment. A bubble that migrates posteriorly indicates the need to create a more stable iris IOL diaphragm. In case the bubble migrates posteriorly, the easiest way to handle this is by doing an iridoplasty in such a way as to cover the IOL adequately enough from all sides. This may also be required in case of a floppy iris, a widely dilated atrophic iris or in case of a broken posterior capsule.

The PDEK graft is then loaded into the injector and the E-DEMK/E-PDEK technique is used to verify the orientation of the graft. Similar to a DMEK graft, the PDEK graft also curls toward the Descemet's membrane so that the endothelium is to the outer side of the role and the Descemet's membrane is to the inner side. The graft is then injected into the anterior chamber

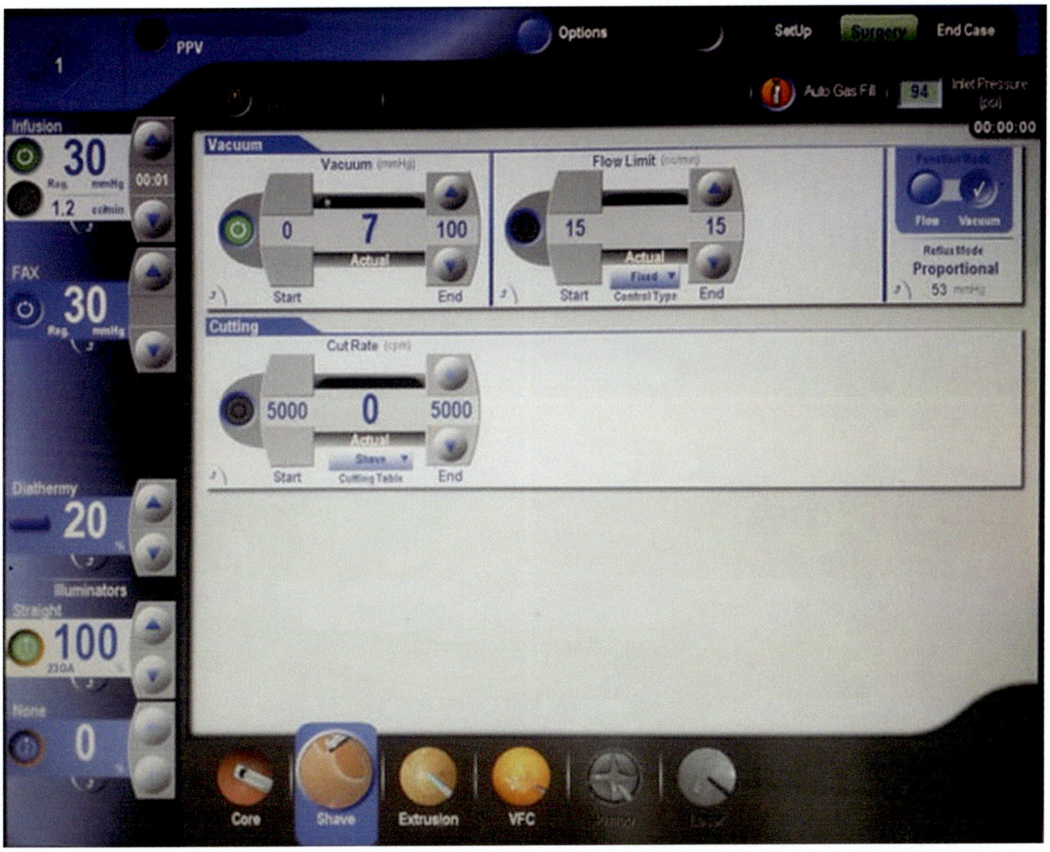


**Fig. 7.2** Air pump assisted PDEK performed using the fluid air exchange system of the vitrectomy machine

and unrolled using standard techniques. It is generally easier to unroll a PDEK graft as it is usually injected into the AC either as a trifold or as a double scroll. Extreme peripheral edge folds can be ignored, and the graft can be floated up once it is almost completely unrolled. However, it is not a must to attain complete unrolling of every single peripheral edge fold before floating it up as peripheral edge folds can be handled with less trauma even after flotation as compared to repeated attempts to unroll every single last edge. Once the graft is mostly unfolded, air is injected into the AC through a cannula connected to a 2 mL syringe. Care should be taken to position the cannula under the graft and also to make sure to inject after positioning the cannula in the central zone over the pupil (Fig 7.4a–d). Once the graft is floated up, the ACM connected to the air pump is again inserted into the AC (with the air off) and air infusion is started after making sure the tip is positioned well below the graft. The incision is then sutured, and the graft checked for centration and any peripheral edge folds. A decentered graft at this stage can be easily centered using the air-pump assisted technique which holds the graft up and prevents AC shallowing while a reverse Sinskey is used to pull the graft into centration. This is done very gently with a single extreme peripheral edge touch point. Next, any peripheral edge folds are also unrolled. This is done carefully with as few touch points as possible and without applying undue pressure on the folds. The continuous pressurized air infusion helps in doing this. It is to be noted that rough handling of the graft is not required for these steps and should be avoided. Minimum possible touch points should be used at as peripheral locations as possible. Once graft positioning

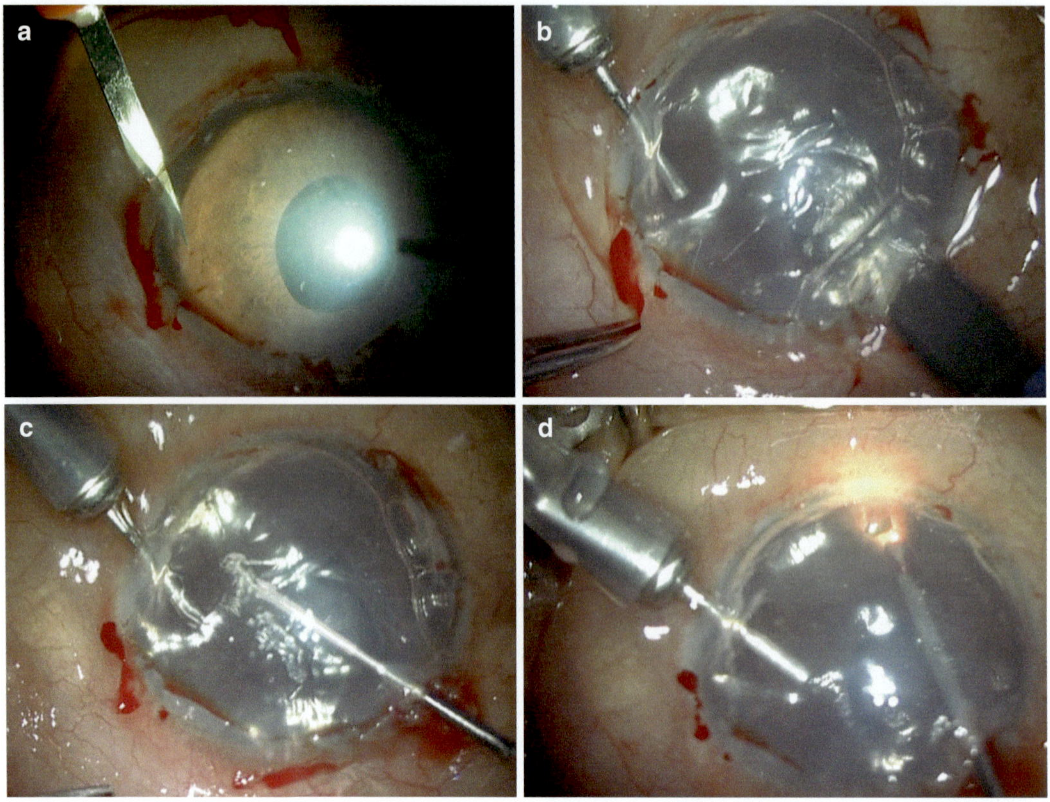


**Fig. 7.3** Air pump assisted PDEK: (**a**) tangential paracentesis made; (**b**) anterior chamber maintainer inserted, main port incision created; (**c**) Descemetorhexis done under air; (**d**) peripheral iridectomy done under air

and unfolding are completed, it is generally seen that the continuous pressurized air infusion also helps in increasing graft attachment in the intraoperative period itself. Finally, the ACM is removed and in case of any leakage from the incisions, sutures may be applied (Figs. 7.5a–d and 7.6). An 80% air fill is maintained taking care to leave a thin film of fluid over the IOL.

### 7.2.2 Air Pump Pressure Used

The infusion pressure that is read on the machine does not correspond to the actual intracameral pressure as the air constantly leaks from the incisions. Therefore, despite a higher pressure reading on the machine, the intracameral pressure can be felt to be much lower.

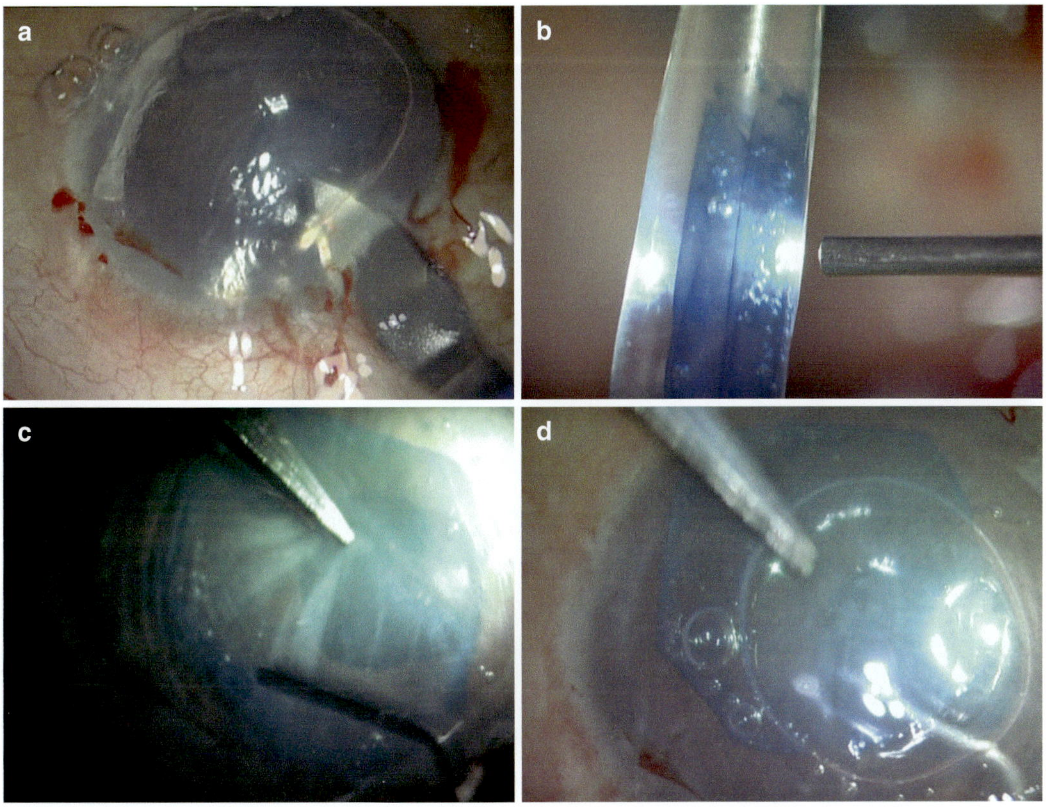

**Fig. 7.4** Air pump assisted PDEK: (**a**) bubble test shows a well maintained, non-migrating bubble within the anterior chamber (AC); (**b**) E-PDEK [5] using the endoilluminator for determining graft orientation within the injector as well as within the AC; (**c**) anterior chamber maintainer removed and graft unrolled; (**d**) air injected to float the graft up

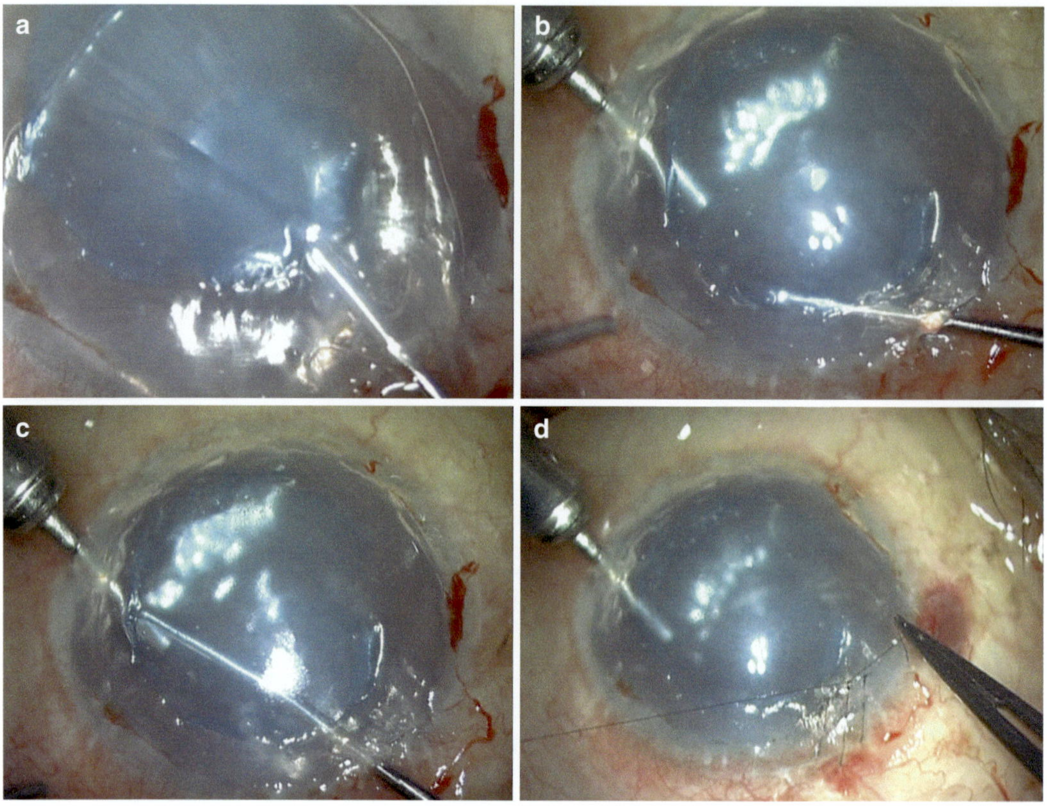


**Fig. 7.5** Air pump assisted PDEK: (**a**) graft pulled into position under air; (**b**, **c**) peripheral edge folds unfolded under air; (**d**) a well centered and completely unrolled graft is seen lying in apposition with overlying cornea

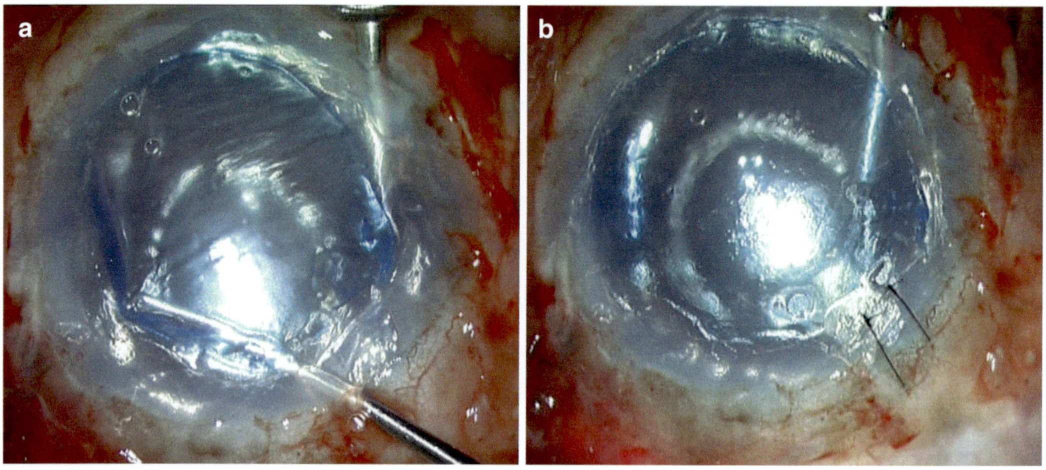


**Fig. 7.6** Air pump assisted PDEK: (**a**) peripheral edge fold unfolded under air; (**b**) a well centered and completely unrolled graft is seen lying in apposition with overlying cornea

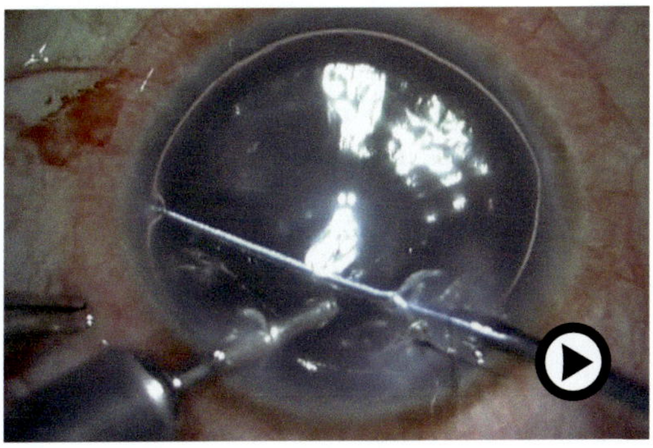

Air pump assisted Descemetorhexis and graft opening (https://doi.org/10.1007/000-dhb)

## 7.3 Advantages

The air pump assisted technique has numerous advantages: [6]

1. It helps in maintaining space within the anterior chamber and acts as a third hand in many situations. It therefore prevents graft detachment/graft trauma by maintaining a well-formed anterior chamber during various steps, especially those involving graft centration and peripheral edge unfolding.
2. It prevents bleeding into the anterior chamber from various sources such as during creation of the PI or secondary to breaking any peripheral anterior synechiae or during an iridoplasty. It also prevents blood from oozing into the anterior chamber from outside such as from incisions created in a case with long standing bullous keratopathy with peripheral corneal neovascularization.
3. Prevention of bleeding helps maintain a non-fibrinous atmosphere within the anterior chamber. This makes surgery easier, allows free movements of the graft within the anterior chamber, prevents the graft from being trapped by fibrin strands, prevents blood from entering the interface between graft and host stroma and decreases post-operative hyphema and inflammation.
4. It helps perform the Descemetorhexis more easily by making the tearing edge of the rhexis clearly visible. It also allows better control of the rhexis, thus allowing greater predictability in size, centration, and location.
5. It helps to hold the floated graft up against the stroma while the graft is pulled into centration.
6. It also helps unfold extreme peripheral edge folds in the graft and helps uncrease the graft.
7. It helps remove wrinkles and creases in the graft, thus ensuring better graft adhesion as well as undistorted vision in the post-operative period.
8. It helps rapid expression of fluid trapped in the interface and thus allows rapid adherence of the graft to the overlying stroma. This allows faster and firmer adherence of the graft, thus decreasing incidence of partial or total graft detachment.
9. It helps perform PDEK in complex eyes such as those with aphakia, secondary IOL fixation, deep anterior chambers, glaucoma drainage devices, etc. by allowing greater flexibility in floating up a graft that may not be perfectly centered and before attaining 100% graft unrolling. It also increases graft adherence intra-operatively, thus decreasing the risk of graft detachment in the post-operative period in these complex cases.
10. It makes surgery faster as time need not be spent in making sure extreme edge folds are removed and that the graft is perfectly centered.
11. It decreases endothelial cell loss secondary to repeated attempts to unscroll the graft completely. Similarly, trying to exactly center a mostly unfolded graft before floatation can sometimes cause the graft to scroll up again resulting in increased intra-ocular manipulation. The resulting increased intra-ocular maneuvering and more surgical time taken by such attempts can contribute to increased endothelial cell loss. This is avoided by the air pump technique by removing peripheral edge folds and by achieving perfect centration of graft after floatation.
12. Host Descemetic scaffolding: The perfectly open and non-collapsing anterior chamber allows the surgeon to perform the host

Descemetic scaffolding technique with ease, thereby decreasing the risk of graft detachment and dislocation. This is done by making a Descemetorhexis that is smaller than the graft (in few quadrants) and then using the host's Descemet's membrane as a scaffold to hold the graft in position against the host stroma. Wound scaffolding may also be performed for the same purpose. For more details, see Chap. 11.

13. Its ability to act as a third hand holding the graft up makes possible instruments to be introduced and maneuvers to be performed safely within the AC even after PDEK graft floatation without causing any graft damage or chamber collapse. For example, any excess Descemet's tags can be removed with a reverse Sinskey or microforceps, an oversized graft or graft tags can be cut with microscissors, vitrectomy can be performed under air, pupilloplasty can be performed under air, etc.

## 7.4 Conclusion

The air pump assisted technique is very useful and allows various steps of the procedure to be performed safely. The tough resilient nature of the PDEK graft allows easy manipulation even after floatation. However, the graft should nevertheless be unfolded maximally before floatation to avoid excessive manipulation. It is also important that the graft is handled only to the minimum possible and only at peripheral edge points. Rough and excessive handling should be avoided. The air pump assisted technique can also be used for DMEK for all steps except for graft centration as the DMEK graft being fragile, may tear from such manipulation. Small peripheral edge folds may however be removed from a DMEK graft using this technique. Other benefits of air pump assisted technique may also be used in DMEK such as tamponading iris stromal bleeding during peripheral iridectomy or synechiolysis, preventing blood oozing into the AC from peripheral neovascularization, increasing surgical space, and preventing AC depth fluctuations.

## References


1. Dua HS, Faraj LA, Said DG, Gray T, Lowe J. Human corneal anatomy redefined: a novel pre-Descemet's layer (Dua's layer). Ophthalmology. 2013;120(9):1778–85.
2. Agarwal A, Dua HS, Narang P, Kumar DA, Agarwal A, Jacob S, Agarwal A, Gupta A. Pre-Descemet's endothelial keratoplasty (PDEK). Br J Ophthalmol. 2014;98(9):1181–5.
3. Jacob S, Narasimhan S, Agarwal A, Agarwal A, Saijimol AI. Air pump-assisted graft centration, graft edge unfolding, and graft uncreasing in young donor graft pre-Descemet endothelial keratoplasty. Cornea. 2017;36(8):1009–13.
4. Jacob S. Use of pressurized air infusion for pre Descemet's endothelial keratoplasty (PDEK)—the air pump assisted PDEK technique. Open Ophthalmol J. 2018;12:175–18.
5. Jacob S, Agarwal A, Agarwal A, Narasimhan S, Kumar DA, Sivagnanam S. Endoilluminator-assisted transcorneal illumination for Descemet membrane endothelial keratoplasty: enhanced intraoperative visualization of the graft in corneal decompensation secondary to pseudophakic bullous keratopathy. J Cataract Refract Surg. 2014;40(8):1332–6.
6. AIR PUMP ASSISTED PDEK Soosan Jacob 6 2 min with audio final. https://www.youtube.com/watch?v=onK1R0DG-ow. Accessed 19 Aug 2020.

# 8 Visualization and Determining Graft Orientation: Stamping, Endo-illuminator and Other Techniques

Tanya Trinh, David S. Rootman, and Clara C. Chan

## 8.1 Introduction

Visualization of graft orientation in the oedematous cornea can be challenging. Endothelial keratoplasty success ultimately depends on attaining the correct orientation of the graft within the anterior chamber with minimal intraoperative manipulation and endothelial cell loss. Both primary success and rebubbling success are dependent on these factors as well. This chapter aims to provide an overview of the milieu of techniques used to identify proper orientation of the graft tissue from inking and stamping techniques to tissue modification, use of external instrumentation to aid visualization such as the hand-held slit lamp, chandelier or endo-illuminator probes, and intraoperative anterior segment ocular coherence tomography.

**Supplementary Information** The online version contains supplementary material available at https://doi.org/10.1007/978-981-97-3469-6_8. The videos can be accessed individually by clicking the DOI link in the accompanying figure caption or by scanning this link with the SN More Media App.

T. Trinh
Mosman Eye Centre, Mosman, NSW, Australia

Sydney Eye Hospital, Sydney, NSW, Australia

D. S. Rootman · C. C. Chan (✉)
Department of Ophthalmology and Vision Sciences, University of Toronto, Toronto Western Hospital, Toronto, ON, Canada

TLC Yonge-Eglinton, Toronto, ON, Canada

## 8.2 Techniques

DMEK and PDEK donor tissue stained with trypan blue typically display a characteristic appearance with rolled edges and endothelial cells on the outside of the curve [1]. Attaining correct orientation can be challenging due to the inherent tendency of the donor tissue to scroll and rotate during insertion and unfolding within the anterior chamber. This is made even more difficult in the presence of corneal edema. In the first instance, visibility may often be enhanced by the use of dehydrating substances on the cornea preoperatively, epithelial debridement, anterior chamber air tamponade prior to graft injection, and graft staining. Prevention of endothelial cell loss (ECL) is of vital importance to prevent primary graft failure.

Correct orientation of the DMEK donor tissue during surgery is a critical step, as accidental graft inversion leads to graft detachment, which in turn is a leading contributing factor to primary graft failure and also is the most common complication [2]. Classically, the management of graft detachment is rebubbling; however, if the graft tissue is incorrectly orientated, then resolution of corneal clarity is impeded.

Many techniques have been described to better visualize and ensure correct graft orientation,



S. Jacob (ed.), *Mastering DMEK and PDEK*, https://doi.org/10.1007/978-981-97-3469-6_8

ranging from stamping, modification of the DMEK tissue itself, use of the hand held slit lamp, chandelier or endo-illuminator probes, and intraoperative assisted anterior segment ocular coherence tomography. This chapter explores the variety of published methods and techniques to determine DMEK and PDEK graft orientation.

## 8.3 Moutsouris Sign

The Moutsouris sign involves the manipulation of a cannula inside the peripheral curl of the graft scroll within the anterior chamber so as to check the orientation of the stained and scrolled graft tissue. A positive Moutsouris sign is seen if there is a change in colour between the shaft and tip of the cannula—the cannula tip should look blue due to its encapsulation within the peripheral roll of stained tissue in contrast to the silver colour of the rest of the shaft. Conversely, a negative Moutsouris sign shows no change in colour between the shaft and cannula tip. Caution must be taken as the manoeuvre may result in traumatic endothelial cell loss and requires entry into the anterior chamber [1]. Advanced corneal edema may impact on the utility of this sign.

## 8.4 Inking and Stamping Techniques

Inspired by the success of the S-stamping practice in DSAEK tissue, Veldman et al. pioneered the ex-vivo technique of using a commonly available non-mirror-reversible letter shaped S-stamp (Moria, Antony, France) to mark the stromal side of the DMEK tissue (the letter S) via the use of gentian violet dye [3]. This technique was found to allow for an acceptable level of ECL (additional 0.6%) from the stamp itself [3]. Subsequently, the same group reported in vivo results with the use of a surgical marking pen containing gentian violet dye (P-3; Accu-line, Hyannis, MA) after allowing evaporation of the alcohol carrier in order to minimize ECL and showed a reduction in incidence of upside-down grafts from 9.4 frequency to 0%. Other letters such as the F-stamp (Bausch and Lomb) have since been reported for the same purpose [4].

Not only were they useful in reducing the risk of primary graft failure by prevention of incorrect graft orientation [5], they were also useful as a visual marker to identify the rare case of accidental upside-down graft orientation intraoperatively after SF6 injection and allowed the surgeon to rescue the graft into the correct position and proceed to case completion with successful corneal clearance and improved visual acuity. Furthermore, there was no difference in graft failure, rebubble or rejection rates but slightly higher 6 month endothelial cell loss due to intraoperative manipulation [6].

With all stamping techniques, it should be noted that focal ECL in the area of the stamp can be quite dramatic, with all cells within the actual stamped area being lost. Anecdotal feedback suggests areas of focal edema at the site of the S-stamp in eye-bank prepared tissue, so this may still act as a nidus for localized detachment and may necessitate a rebubble.

Other alternate methods of marking an "F" shape in the absence of a stamp involve the use of the Sinskey hook [7], Fogla hook, or any other readily available surgical instrument with fine edges (Figs. 8.1 and 8.2). These techniques differ from stamps in that they require touching of the graft tissue multiple times to create the "F" shape, which hypothetically may increase ECL, and still require the use of ink transfer with alcohol. A modified F sign (Fig. 8.3) pioneered by Rootman and colleagues involves less ink by way of a simplified radially oriented line with a single dot placed always to the right of the line (Figs. 8.4 and 8.5).

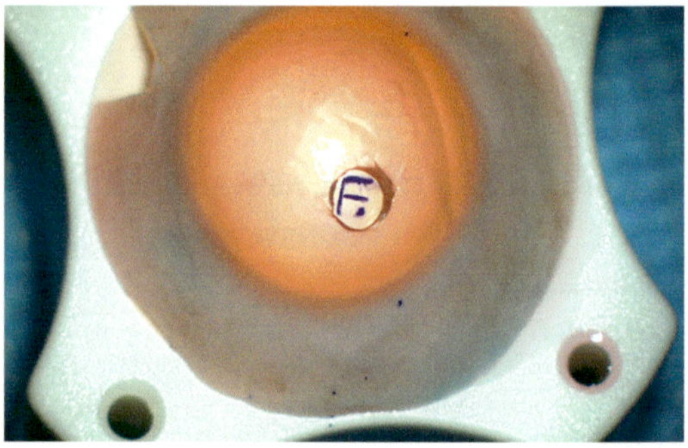

**Fig. 8.1** The F sign

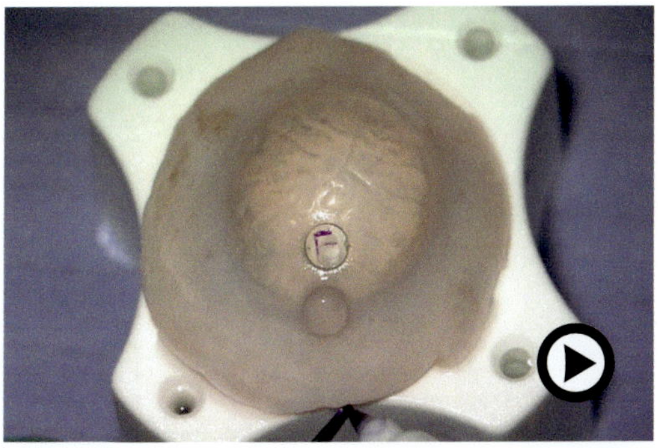

**Fig. 8.2** The F sign (https://doi.org/10.1007/000-dhe)

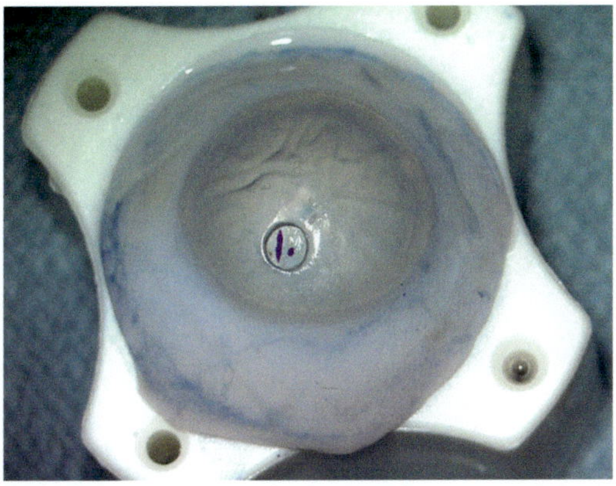

**Fig. 8.3** The modified F sign

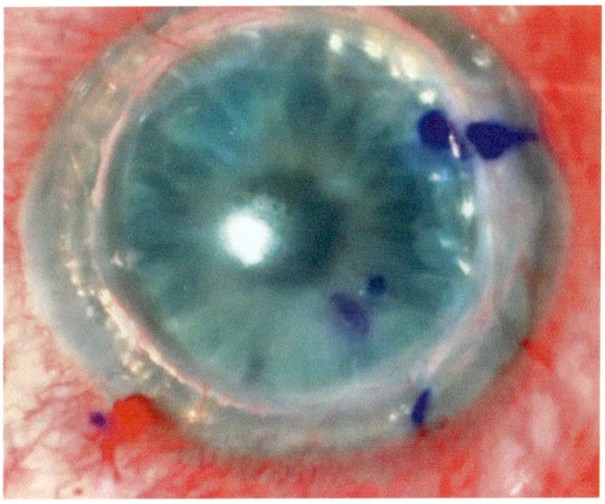

**Fig. 8.4** The modified F sign in situ

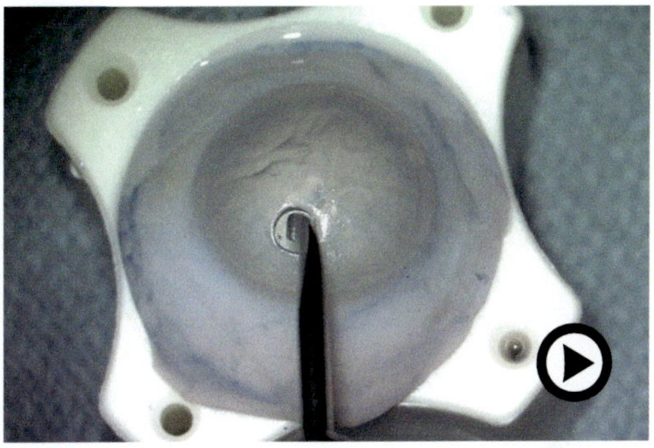

**Fig. 8.5** Modified F technique (https://doi.org/10.1007/000-dhd)

Asymmetric marking (Fig. 8.6) is performed in the form of a three dot technique which is easier to perform and only requires the marker and no second instrument. Care must be taken not to place the dots equilaterally because the asymmetry of the dots is the key to success—two dots at the "base" are placed close together and the third dot forms the "apex" of the "arrowhead" which should be performed in a consistently clockwise or anticlockwise manner (surgeon choice) to avoid confusion (Figs. 8.7 and 8.8). Asymmetric marking allows less ink to be used on the tissue and therefore less ECL loss.

Marking and inking techniques can be impeded by a small aperture within which to mark, so the "infinity" punch pioneered by Chan and colleagues allows a workaround by way of overlapping a 2 mm punch to form an figure of 8 or "infinity" sign (Fig. 8.9).

**"Ghost DMEK" marking** was described in 2019 by Livny and colleagues involving the inking of the periphery of the donor tissue. The technique involves stripping the donor DMEK tissue approximately 50% off the stromal bed, endothelial side up, upon the punch block. The interior margin of the donor punch is then marked with a gentian violet marker until a violet mark is seen, and the alcohol is allowed to evaporate to minimize endothelial cell toxicity. The usual partial thickness trephination is performed, and the tissue then irrigated copiously to remove excess dye. The graft is then peeled away completely and loaded into a glass injector tube. Graft orientation is easily visualized in the anterior chamber due to the contrast between the stained borders of the graft and the rest of the non-stained graft tissue, allowing for instantaneous recognition of the curling direction of the graft tissue. Benefits of

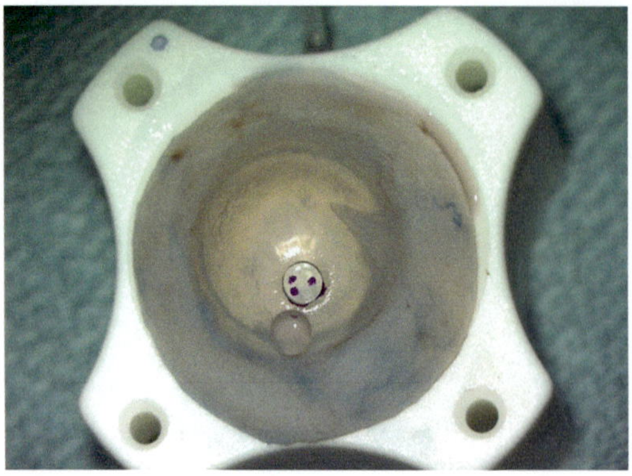

**Fig. 8.6** Asymmetric dots in tissue preparation

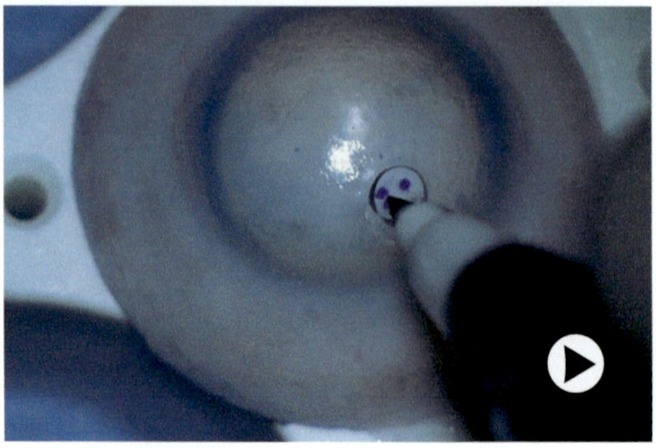

**Fig. 8.8** Asymmetric dots technique (https://doi.org/10.1007/000-dhc)

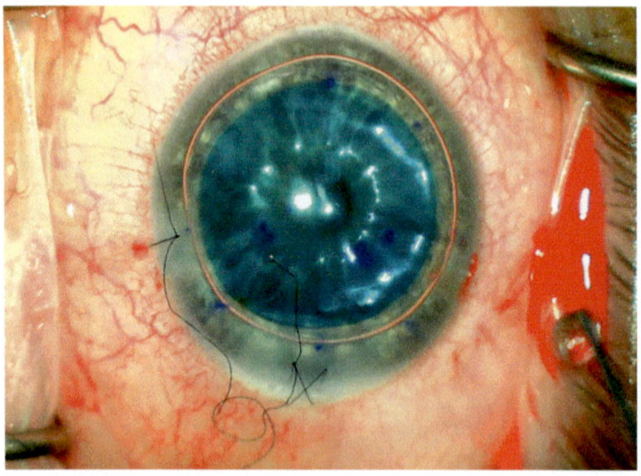

**Fig. 8.7** Asymmetric dots in situ

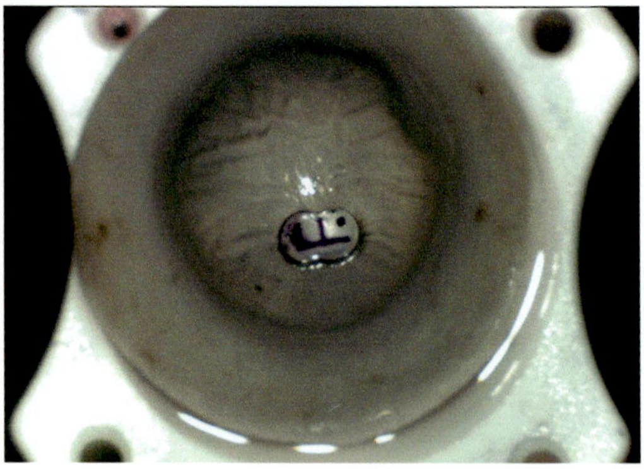

**Fig. 8.9** Infinity sign

this technique are that the staining is readily apparent and does not fade away during surgery, avoids graft or iris trauma that can occur with other invasive techniques, and avoids costs of a microscope mounted AS-OCT [8].

## 8.5 Tissue Modification Methods

### 8.5.1 Bachmann Technique

Bachmann et al. reported on the use of three asymmetric peripheral markings using a 1 millimetre–diameter dermatological biopsy trephine. Prior to transplantation, the punched 8 mm Descemet membrane layer graft is completely stripped from the stroma. Next, to aid anterior-posterior orientation, the 1 mm dermal biopsy trephine is used to excise three separate semicircles at the periphery endothelial tissue edge. Two semicircles are positioned closely, and the third is positioned at a recognizable distance away (Fig. 8.10). The graft tissue is then elevated from the stroma, stained with trypan blue solution 0.06% (VisionBlue; D.O.R.C. International, Zuidland, Netherlands) and transferred into an injector cartridge (Acri.Tec GmbH, Hennigsdorf, Germany) [9].

### 8.5.2 Matsuzawa Technique

Matsuzawa et al. reported the use of 2 different sized punches of 1 mm and 1.5 mm diameter (Kai Industries, Seki, Japan), respectively, to create four semicircular marks. The 1 mm semicircular marks were set at 180° to each other, and likewise for the 1.5 mm punch (Fig. 8.11). This pairing on opposite sides of the graft enables correct graft orientation. The

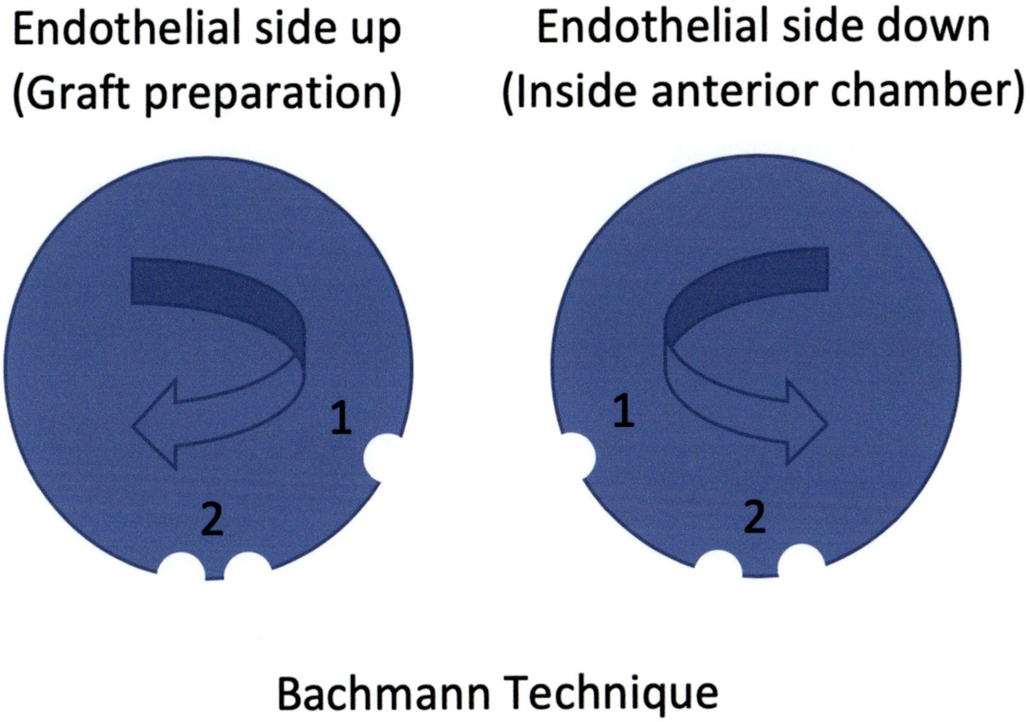


**Fig. 8.10** Bachmann technique

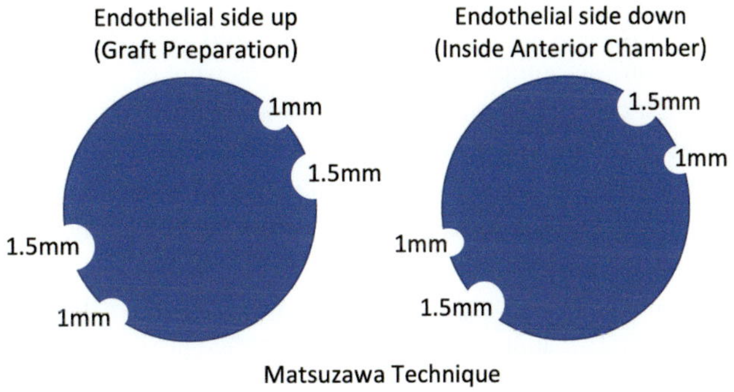


**Fig. 8.11** Matsuzawa technique

surgeon observes the semicircular marking positions intraoperatively and notes that the larger and smaller markings should always be observed in the opposite order than that in which they were created endothelial side up. Should the graft be upside-down, the marking pairs would appear in the same order that they were observed during preparation. This technique was associated with a slightly higher rate of ECL [10].

**Bhogal et al.** described a technique using a single peripheral triangular mark to ensure correct graft orientation. The graft is stripped 50% initially and replaced flat. After trephination with an 8–8.75 mm trephine, a 30° incision knife is used to excise a small right-angled triangle shaped segment of the graft from the graft edge 180° to the initiated peel edge (i.e. where the graft is still attached to the trephined edge). The rest of the peel is then completed under balanced salt solution to reduce the risk of radial tear from the excised portion. The graft is then stained and loaded as per the usual technique [11].

## 8.6 Intraoperative Anterior Segment Optical Coherence Tomography

Intraoperative anterior segment optical coherence tomography (AS-OCT) has also been shown to be a useful modality to determine graft orientation in DMEK. The initial studies of AS-OCT use for DMEK were reported by Saad and colleagues in 2013. The correct orientation of the graft tissue was demonstrated in the early post-operative period by the inward scroll of the peripheral edges of the graft towards the stroma on AS-OCT. Conversely, inverted graft orientation was also shown by the graft tissue curling outwardly towards the anterior chamber. The authors suggested that AS-OCT be performed at the first post-operative week to determine the need for rebubbling [12].

With the advent of OCTs coupled to a surgical microscope, Steven et al. reported enhanced graft visibility of graft orientation and unfolding with intraoperative OCT at all surgical steps [13]. Saad et al. also reported on the use of intraoperative AS-OCT in DMEK surgery to visualize and assess graft orientation. They found that in cases of severe corneal oedema where direct graft visualization was compromised, OCT images were of enough clarity to permit correct evaluation of the graft orientation, thus avoiding excessive manipulation. Time to correct graft positioning was also shorter in the presence of severe corneal edema [14]. Cost reported similar findings [15]. The use of hand-held spectral domain AS-OCT as an intraoperative adjunct has also been reported [16].

## 8.7 Hand-Held Slit Lamp

Hand-held slit lamps have also been reported as useful intraoperative adjuncts to DMEK surgery. Burkhart et al. described a technique of using the Eidolon model 510 L hand-held slit lamp (Eidolon Optical LLC) to identify the orientation of inserted graft tissue prior to unrolling in the anterior chamber [17]. The technique is enhanced further with trypan blue staining of the donor tissue. Sterility is maintained by the placement of the portable slit lamp into a sterile glove. Overhead and microscope lights are extinguished, and the slit beam is directed into the anterior chamber. Correct graft positioning with endothelium facing downwards is seen as two adjacent arcs representing two scrolls, with a short "connector" beam in between them posterior to the arcs (best seen over the pupil). Should the graft be inverted, the slit lamp beam shines onto the "connector" appearing as a single broad arc below the host cornea.

## 8.8 Endo-illuminator Technique (E-DMEK and E-PDEK)

Jacob et al. [18, 19] reported a technique of using the endo-illuminator to identify graft orientation as well as enhancing the three-dimensional depth perception within the anterior chamber. After graft injection into the anterior chamber, the microscope light is switched off and the endo-illuminator probe of the 20-, 23-, or 25-gauge variety is used to enhance visualization by its oblique light source. The probe is held by the surgeon for confirmation of orientation. Switching off the microscope light at this point aids visualization further. The probe tip can be moved around the limbus with the light directed tangentially to optimize visualization and utilize the light reflexes from the rolled edges and scrolls of the graft. With this technique, the three-dimensional aspects of graft folds, position, detail, and orientation can be easily visualized and confirmed. Confirmation of correct orientation can further be ensured by the gentle tapping onto the host cornea which reveals light reflexes created from the light reflected off the graft edges, the dynamic movement of the graft tissue, and the fact that the graft edges should appear to scroll upwards (Figs. 8.12 and 8.13).

Advantages included entire graft visualization despite poor corneal clarity leading to better understanding of anterior chamber dynamics and graft orientation, positioning, and morphology. In addition, the final graft location is also easily visualized by the endo-illuminator. Once orientation is confirmed, the remaining surgery may be carried out using the microscope light. If the cor-

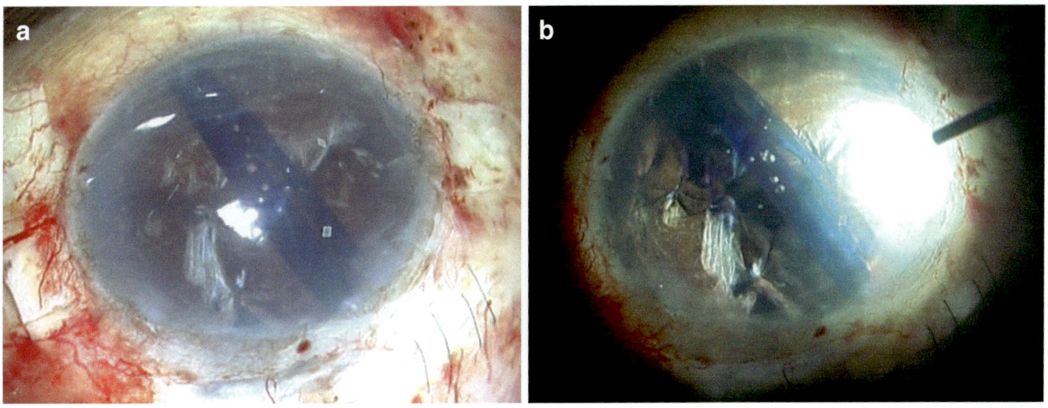


**Fig. 8.12** E-DMEK: (**a**) poor visibility and orientation under microscope light; (**b**) good visibility and orientation with E-DMEK technique (Courtesy Dr. Soosan Jacob, MD)

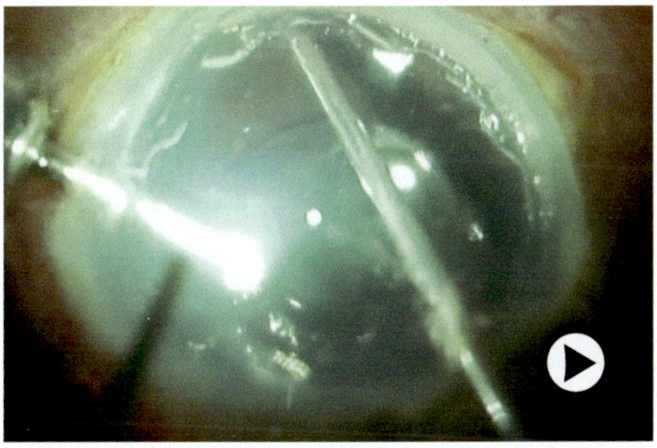

**Fig. 8.13** E-PDEK and E-DMEK (https://doi.org/10.1007/000-dhf)

nea is very edematous and the view is poor, the surgeon may also continue with unrolling under the endo-illumination light with the assistant holding the light source.

## 8.9 Berrospi's Sign

This method relies on the observation of light reflections on the donor tissue after injection into the anterior chamber. The tissue should be encouraged to form a double scroll if not already by a combination of the Dirisamer or Dapena techniques. Inspection of the graft in this conformation reveals subtle linear light reflections on the apex of each scrolled curl, aiding evaluation of graft orientation prior to unfolding, termed Berrospi's sign. When in the correct orientation and well stained, the curls face up to the donor stroma with the endothelial cells facing the iris surface and the linear reflections are visible. When inverted, a diffuse central reflection is observed, and the linear reflections are absent [20].

## 8.10 Chandelier Illumination Techniques

Posterior chandelier illumination techniques have also been described [21]. The principle is borrowed from other uses of chandelier illumination, for example, from cataract surgery in eyes with advanced bullous keratopathy or corneal stromal scarring. The diffuse retroillumination from the vitreous cavity aids in visualizing anterior chamber structures better than that which can be seen at the surgical microscope. The chandelier illuminator is inserted transconjunctivally into the vitreous cavity from a pars plana approach with a 25 g trocar (3.5 mm posterior to the corneal limbus). The donor DMEK tissue is injected into the anterior chamber, and the chandelier is activated. The donor graft is then allowed to unfold using a "no-touch technique" under retroillumination and also allows the surgeon to operate bimanually as the chandelier is hands free. Caution should be used with this method as the pupil is not miotic, to allow the illumination of the graft in the anterior chamber. Thus the donor tissue can be damaged by inadvertent contact with the intraocular lens, can be lost behind a dilated pupil and the DMEK unfolding may be more difficult when the anterior chamber is deeper. Costs associated with chandelier illumination should also be taken into account [18].

## 8.11 Conclusion

In conclusion, a key component to successful DMEK surgery involves ensuring proper graft orientation prior to complete graft unscrolling and anterior chamber air or gas fill. There are a plethora of techniques which can be used to aid graft visualization, orientation, and positioning. Knowledge and judicious use of such methods will be of immense value to a DMEK surgeon's arsenal in the difficult visualization case.

**Acknowledgments** The authors would like to thank Dr. Hall Chew and Dr. Neera Singal for their assistance in obtaining some of the images and techniques used in this chapter.

## References

1. Dapena I, Moutsouris K, Droutsas K, Ham L, van Dijk K, Melles GRJ. Standardized "no-touch" technique for descemet membrane endothelial keratoplasty. Arch Ophthalmol (Chicago, Ill 1960). 2011;129(1):88–94.
2. Ham L, van der Wees J, Melles GRJ. Causes of primary donor failure in descemet membrane endothelial keratoplasty. Am J Ophthalmol. 2008;145(4):639–44.
3. Veldman PB, Dye PK, Holiman JD, et al. Stamping an S on DMEK donor tissue to prevent upside-down grafts: laboratory validation and detailed preparation technique description. Cornea. 2015;34(9):1175–8.
4. Newman LR, Tran KD, Odell K, et al. Minimizing endothelial cell loss caused by orientation stamps on preloaded Descemet membrane endothelial keratoplasty grafts. Cornea. 2019;38(2):233–7.
5. Veldman PB, Dye PK, Holiman JD, et al. The S-stamp in Descemet membrane endothelial keratoplasty safely eliminates upside-down graft implantation. Ophthalmology. 2016;123(1):161–4.
6. Veldman PB, Mayko ZM, Straiko MD, Terry MA. Intraoperative S-stamp enabled rescue of 3 inverted Descemet membrane endothelial keratoplasty grafts. Cornea. 2017;36(6):661–4.
7. Cronin B. DMEK tips and tricks-"F" marking for correct orientation. 2016.
8. Livny E, Bahar I, Nahum Y. "Ghost DMEK" technique: circular peripheral staining of Descemet's membrane endothelial keratoplasty grafts. Cornea. 2019;38(2):252–5.
9. Bachmann BO, Laaser K, Cursiefen C, Kruse FE. A method to confirm correct orientation of Descemet membrane during Descemet membrane endothelial keratoplasty. Am J Ophthalmol. 2010;149(6):922–925.e2.
10. Matsuzawa A, Hayashi T, Oyakawa I, et al. Use of four asymmetric marks to orient the donor graft during Descemet's membrane endothelial keratoplasty. BMJ Open Ophthalmol. 2017;1(1):e000080.
11. Bhogal M, Maurino V, Allan BD. Use of a single peripheral triangular mark to ensure correct graft orientation in Descemet membrane endothelial keratoplasty. J Cataract Refract Surg. 2015;41(9):2022–4.
12. Saad A, Sabatier P, Gatinel D. Graft orientation, optical coherence tomography, and endothelial keratoplasty. Ophthalmology. 2013;120(4):871–871.e3.
13. Steven P, Le Blanc C, Velten K, et al. Optimizing Descemet membrane endothelial keratoplasty using intraoperative optical coherence tomography. JAMA Ophthalmol. 2013;131(9):1135–42.
14. Saad A, Guilbert E, Grise-Dulac A, Sabatier P, Gatinel D. Intraoperative OCT-assisted DMEK: 14 consecutive cases. Cornea. 2015;34(7):802–7.
15. Cost B, Goshe JM, Srivastava S, Ehlers JP. Intraoperative optical coherence tomography-assisted Descemet membrane endothelial keratoplasty in the DISCOVER study. Am J Ophthalmol. 2015;160(3):430–7.
16. Ang M, Dubis AM, Wilkins MR. Descemet membrane endothelial keratoplasty: intraoperative and postoperative imaging spectral-domain optical coherence tomography. Case Rep Ophthalmol Med. 2015;2015:506251. https://doi.org/10.1155/2015/506251.
17. Burkhart ZN, Feng MT, Price MO, Price FW. Handheld slit beam techniques to facilitate DMEK and DALK. Cornea. 2013;32(5):722–4.
18. Jacob S, Agarwal A, et al. Endoilluminator-assisted transcorneal illumination for Descemet membrane endothelial keratoplasty: enhanced intraoperative visualization of the graft in corneal decompensation secondary to pseudophakic bullous keratopathy. J Cataract Refract Surg. 2014;40(8):1332–6.
19. Jacob S, Agarwal A, Kumar DA. Endoilluminator-assisted Descemet membrane endothelial keratoplasty and endoilluminator-assisted pre-Descemet endothelial keratoplasty. Clin Ophthalmol. 2015;9:2123–5.
20. Berrospi RD, Galvis V, Bhogal M, Tello A. Double-line reflection pattern as a simple method to determine graft orientation of Descemet membrane endothelial keratoplasty. Cornea. 2019;38(6):768–71.
21. Shimizu T, Hayashi T, Yuda K, et al. Chandelier illumination for Descemet membrane endothelial keratoplasty. Cornea. 2017;36(9):1155–7.

# 9 DMEK in Complex Cases

Mohamed Gamal Elghobaier, Marianne O. Price, and Francis W. Price

## 9.1 Introduction

Descemet Membrane Endothelial Keratoplasty (DMEK) is gaining popularity among cornea specialists and for many is the surgical treatment of choice for corneal endothelial dysfunction [1]. A learning curve is expected for surgeons who have never done endothelial keratoplasty (EK) before or even for surgeons who are in the transition period from Descemet's Stripping Endothelial Keratoplasty (DSEK) [2, 3].

A successful DMEK depends on air/ gas tamponade which secures the graft in place until the endothelial pump starts to work for attachment to the back of the recipient cornea. Abnormalities of the lens, iris, or anterior chamber (AC) may impair the stability of this tamponade and jeopardize the graft attachment. Moreover, cases previously operated for glaucoma, vitrectomy, or keratoplasty will add to the complexity of the case. Case selection is advisable, particularly for beginning surgeons, and other treatment options, such as DSAEK or PK, should also be considered for challenging cases.

**Supplementary Information** The online version contains supplementary material available at https://doi.org/10.1007/978-981-97-3469-6_9. The videos can be accessed individually by clicking the DOI link in the accompanying figure caption or by scanning this link with the SN More Media App.

M. G. Elghobaier · M. O. Price · F. W. Price (✉)
Price Vision Group, Indianapolis, IN, USA
e-mail: mprice@cornea.org; fprice@pricevisiongroup.net

## 9.2 Crystalline Lens/IOL Abnormalities

### 9.2.1 Aphakia

DMEK can be performed in phakic eyes, pseudophakia, and aphakia after posterior chamber secondary IOL implantation and in eyes requiring combined phacoemulsification with IOL implantation [4–8]. Aphakic bullous keratopathy can be an indication for DMEK for the treatment of complications after cataract surgery. Aphakic cases have more challenges to be considered before performing DMEK; the graft can easily dislocate to the posterior chamber through the pupil with changes in pressure between the anterior and posterior chamber that lead to fluid movement to the back of the eye. Unless the pupil is very small, the absence of a lens/IOL diaphragm also allows the air tamponade to escape from the AC to the bigger vitreous cavity, leading to loss of graft support and the risk of early graft detachment or dislocation [9, 10].

Forming the iris/ lens diaphragm by implanting a posterior chamber intraocular lens (IOL) is an important step not only for visual results but also for successful DMEK. The posterior chamber IOL can be fixated to capsule remnants, fixated in the sulcus, or supported by fixation to the iris or sclera [11, 12].



S. Jacob (ed.), *Mastering DMEK and PDEK*, https://doi.org/10.1007/978-981-97-3469-6_9

Hydrophilic IOLs are not recommended with DMEK because the prolonged contact with an air bubble under high pressure can lead to IOL opacification and require IOL exchange [13, 14].

Secondary IOL implantation can be combined with DMEK or staged with DMEK performed 1 month later. A staged procedure allows the IOL to be secured by healing which allows the IOL to bear more pressure from the air tamponade with less risk of posterior IOL dislocation. Another advantage of a staged procedure is avoiding the possibility of hypotony or a soft eye in the early postoperative period secondary to wound leakage around the PPV ports or IOL fixation sites which could impair DMEK graft attachment.

Poor visualization because of corneal edema is a main concern in managing such cases. Epithelial debridement, intraoperative topical glycerin, and operating under air pump [15] are good techniques to facilitate visualization. If DMEK was planned concurrently, we advise dense staining of the graft with trypan blue 0.06% (VisionBlue, DORC international, Netherlands), and use of intraoperative OCT [16], handheld slit beam [17], or endoilluminator to facilitate graft visualization in the AC [18] (Video 9.1).

Alternatively, DSEK with a pull through technique, either with an intraocular forceps or using 10/0 polypropylene, is a good option and the graft can be secured to the host cornea with the suture [19].

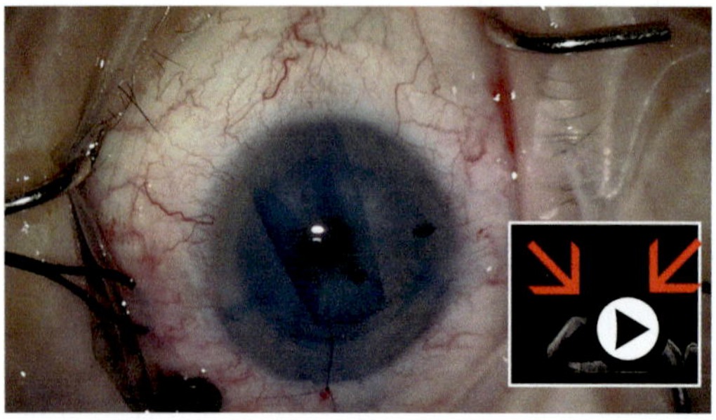

**Video 9.1** iOCT in DMEK (https://doi.org/10.1007/000-dhj)

### 9.2.2 IOL Subluxation/Dislocation

Pseudophakic bullous keratopathy (BPK) is a common indication for DMEK. Complications of cataract surgery can result in various types of IOL malposition such as subluxation with or without pupil capture, or anterior or posterior dislocation. If the IOL is malpositioned in the AC, partially or completely, it can lead to crowding of the AC and difficulties with graft manipulation, whereas if it is dislocated posteriorly, the IOL needs to be either replaced or repositioned prior to proceeding with surgery.

Proper IOL repositioning or exchange should be performed before DMEK either at the same setting or as a staged procedure. The best anatomical position for an IOL is to be placed in the bag if possible. If not possible, the IOL should be placed in the posterior chamber (PC) with fixation in the sulcus, or to the iris, capsule, or scleral supported.

A malpositioned IOL has its own complications such as UGH syndrome (uveitis, glaucoma, and hyphema), poor refractive outcome due to IOL tilt, and retinal traction, especially if associated with vitreous prolapse. A thorough PPV should be performed before IOL manipulation to decrease retinal traction by the prolapsed vitreous.

## 9.3 Anterior Chamber Abnormalities

### 9.3.1 Very Shallow AC

Even in pseudophakic eyes, hyperopes, nanophthalmic eyes, and Asian eyes have less room for manipulating the graft in the AC, and of course any phakic eye can have a shallow AC. As a rule, we prefer the graft diameter to be at least 2 mm smaller than the horizontal white to white. We usually implant grafts with 8.25 mm diameter, which could be challenging in smaller eyes with a less than 10 mm white to white measurement as it would be difficult to unfold in a shallow and small diameter AC. On the other hand, implanting a smaller graft to facilitate the procedure will provide a smaller number of functioning endothelial cells.

While it is important in all eyes, it is especially important in small or shallow eyes to make sure there is no back pressure so check the intraoperative adjustment of the speculum, eliminate patient squeezing by adjusting anesthesia (facial block might be required), and in severe cases consider a limited pars plana vitrectomy to deepen the anterior chamber. One should always remove the crystalline lens prior to endothelial keratoplasty in shallow anterior chambers. It certainly will not be easy doing a subsequent cataract surgery in such eyes, and there will be a higher chance of damaging the graft. Also one has to consider in small eyes, whether if you leave them phakic there will be room to actually make a corneal incision or scleral incision without damaging the graft. Finally, consider implanting the graft in a trifold configuration as it will decrease unfolding manipulation in the AC [20].

### 9.3.2 Anterior Synechiae

Presence of adhesions between the iris and back of the cornea will decrease the AC volume making graft manipulation more difficult. Anterior synechiae decrease the effective size of the recipient cornea and more importantly might expand to include the graft.

Therefore, synechiolysis must be performed before implanting the graft. The most common intraoperative complication of synechiolysis is hyphema, which should be controlled to decrease the risk of postoperative increase in IOP and graft detachment. The most common postoperative complication is recurrence. A strategy of slightly decentering the graft away from the area of extensive synechiae could be considered.

### 9.3.3 AC IOL

Although a well centered long standing AC IOL is not a contraindication of DMEK [21], it will decrease the effective volume of the AC and will traumatize the graft during intraoperative manipulation [22]. Also all anterior chamber lens designs cause some chronic irritation and inflammation in the eye, and necessitate longer treatment with topical steroids, negating one of the best advantages of DMEK which is requiring less steroids to prevent rejection than other keratoplasty procedures.

### 9.3.4 Vitreous Prolapse (Fig. 9.1)

A vitrectomy should be performed if vitreous is present in the anterior chamber preoperatively. A PPV is the most effective way to treat preoperative vitreous prolapse and can be performed either prior to DMEK surgery, or in combination with DMEK before graft implantation. Vitreous prolapse can happen during DMEK surgery especially in pseudophakic eyes with prior YAG laser capsulotomy; in that case, one can perform PPV to remove the vitreous, but in many cases if you can get the graft unfolded and positioned correctly, the vitreous will retract once the air fills the AC.

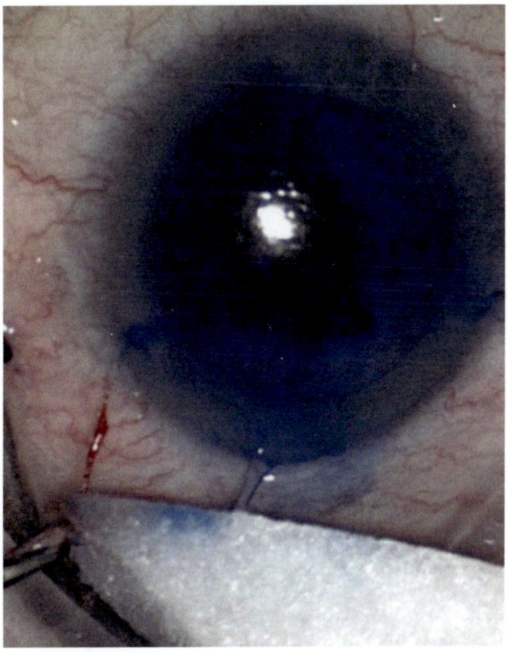

**Fig. 9.1** Vitreous prolapse was detected after stripping DM due to a preoperative defect in the lens posterior capsule

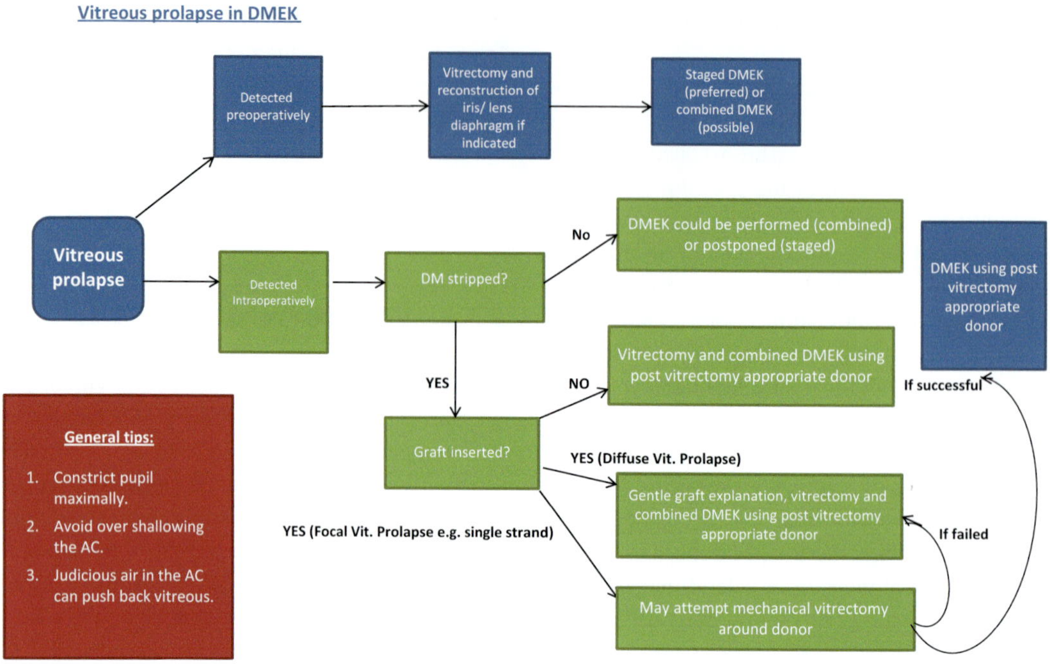


**Fig. 9.2** Decision tree

Vitreous prolapse should be suspected with any case of difficult graft manipulation, difficult aspiration of the air bubble, decentered bubble, or peaked pupil. Intracameral trypan blue may help visualization of the prolapsed vitreous (Fig. 9.2).

### 9.3.5 Very Deep AC

High myopes and patients with megalocornea or buphthalmos have a deep AC which will allow regular sized grafts to rescroll easily. Surgeons prefer implanting a larger graft because the edges can be trapped in the narrow peripheral AC, which helps keep the graft unfolded. Grafts of 9 mm or even more should be considered in such cases. Selecting grafts from old donors (more than 60 years old) is preferable for easier manipulation in a very deep AC.

The most common very deep AC, and one that will not shallow, is an eye with a previous PPV and scleral fixated IOL. A trifold graft configuration with pull in technique for the graft insertion greatly helps in these cases. Once the graft is pulled into the AC, air can be placed underneath it to help hold the graft open and against the cornea. An alternative technique is to compress the cornea to shallow the AC, but that can sometimes make it difficult to get the air bubble under the graft as the graft and cornea are each concave and the bubble can slip out from under the graft.

### 9.3.6 Iris Abnormalities

#### 9.3.6.1 Pupil Abnormalities and Large Iris Defects

An abnormally large pupil (e.g., traumatic mydriasis) should be repaired with pupilloplasty before DMEK. A large pupil could allow the graft and/or the stripped host DM to escape to the posterior chamber. Large iris defects have the same risks as a wide pupil and should be repaired with iridoplasty if possible. We perform a modified Siepser knot (Fig. 9.3), placing the knots on the posterior surface of the iris [23].

If the iris repair was not satisfactory with residual large defects, DSEK would be a better option because it could be implanted without stripping the recipient's DM and it could be sutured to the host cornea to ensure attachment.

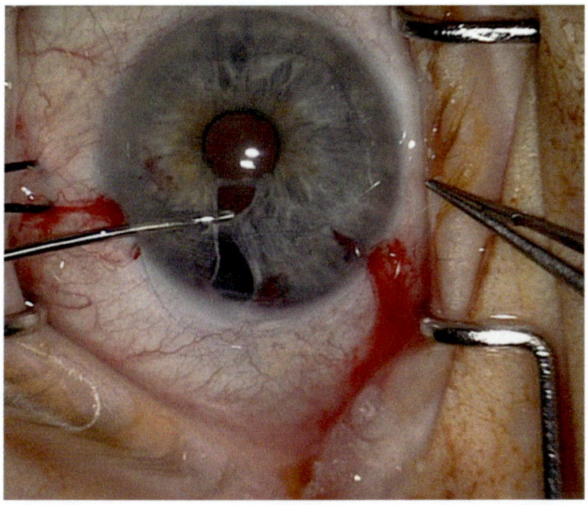

**Fig. 9.3** Suturing a large iris defect before DMEK to guard against graft posterior dislocation

#### 9.3.6.2 Traumatic Aniridia and Iridodialysis

Very severe ocular trauma or surgery could result in very large iris defects, iridodialysis or even complete traumatic aniridia. In such cases, iridoplasty by simply suturing the iris defects is not satisfactory. We prefer implanting an artificial iris implant with or without an IOL to cover the large defect and improve vision [24].Artificial iris implants could be traumatizing to the implanted DMEK graft during intraoperative manipulation and more seriously, the graft could find a passage to the posterior segment around the iris implant. So, DSEK is still a good and safe option for such cases [25]. DMEK and endothelial keratoplasty in general are not a treatment option for congenital aniridia because it is often associated with limbal stem cell dysfunction and corneal scarring including the anterior cornea [26].

## 9.4 Glaucoma Considerations

Eyes previously operated for glaucoma filtering procedures, such as trabeculectomy with or without antimetabolites, filtering tubes, or shunts, are challenging cases for endothelial keratoplasty. Patients with previous glaucoma surgery should be educated about the possibility of graft failure and the likelihood of needing to replace the graft within 5 years [27, 28]. In DMEK, 80–90% AC fill of air or gas is required to secure the graft in place and promote attachment. This could have some considerations in glaucomatous eyes. The air/ gas bubble could easily escape through the filters or tubes once the patient sits up leaving the graft unsupported which could lead to early graft detachment. Overfilling the eye with air or gas to overcome this problem can in some cases increase the IOP and might lead to more optic nerve damage. Gases, e.g., sulfur hexafluoride ($SF_6$ 20%) will remain in the eye longer than air which gives prolonged support to the graft but on the other hand, IOP spikes are more expected with gas than air. The long contact time with an air bubble can in some cases lead to failure of a trabeculectomy bleb.

IOP could increase in the early postoperative period after DMEK for several reasons. Air or gas could block the tube, shunt or trabeculectomy bleb. Hyphema can fill the trabecular meshwork and/or the filtering pathways with blood. As with all intraocular surgery, early postoperative uveitis from prolonged surgery or iris manipulation could fill the AC angle with fibrin and inflammatory cells, and if viscoelastic substances were used, a risk of clogging the filtering tube is present.

IOP can also increase due to failure of the filtering surgery which is possible as the prolonged air/gas tamponade can lead to scarring of the bleb. Aggressive AC air fill can also lead to rupture of the thin encapsulations around a filtering bleb.

In eyes with filters, we usually aim for a full AC air fill intraoperatively because we expect that some of the air will escape through the filtering bleb or tube. If it is difficult to fill the AC intraoperatively in a patient with filtering tube, a small amount of cohesive viscoelastic substance could be put at the tube tip.

We prefer using cohesive viscoelastic to clog the tube because extra maneuvers are not required to reopen the tube. Once the patient resumes sitting in an erect position, gravity will cause the viscoelastic to drop leaving the tube patent again. Importantly, the viscoelastic should only be injected after complete intraoperative graft attachment and positioning to prevent it from entering the graft interface.

If a tube is protruding too far into the AC, it should be trimmed to prevent graft damage. If a tube was malpositioned, it should be repositioned in a staged procedure followed by DMEK 1 month later, because in a combined surgery, aqueous will leak around both the old and new tube tracks resulting in postoperative hypotony and graft detachment.

Minimally invasive glaucoma surgery (MIGS), e.g., iStents (Glaukos, San Clemente, California) is a short procedure that could be combined with DMEK with or without phacoemulsification to control IOP. However, combining the two procedures increases the risk of postoperative hypotony that could impair DMEK attachment.

## 9.5 Corneal Abnormalities

### 9.5.1 Irido-corneal Endothelial (ICE) Syndrome

ICE syndrome can cause some challenges with DMEK because of anterior synechiae, iris defects, shallow AC, and high IOP. Some patients already present with a prior glaucoma surgery which adds to the difficulty of DMEK intraoperatively and graft attachment postoperatively. However, DMEK could be an excellent treatment for ICE syndrome patients who have mild changes or if all the associated conditions were managed appropriately [29, 30].

### 9.5.2 Previous Failed Penetrating Keratoplasty (PK) (Video 9.2)

DMEK could be performed to rescue a failed PK graft (Fig. 9.4) if that graft was satisfactory to the patient before failure [31–33]. In cases of severe corneal edema, even with good DMEK graft attachment, the cornea takes time to thin and regain clarity. Although it could take several months to gain the best visual outcome, DMEK is still better than performing a second PK as the latter will also require a long period of visual rehabilitation and has a much higher complication rate than DMEK.

When performing DMEK to treat a failed PK, some intraoperative precautions should be considered such as scoring and stripping the DM within the PK graft margin to avoid wound dehiscence. Actually for this reason some surgeons prefer doing DSEK for failed PK because DSEK could

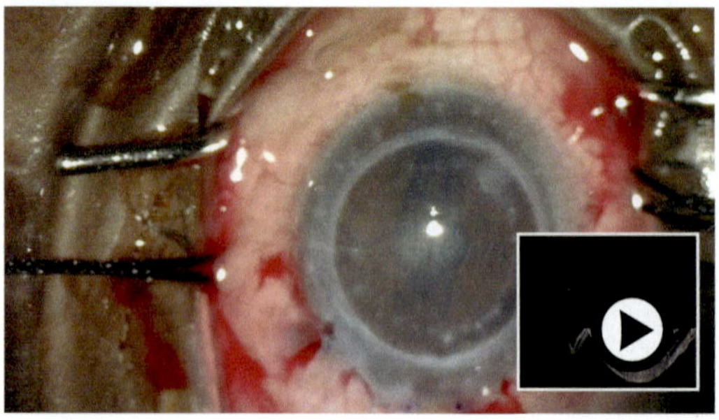

**Video 9.2** DMEK under failed PKP graft (https://doi.org/10.1007/000-dhh)

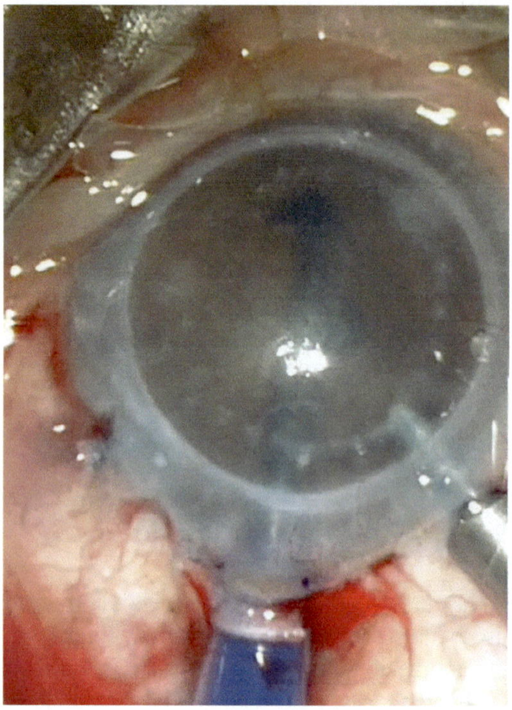

**Fig. 9.4** Insertion of a DMEK graft under an old PK graft after removal of the DM from the PK graft

be performed without DM removal if the center was clear [31, 32, 34]. Using a graft with a smaller diameter than the original PK graft is advisable to avoid the irregular area of the old PK incision scar [35]. A larger DMEK or DSEK graft could conform around the old PK wound scar but the risk of graft detachment and rebubble will be higher [36]. Anterior segment optical coherence tomography (AS OCT) is an important preoperative test to study the posterior surface of the PK graft to determine whether to perform DMEK in cases of smooth inner surface or to consider DSEK if the surface is very irregular. If the posterior surface irregularity is localized to a certain area, decentration of the DMEK graft could be considered and in such cases, host DM scoring and stripping should also be decentered to fit the desired graft position.

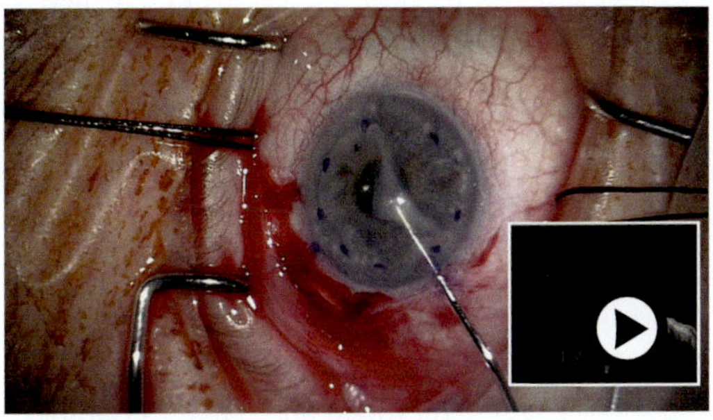

**Video 9.3** DMEK for failed DSEK (▶ https://doi.org/10.1007/000-dhg)

An inferior PI should be performed as usual to prevent pupillary block by the air tamponade. Many cases of previous PK already had a superior PI at the time of the prior PK procedure. If the surgeon decided to depend on this superior PI to prevent pupillary block, the patient should be advised to put his/her head down between knees periodically in the early postoperative period to force the air bubble to move inferiorly, clearing the superior PI, and preventing pupillary block. A laser inferior PI should be considered as a backup if pupillary block happened in the presence of a superior PI.

### 9.5.3 Previous Failed DSEK (Video 9.3)

As with PK, a DMEK graft can be a good solution to restore vision in an eye with a previous DSEK (Fig. 9.5). There are two main considerations when operating on an eye with a previous

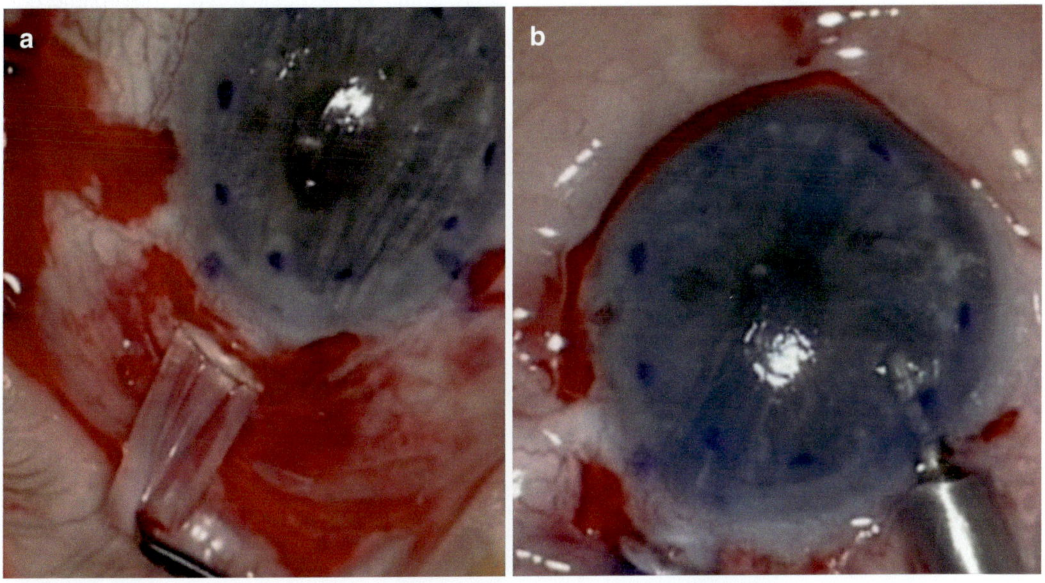

**Fig. 9.5** (**a**) Removal of a decompensated DSEK graft from the eye. (**b**) Insertion of a new DMEK graft

DSEK. First, some surgeons perform DSEK without DM scoring and stripping. A DSEK graft can attach well without DM removal while DMEK will not attach well if implanted without removal of the host DM [35]. So the surgeon should use trypan blue to make sure that the host DM was removed in the previous surgery or carefully remove it before implanting the DMEK regraft. The second consideration is that some surgeons intentionally roughen the stroma to aid DSEK graft attachment. However, this roughening will make DMEK graft attachment more difficult. Staining the stroma with trypan blue will help identify the areas of stromal tags. These should be cut near the stromal base with microscissors not by aspirating them with the bimanual irrigation aspiration system because that could lead to more tearing and disruption of the stromal fibers.

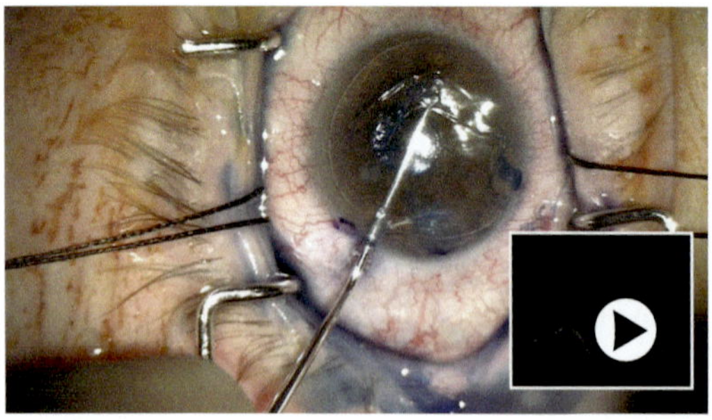

**Video 9.4** Re DMEK for early graft failure (https://doi.org/10.1007/000-dhk)

### 9.5.4 Previous Failed DMEK (Video 9.4)

DMEK regraft is often the best option to replace a failed DMEK graft whether this failure was primary or delayed (Fig. 9.6). Eyes with prior glaucoma surgery or excessive manipulation in the primary DMEK procedure are expected to experience earlier graft failure necessitating a regraft.

The main challenge in replacing a prior DMEK graft is to find the graft edge which is usually strongly attached to the stroma. Trypan blue helps in identifying the old graft, which should be removed completely, by using microforceps to pull out all the old DM fragments attached to the stroma before implanting the new graft. Any remnants from the old DMEK graft will make attachment of the new graft more difficult because they hold the new graft away from the surface of the recipient and make a conduit or channel for fluid to pass into the graft interface. In cases of primary DMEK graft failure, we advise a DMEK regraft at 1–2 months as further delay could be associated with irreversible corneal structural changes that will decrease the visual outcome [37, 38].

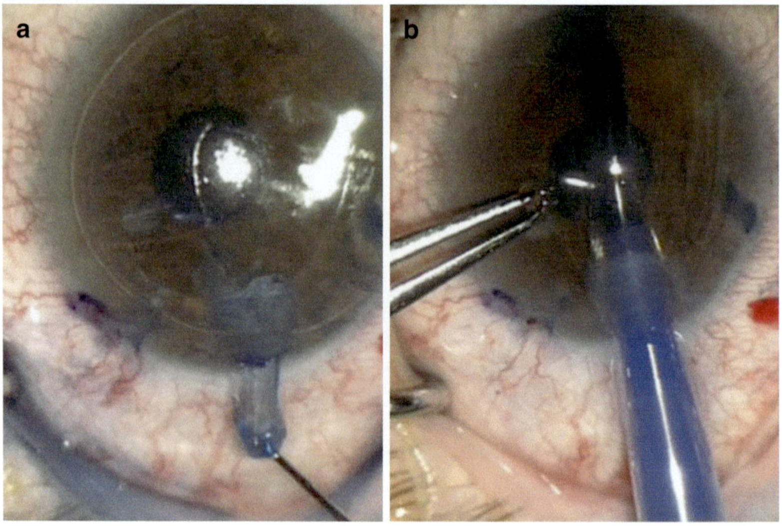


**Fig. 9.6** (**a**) Removal of the decompensated DMEK graft from the eye. (**b**) Insertion of a new DMEK graft

## 9.6 Posterior Segment Considerations

### 9.6.1 Vitrectomized Eyes

A vitrectomized eye combines the previously discussed hazards of a deep AC and aphakia which can allow early dissipation of the air tamponade to the posterior chamber leading to graft detachment.

Air and gases in general obey Laplace's law [2], which means they prefer to escape to larger spaces to minimize surface tension. This can be seen when operating on an aphakic eye: the air/gas bubble sinks to the posterior segment instead of floating up as expected. As described earlier, it is not advisable to attempt DMEK in aphakic eyes; a secondary posterior chamber IOL should be placed prior to DMEK. If the air or gas bubble starts to migrate into the posterior segment, the surgeon should aspirate all air or gas from the vitreous cavity, and refill or even overfill that space with balanced salt solution before placing another bubble in the anterior chamber, and the new bubble should not be over-inflated or it may be forced posteriorly again. It can also be effective to use continuous irrigation through a pars plana infusion cannula inserted through a small sclerotomy, usually 25 G, to be water tight. Any leakage of the sclerotomy site must be sutured to preserve the high posterior segment pressure and guard against intraocular infection.

### 9.6.2 Combined with Injection of Intravitreal Anti-vascular Endothelial Growth Factors (Anti VEGF)

In vitro and in vivo studies showed that bevacizumab as an anti-VEGF is safe for corneal endothelial cells [39, 40]. DMEK and intravitreal injection of anti-VEGF could be combined to treat comorbidity, e.g., to treat endothelial dysfunction and cystoid macular edema.

## 9.7 DMEK in Pediatrics

DMEK could be considered to treat endothelial dysfunction regardless of the patient's age as long as the anterior corneal layers have no or little scarring. Endothelial keratoplasty has been performed in children with endothelial dysfunction secondary to many conditions, e.g., congenital hereditary endothelial dystrophy (CHED), failed PK, DM rupture secondary to forceps trauma, posterior polymorphous corneal dystrophy (PPMD, PPCD), Peters' anomaly, buphthalmos and Kearns-Sayre syndrome [41–47].

Intraoperative challenges include a high chance of iris prolapse and AC shallowing due to high scleral elasticity, difficult scoring and stripping of the thin DM, poor visualization due to the associated severe stromal edema present in most cases, and the fact that most of these children are phakic which requires extra care not to traumatize the crystalline lens.

The main postoperative challenges are failure to obey the appropriate postoperative face up positioning, eye rubbing, and poor compliance which increase the risk of graft detachment and rebubbling.

DMEK should be considered because it provides a great advantage to children who have a strong immunologic system, as it is proved that DMEK is associated with much less risk of immunologic rejection. Rapid visual recovery and better refractive outcome of DMEK in comparison with PK are important in children to guard against amblyopia [48, 49]. Furthermore, DMEK provides better globe stability which is also needed in children because of their expected activity. On the other hand, a DSEK graft will unfold more easily and stick more reliably in these children.

## 9.8 Conclusion

DMEK offers significant advantages over DSEK and PK and should be attempted whenever indicated. In complex eyes, it is important to consider how to manage the complexity and to consider other keratoplasty options such as DSEK or PK. Patients with complex conditions should be educated well about their disease and treatment in order to set reasonable expectations.

## References


1. 2023 Eye Banking Statistical Report. Eye Bank Association of America. ebaa.users.membersuite.com/shop/store. Accessed 07 October 2024.
2. Giebel AW, Price FW. Air management of posterior grafts. In: Price FW, Price MO, editors. DSEK: all you need to know about endothelial keratoplasty. Thorofare: Slack; 2008. p. 149.
3. Price MO, Giebel AW, Fairchild KM, et al. Descemet's membrane endothelial keratoplasty: prospective multicenter study of visual and refractive outcomes and endothelial survival. Ophthalmology. 2009;116:2361–8.
4. Chaurasia S, Price FW Jr, Gunderson L, et al. Descemet's membrane endothelial keratoplasty: clinical results of single versus triple procedures (combined with cataract surgery). Ophthalmology. 2014;121:454–8.
5. Terry MA, Shamie N, Chen ES, et al. Endothelial keratoplasty for Fuchs' dystrophy with cataract: complications and clinical results with the new triple procedure. Ophthalmology. 2009;116:631–9.
6. Price MO, Price DA, Fairchild KM, et al. Rate and risk factors for cataract formation and extraction after Descemet stripping endothelial keratoplasty. Br J Ophthalmol. 2010;94:1468–71.
7. Parker J, Dirisamer M, Naveiras M, et al. Outcomes of Descemet membrane endothelial keratoplasty in phakic eyes. J Cataract Refract Surg. 2012;38(5):871–7.
8. Burkhart ZN, Feng MT, Price FW Jr, et al. One-year outcomes in eyes remaining phakic after Descemet membrane endothelial keratoplasty. J Cataract Refract Surg. 2014;40:430–4.
9. Price MO, Price FW, Trespalacios R. Endothelial keratoplasty technique for aniridic aphakic eyes. J Cataract Refract Surg. 2007;33:376–9.
10. Afshari NA, Gorovoy MS, Yoo SH, et al. Dislocation of the donor graft to the posterior segment in Descemet stripping automated endothelial keratoplasty. Am J Ophthalmol. 2012;153:638–42.
11. McKee Y, Price FW Jr, Feng MT, et al. Implementation of the posterior chamber intraocular lens intrascleral haptic fixation technique (glued intraocular lens) in a United States practice: outcomes and insights. J Cataract Refract Surg. 2014;40:2099–105.
12. Yamane S, Sato S, Maruyama-Inoue M, Kadonosono K. Flanged intrascleral intraocular lens fixation with double-needle technique. Ophthalmology. 2017;124:1136–42.
13. Neuhann IM, Neuhann TF, Rohrbach JM. Intraocular lens opacification after keratoplasty. Cornea. 2013;32:6–10.
14. Werner L, Wilbanks G, Nieuwendaal CP, et al. Localized opacification of hydrophilic acrylic intraocular lenses after procedures using intracameral injection of air or gas. J Cataract Refract Surg. 2015;41:199–207.
15. Chaudhry P, Prakash G, Jacob S, et al. Safety and efficacy of gas-forced infusion (air pump) in coaxial phacoemulsification. J Cataract Refract Surg. 2010;36:2139–45.
16. Price FW Jr. Intraoperative optical coherence tomography: game-changing technology. Cornea. 2021 1;40(6):675–8.
17. Burkhart ZN, Feng MT, Price MO, Price FW. Handheld slit beam techniques to facilitate DMEK and DALK. Cornea. 2013;32(5):722–4.
18. Jacob S, Agarwal A, et al. Endoilluminator-assisted transcorneal illumination for Descemet membrane endothelial keratoplasty: enhanced intraoperative visualization of the graft in corneal decompensation secondary to pseudophakic bullous keratopathy. J Cataract Refract Surg. 2014;40:1332–6.
19. Macsai MS, Kara-Jose AC. Suture technique for Descemet stripping and endothelial keratoplasty. Cornea. 2007;26:1123–6.
20. Busin M, Leon P, D'Angelo S, Ruzza A, Ferrari S, Ponzin D, Parekh M. Clinical outcomes of preloaded Descemet membrane endothelial keratoplasty grafts with endothelium tri-folded inwards. Am J Ophthalmol. 2018;193:106–13.
21. Liarakos VS, Ham L, Dapena I, et al. Endothelial keratoplasty for bullous keratopathy in eyes with anterior chamber intraocular lens. J Cataract Refract Surg. 2013;39:1835–45.
22. Ang M, Li L, Chua D, et al. Descemet's stripping automated endothelial keratoplasty with anterior chamber intraocular lenses: complications and 3-year outcomes. Br J Ophthalmol. 2014;98:1028–32.
23. Schoenberg ED, Price FW Jr. Modification of Siepser sliding suture technique for iris repair and endothelial keratoplasty. J Cataract Refract Surg. 2014;40:705–8.
24. Aldave AJ, Baghdasaryan E, Miller KM. Descemet stripping endothelial keratoplasty after Ophtec 311 iris reconstruction lens implantation. Cornea. 2011;30:405–8.

25. Khor WB, Teo KY, Mehta JS, et al. Descemet stripping automated endothelial keratoplasty in complex eyes; results with a donor insertion device. Cornea. 2013;32:1063–8.
26. Lee HJ, Colby KA. A review of the clinical and genetic aspects of aniridia. Semin Ophthalmol. 2013;28:306–12.
27. Anshu A, Price MO, Price FW. Descemet's stripping endothelial keratoplasty: long-term graft survival and risk factors for failure in eyes with preexisting glaucoma. Ophthalmology. 2012;119:1982–7.
28. Aldave AJ, Chen JL, Zaman AS, et al. Outcomes after DSEK in 101 eyes with previous trabeculectomy and tube shunt implantation. Cornea. 2014;33:223–9.
29. Price MO, Price FW. Descemet's stripping with endothelial keratoplasty for treatment of iridocorneal endothelial syndrome. Cornea. 2007;26:493–7.
30. Chaurasia S, Ramappa M, Garg P, et al. Endothelial keratoplasty in the management of irido-corneal endothelial syndrome. Eye (Lond). 2013;27:564–6.
31. Price FW, Price MO. Endothelial keratoplasty to restore clarity to a failed penetrating graft. Cornea. 2006;25:895–9.
32. Heitor de Paula F, Kamyar R, Shtein RM, et al. Endothelial keratoplasty without Descemet stripping after failed penetrating keratoplasty. Cornea. 2012;31:645–8.
33. Pasari A, Price MO, Feng MT, Price FW Jr. Descemet membrane endothelial keratoplasty for failed penetrating keratoplasty: visual outcomes and graft survival. Cornea. 2019;38:151–6.
34. Price FW, Price MO, Arundhati A. Descemet stripping automated endothelial keratoplasty under failed penetrating keratoplasty: how to avoid complications. Am J Ophthalmol. 2011;151:187–8.
35. Tourtas T, Schlomberg J, Wessel JM, et al. Graft adhesion in Descemet membrane endothelial keratoplasty dependent on size of removal of host's Descemet membrane. JAMA Ophthalmol. 2014;132:155–61.
36. Straiko MD, Terry MA, Shamie N. Descemet stripping automated endothelial keratoplasty under failed penetrating keratoplasty: a surgical strategy to minimize complications. Am J Ophthalmol. 2011;151:233–7.
37. Price FW Jr, Price MO. To intervene or not to intervene: that is the question. Ophthalmology. 2015;122:6–7.
38. Baydoun L, Van Dijk K, Dapena I, et al. Repeat Descemet membrane endothelial keratoplasty after complicated primary Descemet membrane endothelial keratoplasty. Ophthalmology. 2015;122:8–16.
39. Rusovici R, Sakhalkar M, Chalam KV. Evaluation of cytotoxicity of bevacizumab on VEGF-enriched corneal endothelial cells. Mol Vis. 2011;17:3339–46.
40. Weller JM, Tourtas T, Kruse FE. Feasibility and outcome of Descemet membrane endothelial keratoplasty in complex anterior segment and vitreous disease. Cornea. 2015;34(11):1351–7.
41. Ashar JN, Madhavi Latha K, Vaddavalli PK. Descemet's stripping endothelial keratoplasty (DSEK) for children with congenital hereditary endothelial dystrophy: surgical challenges and 1-year outcomes. Graefes Arch Clin Exp Ophthalmol. 2012;250:1341–5.
42. Srinivasan B, Agarwal M, Iyer G, et al. Pediatric Descemet Membrane Endothelial Keratoplasty. Am J Ophthalmol. 2021;227:12–7.
43. Scorcia V, Pietropaolo R, Carnevali A, et al. Results of descemet stripping automated endothelial keratoplasty for the treatment of late corneal decompensation secondary to obstetrical forceps trauma. Cornea. 2016;35:305–7.
44. Sella R, Rootman D, Bahar I. Descemet's stripping automated endothelial keratoplasty for posterior polymorphous corneal dystrophy in an 8-month-old boy. J AAPOS. 2013;17:94–6.
45. Hashemi H, Ghaffari R, Mohebi M. Posterior lamellar keratoplasty (DSAEK) in Peters anomaly. Cornea. 2012;31:1201–5.
46. Beltz J, Madi S, Santorum P, et al. Descemet stripping automated endothelial keratoplasty for endothelial decompensation in buphthalmos. Am J Ophthalmol. 2013;156:608–615.e1.
47. Gonnermann J, Klamann MK, Maier AK, et al. Descemet membrane endothelial keratoplasty in a child with corneal endothelial dysfunction in Kearns–Sayre syndrome. Cornea. 2014;33:1232–4.
48. Anwar HM, El-Danasoury A. Endothelial keratoplasty in children. Curr Opin Ophthalmol. 2014;25:340–6.
49. Trief D, Marquezan MC, Rapuano CJ, Prescott CR. Pediatric corneal transplants. Curr Opin Ophthalmol. 2017;28(5):477–84.

# PDEK in Complex Cases 10

Soosan Jacob

Pre-Descemet's Endothelial Keratoplasty or PDEK refers to transplantation of the Pre-Descemet's layer or Dua's layer, Descemet's membrane and endothelium [1, 2]. This surgery has certain advantages, especially in complex cases as the PDEK graft is tougher, resilient as well more resistant to tearing than the DMEK graft. This allows the easier use of a technique that has been described by the author—"the air pump assisted PDEK/ DMEK technique" for surgery and therefore allows one to harness all the advantages of this technique, even in complex cases [3–5]. The air pump assisted PDEK technique has many advantages and can be used for various purposes in PDEK surgery such as to make the Descemetorhexis easily, to remove host Descemet's membrane tags, to tamponadc bleeding from the peripheral iridectomy or from synechiolysis, to allow graft edgc unfolding, centration and uncreasing of the graft (Fig. 10.1), to maintain a formed AC and to act like a third hand supporting the graft from beneath. Though the technique can be harnessed in DMEK as well, for some of the steps, it cannot be used for edge unfolding or centration as the DMEK graft, unlike the PDEK graft is much more delicate and can tear with these maneuvers. However, the ability to use this technique is a major advantage for PDEK over DMEK, especially in complex cases.

Two other techniques that have been described by the author also aid in increasing the success rates of PDEK in these complex situations—the Endoilluminator-assisted PDEK [6, 7] (Fig. 10.2) and Host Descemetic Scaffolding [8] (Fig. 10.3 See Chapters 8 and 11). The air pump-assisted technique as well as these two techniques can therefore be used to allow successful PDEK in a variety of complex situations, some of which are discussed below.

---

**Supplementary Information** The online version contains supplementary material available at https://doi.org/10.1007/978-981-97-3469-6_10. The videos can be accessed individually by clicking the DOI link in the accompanying figure caption or by scanning this link with the SN More Media App.

S. Jacob (✉)
Dr. Agarwal's Refractive and Cornea Foundation, Chennai, India

Dr. Agarwal's Eye Hospital and Eye Research Centre, Chennai, India



S. Jacob (ed.), *Mastering DMEK and PDEK*, https://doi.org/10.1007/978-981-97-3469-6_10

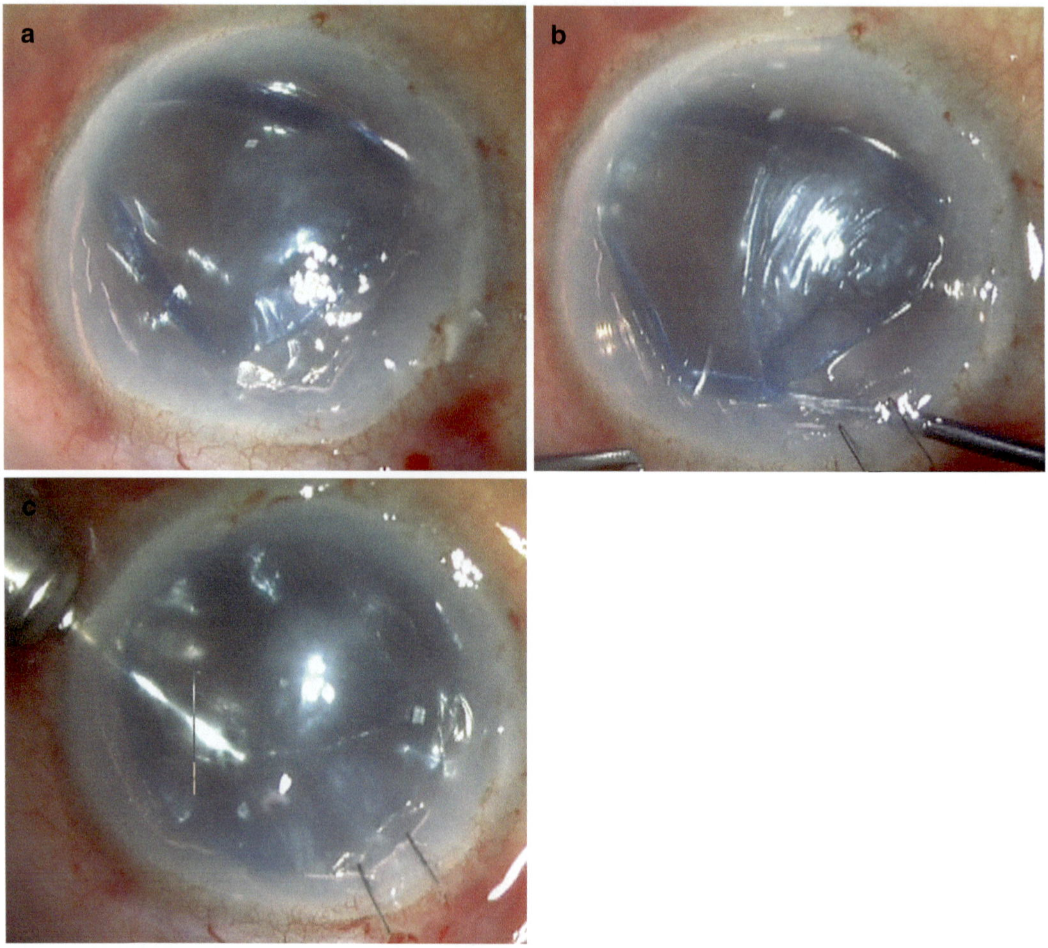

**Fig. 10.1** Air pump-assisted PDEK technique: (**a**) The PDEK graft is floated up; (**b**) The graft is centered; (**c**) The ACM is inserted and edge folds are removed under gentle air infusion so as to avoid collapse of the AC. This technique was described by the author (Soosan Jacob)

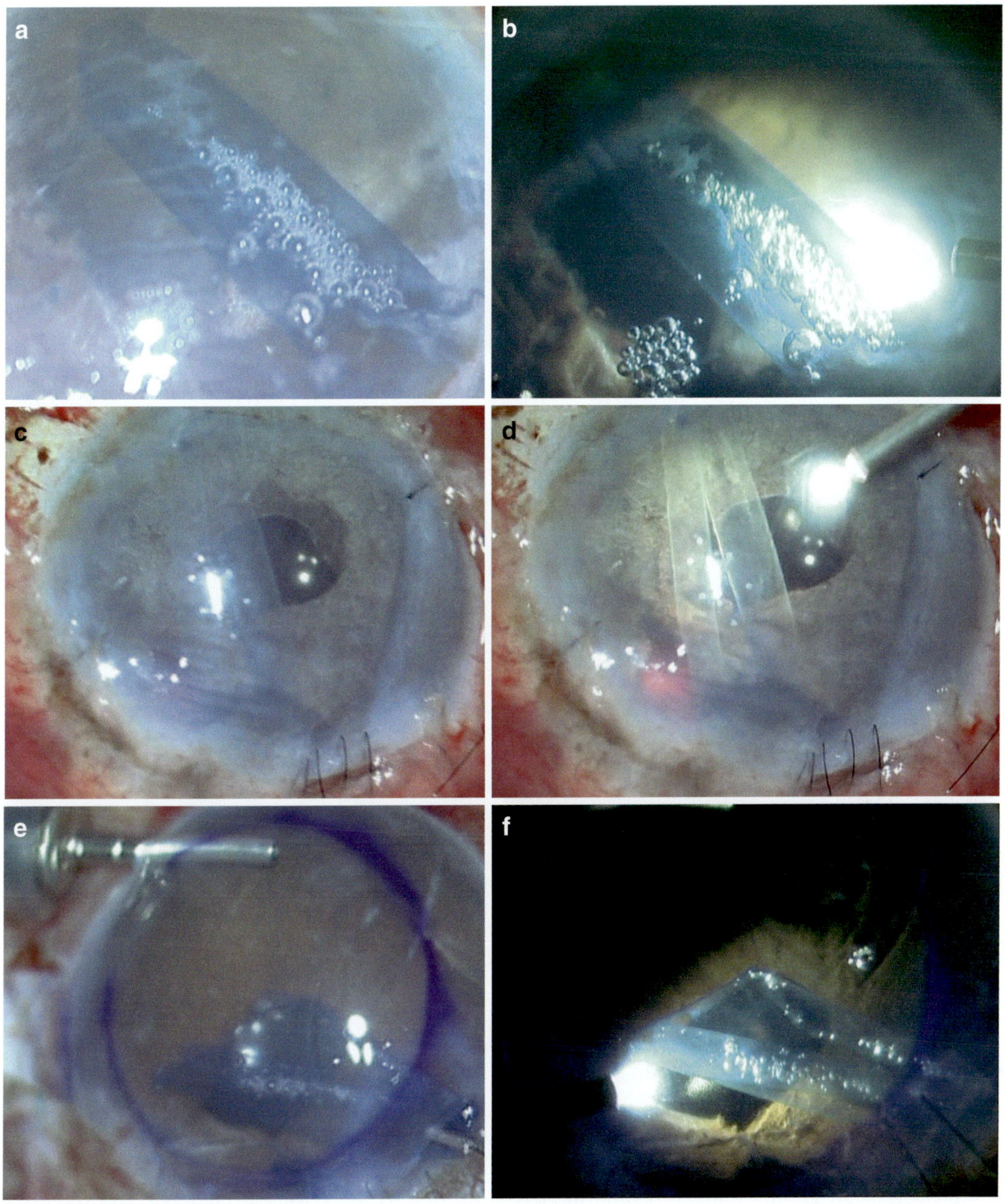


**Fig. 10.2** E-PDEK/E-DMEK—The endoilluminator-assisted PDEK/DMEK technique described by the author—(**a**, **c**, **e**) View through the operating microscope; (**b**, **d**, **f**) Corresponding view after switching off the microscope light and using endoilluminator light shown obliquely

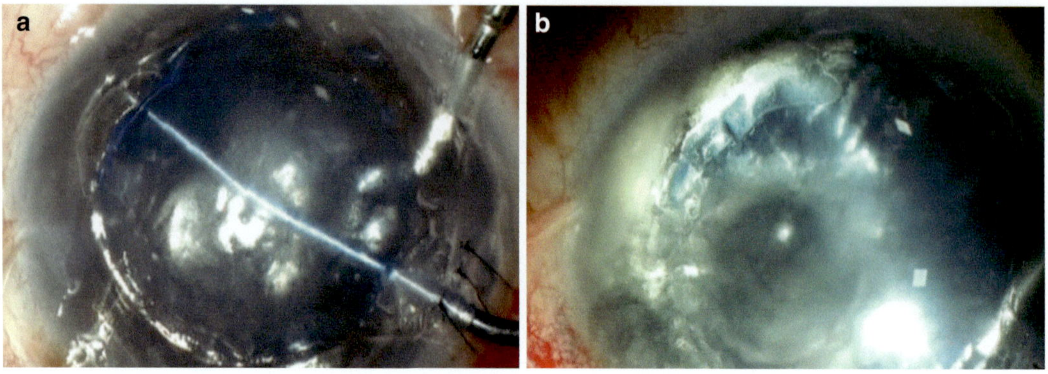


**Fig. 10.3** Host Descemetic scaffolding technique: Described by the author (Soosan Jacob). (**a**) The peripheral rim of host Descemet's membrane is teased out to lie under the graft: (**b**) The peripheral rim of host Descemet's membrane is seen lying posterior to the graft supporting and scaffolding it from beneath

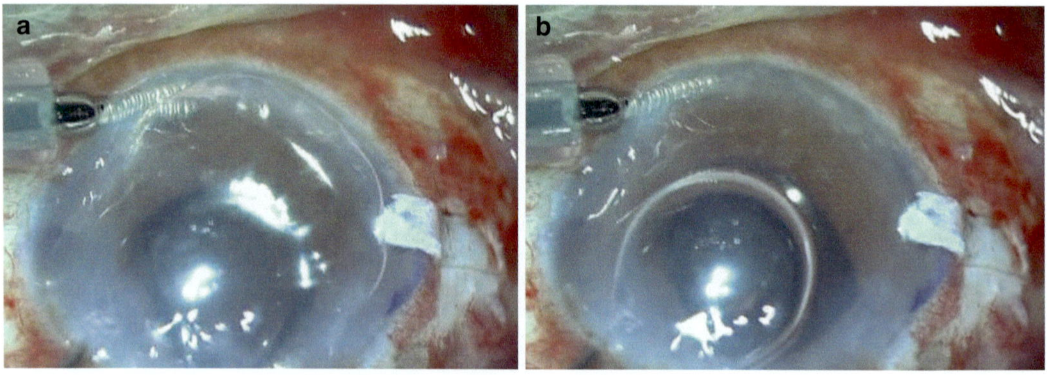


**Fig. 10.4** Bubble test: (**a**) A full air bubble is injected into the AC and its behavior noted; (**b**) Posterior migration or an unstable bubble may indicate the need for a pupilloplasty. This test was described by the author (Soosan Jacob). It can be done either after simply turning off the pressurized air infusion or after removing the anterior chamber maintainer

## 10.1 Floppy Iris Syndrome

A floppy iris results in iris prolapse through the wound, distortion of the pupil as well as increases the chance of air getting trapped behind the iris and causing pupillary block either intraoperatively or postoperatively. This is managed by doing a pupilloplasty in order to make the iris diaphragm taut followed by what the author refers to as the "bubble" test (Fig. 10.4) [9, 10]. This test essentially consists of injecting a full air bubble into the AC before injecting the graft and watching the bubble dynamics [10]. This helps one understand whether or not the bubble will migrate to the posterior chamber and therefore allows management of the iris-capsular bag-IOL diaphragm prior to injecting the graft, thus decreasing risk of damage to the graft endothelium by avoiding unnecessary manipulations after the graft is injected in.

## 10.2 Shallow AC

Shallow anterior chamber can be pre-existing or can occur intraoperatively due to progressive hydration of the vitreous. Though the AC is shallowed intentionally during DMEK/PDEK to help unroll the graft, a very shallow AC can be challenging to operate on, especially if associated with positive vitreous pressure. The graft can be difficult to inject within the AC and may sometimes shoot out of the incision when the cartridge/injector system is withdrawn from the incision. In addition, the graft may crumple up within the AC and the tight space may not allow it to be opened out, thereby making unrolling and centering the graft difficult (Fig. 10.5). Floatation also becomes difficult as the cannula rubs against the iris when it is introduced into the AC under the graft to inject air. This can result in iris pigment release and muddying of the aqueous or even an iridodialysis and bleeding from the iris. Postoperative inflammation is increased because of increased release of inflammatory mediators. The iris pigments may enter the graft host interface and persist as interface debris. When present over the visual axis, this can lead to a degradation of the visual acuity. A shallow AC is tackled by first identifying the etiology. Topical anesthesia should be avoided. A peri-bulbar block is preferred to prevent lid squeezing, pain from possible iris touch and unwanted ocular movements. Preoperatively, a Pinkie ball is applied to shrink the vitreous and make the eye softer. An overly tight speculum can cause a shallow AC and this should be loosened. Similarly, if required, a lateral canthotomy may be performed. Intraoperatively, if the AC is still shallow despite all precautions, a limited dry vitrectomy may be performed through a pars plana trocar and the AC allowed to deepen. This may also be required in case fluid passes posteriorly into the vitreous cavity through a posterior capsular rent/zonulodialysis. Once the tight, shallow AC is made deeper and softer, surgery can be carried on as usual, taking precautions however that posteriorly directed fluid does not again cause forward movement of the iris-IOL diaphragm resulting once again in a tight AC. The dry vitrectomy may need to be repeated in this situation.

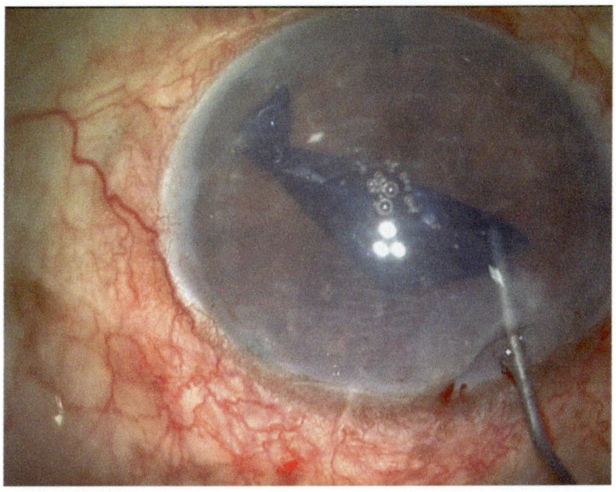

**Fig. 10.5** A shallow AC makes graft unrolling difficult within the AC

## 10.3 Deep AC

A deep AC is the other end of the spectrum and may be seen in aphakic eyes, vitrectomized eyes and eyes with low scleral rigidity. Graft unscrolling and unrolling is difficult in this case since unrolled edges tend to spontaneously roll up again. Different options exist to address this problem. Gentle pressure on the side of the globe applied at the correct angle can shallow the AC. Another option is to depress the cornea down to hold the opened edge of graft in place while fluid is expressed from the opposite paracentesis to make the other half of the AC as shallow as possible while also simultaneously trying to open the rest of the graft. The cornea may also be depressed down in the center to hold the graft centrally. The AC on either side is then shallowed by expressing fluid and the rolled edges on either side are opened. Alternately, fluid may be used gently to open the graft up. Air pump-assisted PDEK has an especially beneficial role in these cases as the graft can be floated up even in the presence of minimal edge folds and a decentered position (Figs. 10.6 and 10.7). This is unlike in a DMEK where it is very essential to have the graft unfolded completely as well as centered in position before the graft is floated up. At the end of surgery, an adequate sized and stable air bubble must be ascertained to prevent postoperative detachments [11].

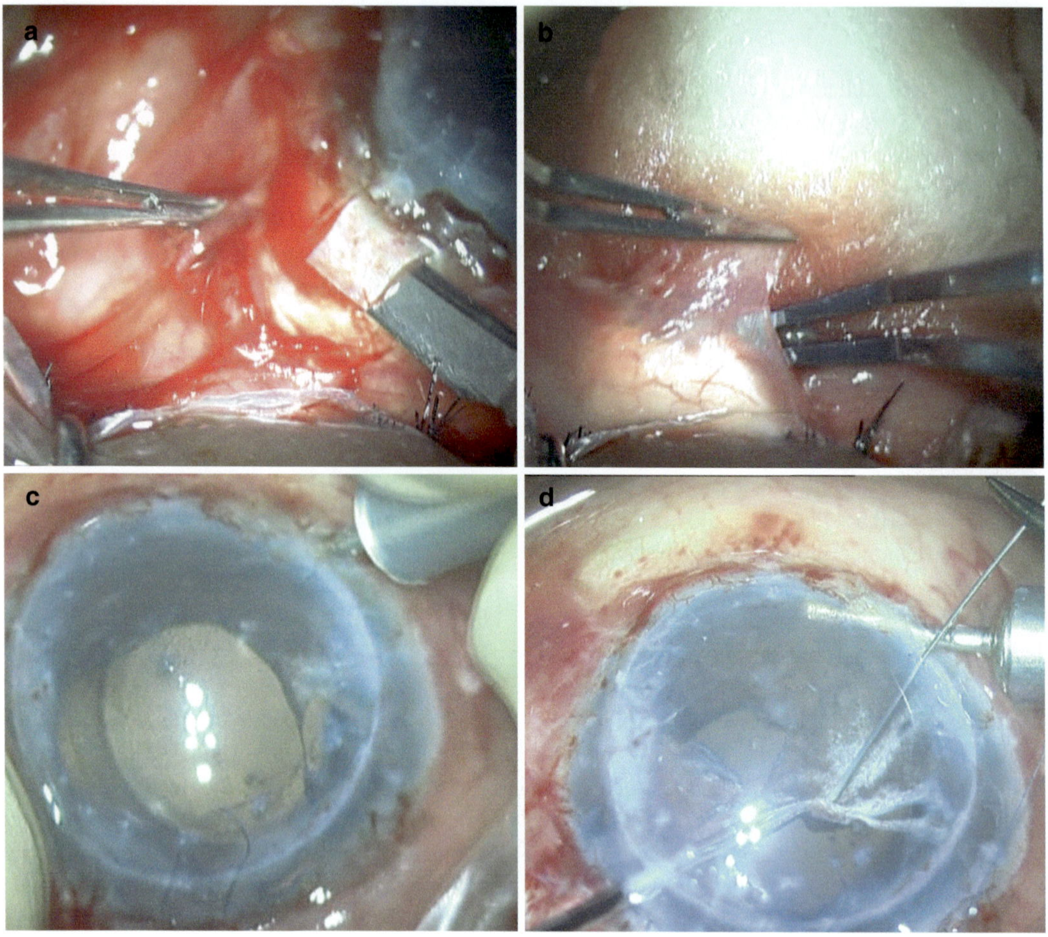


**Fig. 10.6** PDEK using air pump-assisted, E-PDEK, and Host Descemetic scaffolding techniques in complex eye with multiple risk factors: a failed decompensated graft, large sector iridectomy, glued IOL, vitrectomized mono-cameral eye, deep anterior chamber, and post-penetrating keratoplasty glaucoma. This eye has multiple high risk factors for graft detachment and would traditionally be considered a poor indication for PDEK or DMEK. (**a**) A superficial scleral flap is made for trabeculectomy; (**b**) Mitomicin-C soaked sponge is placed under the scleral and conjunctival flaps; (**c**) An anterior chamber maintainer (ACM) is inserted and BSS irrigation is started; (**d**) Pupilloplasty is performed for bringing down the size of the pupil to decrease chances of air migrating posteriorly. Continued in next figure

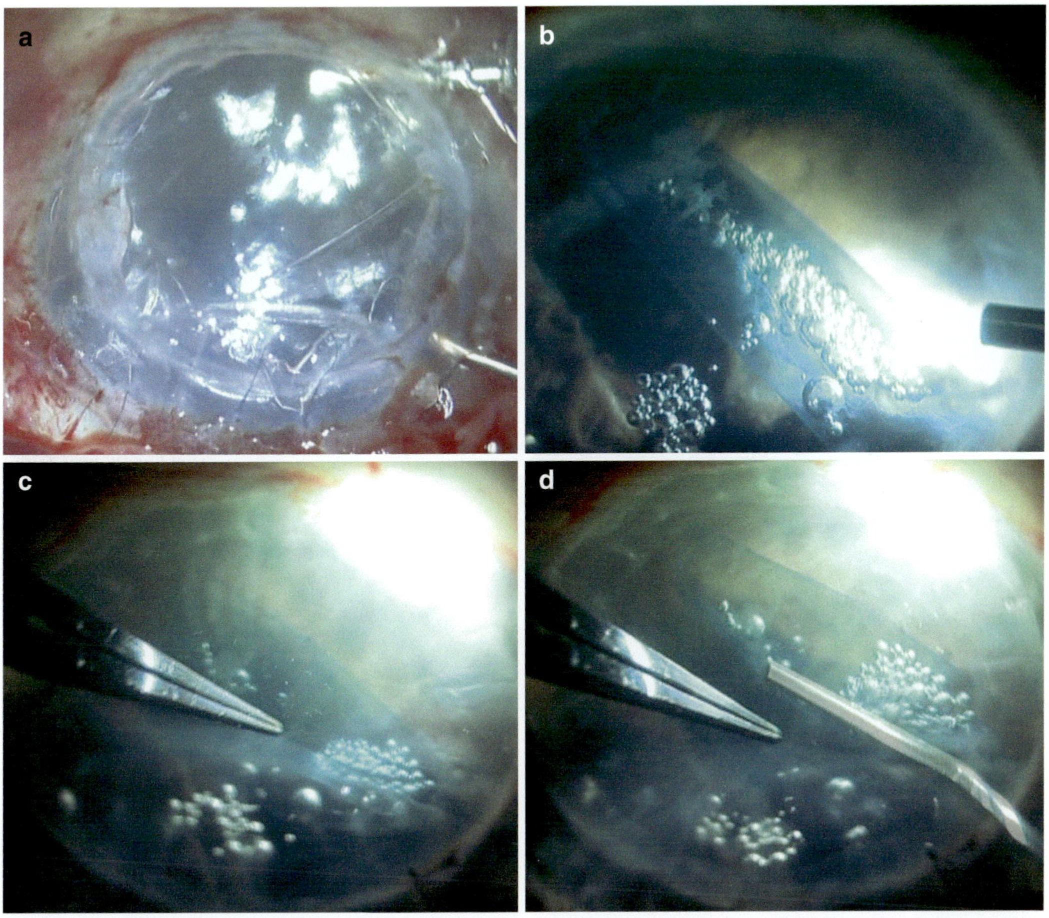

**Fig. 10.7** Same case as Fig. 10.6 (Contd): (**a**) Air infusion is started through the ACM and Descemetorhexis is done leaving small rim of host Descemet's membrane in few areas to use as scaffold at a later stage. Care is taken not to dig into the graft host junction; (**b**) PDEK graft is inserted and E-PDEK technique is used to verify orientation of the graft; (**c**, **d**) The graft is unfolded by using a combination of maneuvers as described in text. Continued in next figure

## 10.4 Difficult Unrolling and Centration of Graft

As discussed, the air pump-assisted technique can be used in these cases to complete the surgery successfully as well as with good results. Excessive manipulations and repeated rubbing of the graft on the iris in attempts to open up fully or to center the graft can be avoided using this technique. This is because extreme peripheral edge folds are acceptable as is a decentered graft and both these can be rectified later in the surgery. Once the graft has been floated up, the anterior chamber maintainer is re-inserted and continuous pressurized air infusion is started. The graft is then centered using a reverse Sinskey hook. This is followed by unfolding of any peripheral edge folds as well as straightening out of any creases or wrinkles, again using the reverse Sinskey hook (Figs. 10.8 and 10.9). The continuous pressurized air infusion from the air pump-assisted technique maintains the AC open and prevents it from collapsing during these maneuvers. It thereby prevents graft detachment as well as damage while inserting instruments into the AC. Continuing the pressurized infusion while closing the eye allows the graft to start adhering well in the intraopera-

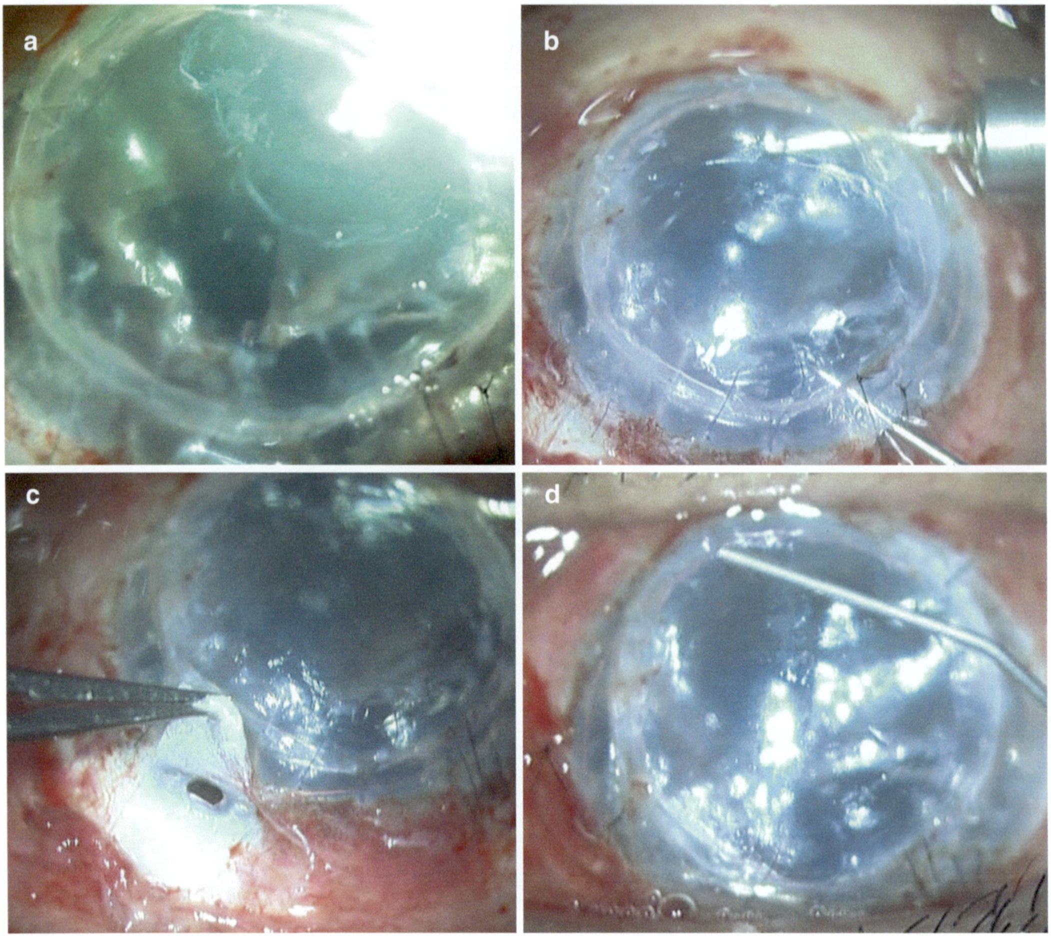


**Fig. 10.8** Same case as Fig. 10.6 (Contd): (**a**) The graft is floated up even though decentered; (**b**) Using the air pump-assisted technique, the graft is then centered, edge folds removed, and host Descemetic scaffolding performed. This avoids the need for excessive manipulations that are required for perfect centration and edge unfolding and that may often be unattainable in such complex eyes; (**c**) The trabeculectomy is then completed by taking a scleral punch. This is done under air infusion; (**d**) The scleral and conjunctival flaps of the trabeculectomy are closed and all incisions are also sutured to get air-tight seal. The eye pressure is left at near-normal levels. The air pump gives intraoperative adhesion of the graft and the host Descemetic scaffolding technique further decreases risk of postoperative graft detachment. Continued in next figure

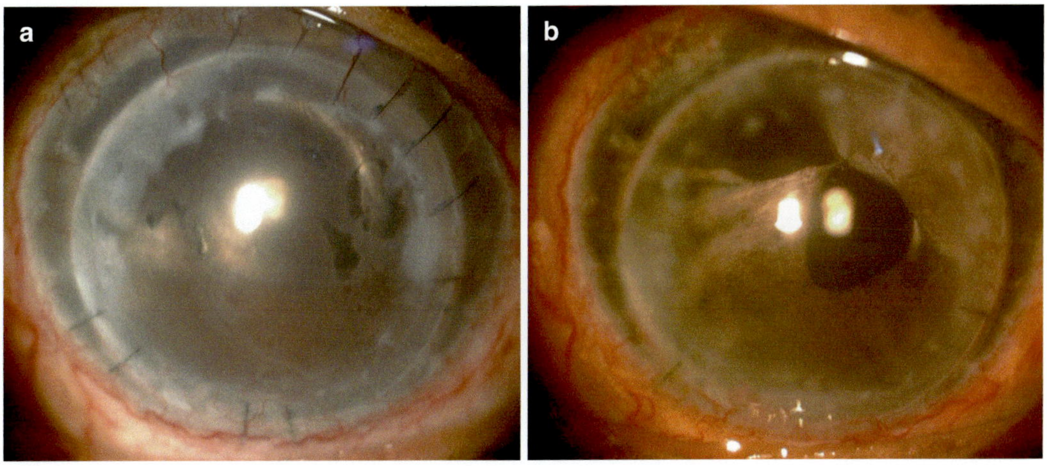


**Fig. 10.9** Same case as Fig. 10.6 (Contd): (**a**) Preoperative slitlamp image of the eye; (**b**) Postoperative image of eye showing a well-attached PDEK graft and clear cornea. The IOP remained under control

tive period itself as seen by a greater difficulty in moving the graft with the reverse Sinskey hook after some time with the air pump on [12].

## 10.5 Aphakia

A secondary IOL is preferably fixed in an aphakic eye in order to get a stable iris-IOL diaphragm that will allow a stable, non-migrating air bubble to support the graft in the postoperative period. This may be done using a iris retro-fixated claw lens or a scleral fixated IOL (glued or Yamane). The author personally prefers the glued IOL technique for secondary IOL fixation. Modifications in the glued IOL that help better graft adhesion include placing the IOL closer to the iris in order to avoid large antero-posterior gap between the iris and the IOL since a large gap can result in the air bubble migrating posteriorly. The importance of a stable iris-IOL diaphragm was stressed by the author for DMEK [9] and the same principles apply for PDEK as well (Figs. 10.4 and 10.6). A pupilloplasty should therefore be done in those cases where the iris-IOL-capsular bag complex is not providing a diaphragm for supporting the air bubble postoperatively [13].

## 10.6 Secondary IOLs

Corneal decompensation can occur in the presence of anterior chamber IOL, iris retro-fixated IOL or scleral fixated IOL. Though a well-fixated and well-sized ACIOL does not cause corneal decompensation, a choice has to be made between explanting it followed by implanting an iris or scleral fixated IOL or retaining the ACIOL. In the case of a poorly positioned or sized ACIOL or a shallow AC with ACIOL, it is better to explant the ACIOL. Opening the graft in the presence of an ACIOL can be challenging and excessive attempts can lead to rubbing of the endothelium over the IOL. In addition, care must be taken to ensure that the ACIOL was in fact not the cause of the primary decompensation as if it was, it could lead on to a decompensation of the implanted graft as well. If the ACIOL is made of PMMA, it requires a larger incision to explant it and unless care is taken to ensure that the incision is closed well in a leak-proof manner, it can lead to an increased risk of graft detachment. If required, surgery can also be performed in a staged manner. ACIOL explantation with (in the author's preference), glued IOL in the first stage (or other manner of secondary scleral fixated IOL, such as Yamane or iris fixated IOL); followed by a PDEK in the second stage once the wounds have become stable. The author however prefers a single stage surgery, using a small scleral frown incision for explanting the ACIOL. This combined with sutures to close the scleral incision, closure further reinforced if required by glue, is generally sufficient to get good non-leaking wound closure.

## 10.7 Lack of Iris IOL Diaphragm

This can be a risk factor for graft detachment and every attempt should be made to get a stable base that allows a stable and non-migrating air bubble tamponade within the AC. This is checked before injecting the graft by performing "the bubble test" that has been described earlier by the author. The iris may require a pupilloplasty or in case of an iridodialysis, a dialysis repair or sometimes a combination of the two till a stable diaphragm is obtained. A thickened and fibrotic capsular bag if present is also sufficient and provides good support to the air bubble postoperatively (Figs. 10.4 and 10.6). Artficial iris implants may also be used to create an iris diaphragm.

## 10.8 Aniridia

Though this is challenging to perform a TMEK in, the air pump-assisted technique can make it possible. An aniridia IOL is implanted and the wound secured in an air tight manner. The PDEK graft is injected carefully, making sure that it does not slip into the vitreous cavity. The PDEK graft can then be scrolled open as much as possible without heavily pressing down on the graft. Air in then injected to float the graft up against the overlying stroma. Once floated up, the air pump is started at a low pressure to continue the rest of the surgery using the air pump-assisted technique. Edge folds are removed and centration is achieved using the pressurized air to hold the graft up. Air pressure can be raised once the graft is centered and edge folds removed (Fig. 10.10). The author has also put a rescue suture on the PDEK graft to prevent graf drop into the vitreous in eyes with large aphakic spaces.

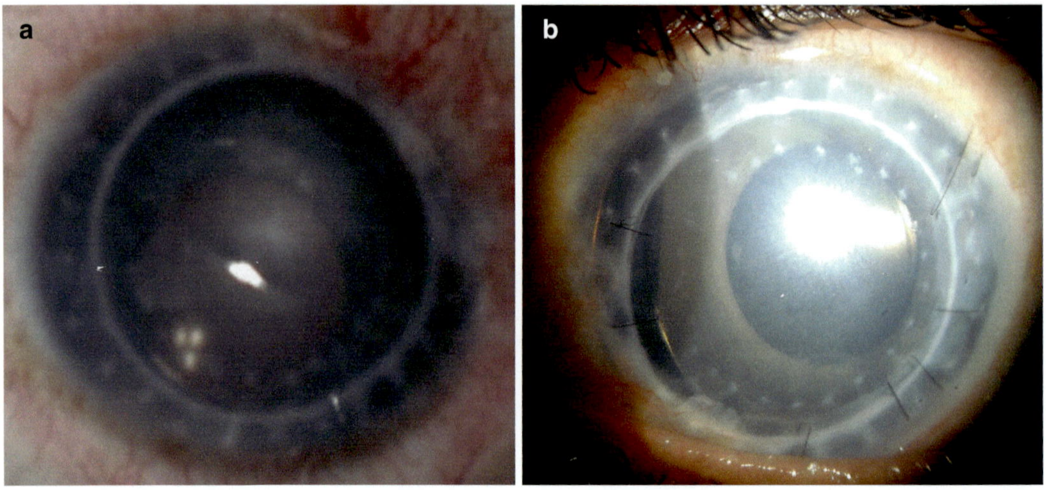


**Fig. 10.10** PDEK in aniridia: (**a**) Traumatic aniridia with aniridia IOL and failed penetrating keratoplasty: (**b**) Post PDEK clear graft seen

## 10.9 Previous Failed DSAEK

Eyes with a failed DSAEK graft are reasonably easy to perform PDEK on (Fig. 10.11). The DSAEK graft can be easily detached except at its edges where the adhesions are stronger. Once it is detached and removed from the anterior chamber, the host Descemetorhexis margins are checked to make sure there will be no overlap between host DM and the PDEK graft. The rest of the surgery proceeds as is generally done for a PDEK [14].

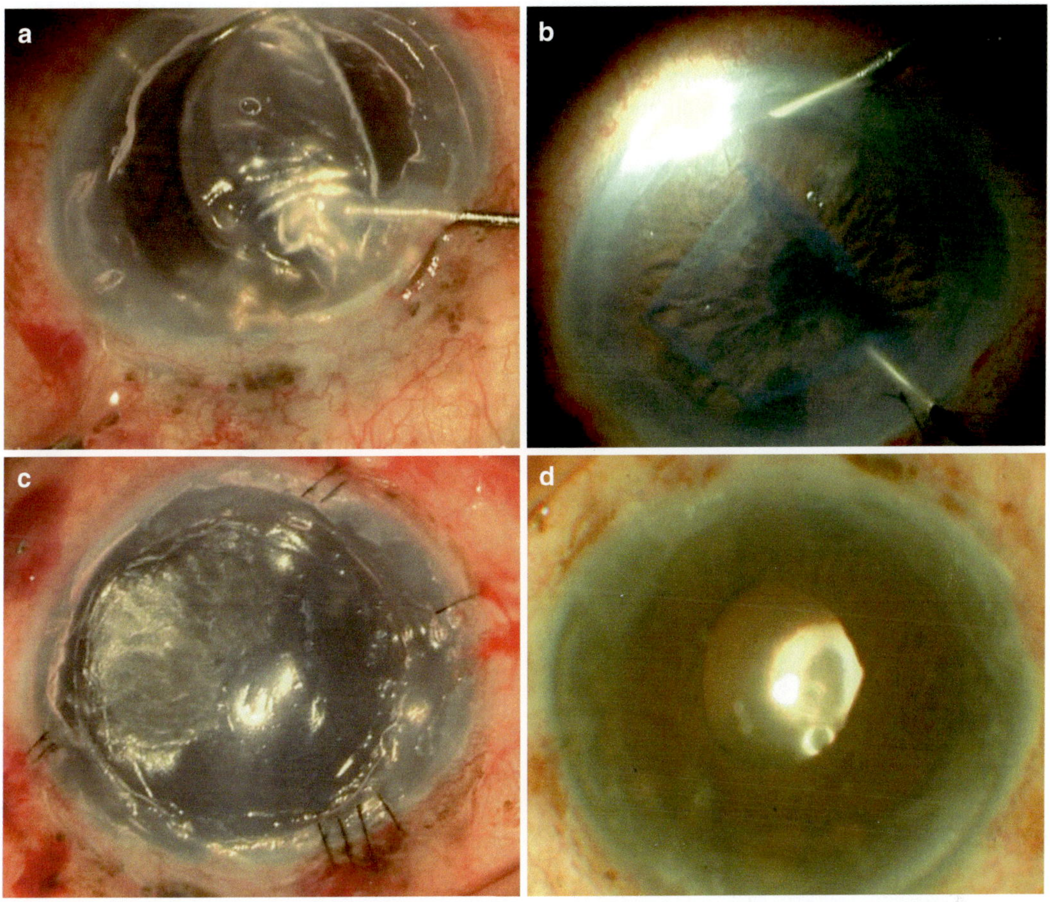


**Fig. 10.11** PDEK for failed DSAEK: (**a**) Failed DSAEK graft removed; (**b**) PDEK graft injected and unrolled using E-PDEK technique; (**c**) Graft floated up using air pump-assisted technique; (**d**) Postoperative clear cornea seen

## 10.10 Failed Penetrating Keratoplasty

Air pump-assisted PDEK can successfully be performed in failed penetrating keratoplasties (Figs. 10.6, 10.7, 10.8, 10.9, and 10.10). The author prefers to make a scleral incision for inserting the graft in order to avoid injuring the graft host junction. The Descemetorhexis should be carried out with care and disruption of the graft host junction should be avoided by not digging deeply into the junction. The author initiates Descemetorhexis in a size smaller than the edges of the graft. The left over host DM within the graft can then be easily stripped completely up to the graft edge by using a microforceps passed through the paracentesis. Care should be taken to keep the graft size smaller than the size of the old full-thickness graft. This can be done by using an appropriately sized trephine to cut the graft in such cases instead of using scissors. Overlapping and crossing of the graft over onto the host cornea can result in a graft detachment at that site which may sometimes progress into complete graft detachment. This is more of a problem with DMEK than PDEK since PDEK grafts can easily be centered using the air pump assisted technique. In the eventuality that the graft is oversized, with the air-pump on, radial trans-graft sutures may be taken across the graft host junction at one or more sites [15].

## 10.11 Trabeculectomies

Trabeculectomies and tube shunts are risk factors for an increased rate of detachment after any kind of endothelial keratoplasty. This is because the air bubble within the AC can leak out through the ostium and result in inadequate postoperative air tamponade as well as a soft eye. The use of the air pump-assisted technique allows better intraoperative graft attachment, thereby decreasing the risk of detachment postoperatively. In addition, if the air does not remain within the AC at all, trans-graft corneal mattress sutures can also be applied that hold the graft in place postoperatively. The air pump can sometimes create a leak in the conjunctival covering of very thin, cystic, and avascular blebs. This risk can be decreased by applying some viscoelastic over the bleb to prevent desiccation and also by compressing the trabeculectomy bleb for the duration of the surgery with a thin lamella of stroma dissected from the donor corneo-scleral rim. Postoperatively a very tight AC should be avoided in order to prevent progressive visual field loss. The AC should be kept at physiological intra-ocular pressure (IOP) at the end of surgery. The patient should also be monitored frequently in the postoperative period to assess the IOP (Figs. 10.6, 10.7, 10.8, and 10.9).

## 10.12 Tube Shunts

In addition to the pertinent precautions mentioned above, an additional problem in case of decompensated cornea after a glaucoma valve is often the position or length of the tube that is present within the AC. An anterior position, a mobile tube or an excessively long tube could have been the reason for the corneal decompensation in the first place, and this should be handled by trimming the tube if required, repositioning the tube more posteriorly against the iris or into the posterior chamber in a pseudophakic eye. The author's personal preference is put the tube in the posterior chamber behind the iris and in front of the anterior capsule in a pseudophakic eye (Fig. 10.12). In a phakic eye, the author prefers to do a phacoemulsification and then place the tube in the posterior chamber. Postoperative air tamponade that is often used in endothelial keratoplasties can lead to anterior capsular cataract formation and long-term steroid use can lead to posterior sub-capsular cataract formation. Having performed the phacoemulsification at the time of the PDEK therefore also avoids the risk of having to do a cataract surgery later in a grafted eye. Tube ligation in the immediate post-operative period till the graft is attached is one means of retaining air in the anterior chamber. The air-pump assisted technique also helps enhance intra-operative graft attachment.

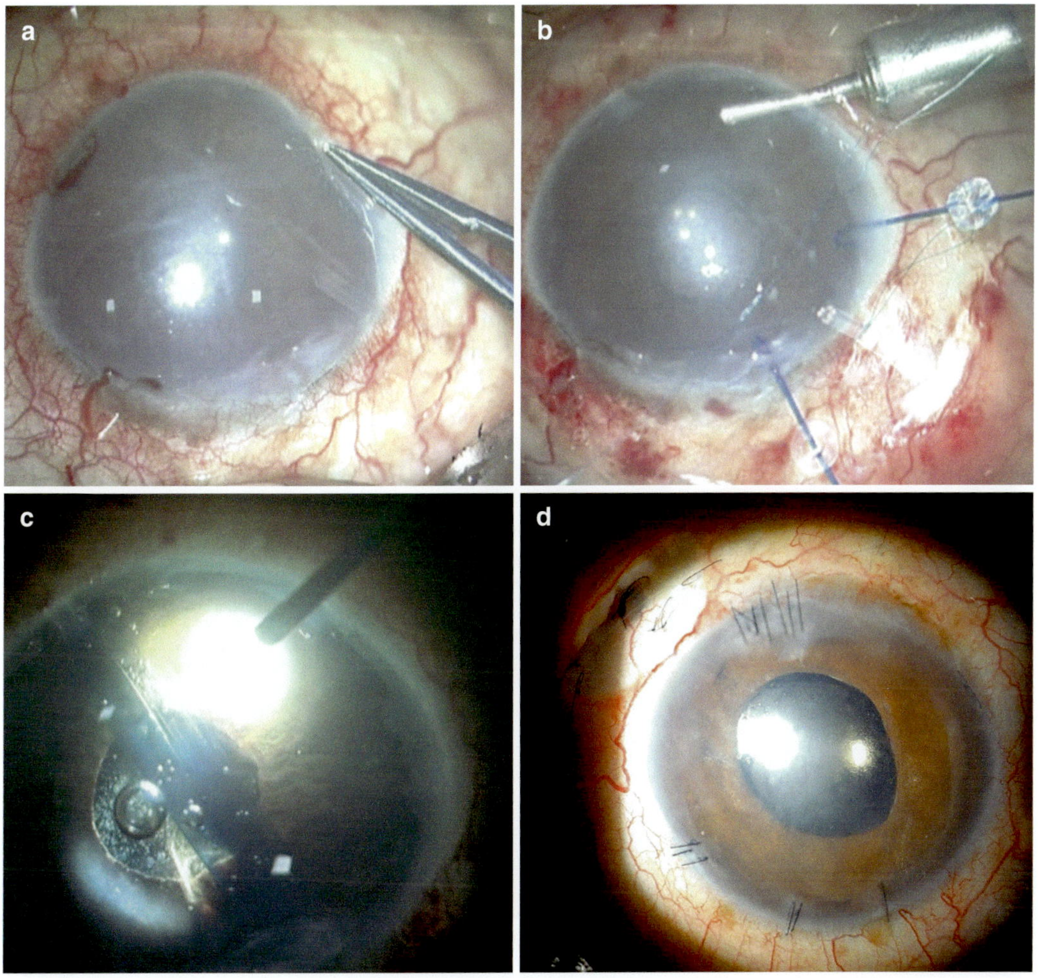


**Fig. 10.12** PDEK for corneal decompensation secondary to Ahmed glaucoma valve tube: (**a**) Tube seen in AC; (**b**) Tube removed and trimmed to reposition behind iris in front of PCIOL. Iris hooks used to improve visualization; (**c**) PDEK graft injected; E-PDEK technique used to determine graft orientation; (**d**) Postoperative clear cornea seen. Ahmed valve is seen in supero-temporal quadrant

## 10.13 Phakic PDEK

Though the author personally prefers to do a phacoemulsification combined with PDEK, depending on the surgeon's choice, PDEK may also be done in a phakic eye. Inadvertent intraoperative damage to the crystalline lens should be avoided and intracameral Miochol should therefore be used to protect it. A complete air fill as well as long-acting gas should be avoided to prevent cataractous changes from developing. Excessive steroids in the long term may also induce cataract formation and a close watch should be kept for this.

## 10.14 PDEK Combined with Phaco

The biggest challenge in performing cataract surgery in an eye requiring endothelial keratoplasty is poor visualization. Every step can become a challenge, right from construction of the rhexis to cortex aspiration. Visualization can be aided by removing the edematous epithelium. Trypan blue staining of the anterior capsule can also help to see better. A strong coaxial light from a good operating microscope aids further. In addition, an endoilluminator or light pipe used in vitreoretinal surgeries can be used to provide oblique illumination in order to see better. During nucleus emulsification or cortex aspiration, it can often be seen that as soon as the irrigation handpiece is introduced into the AC, the cornea hydrates from the pressure of the irrigating fluid making visualization worsen further. In case of very poor visualization, putting off the microscope light and working with oblique illumination from the endoilluminator can help. Even in dense cataracts, it is preferable to work closer to the endothelium as endothelial damage from phaco power is not relevant in these cases since the endothelium is planned to be stripped after phacoemulsification. Working close to the posterior capsule and risking a posterior capsular rent should be avoided as this increases the chances of poor bubble stability and thereby graft detachment. In case of a posterior capsular rent, it is advisable to perform a vitrectomy and perform an optic capture through the rhexis margin to obtain stable IOL fixation and a complete separation of the anterior chamber and vitreous cavity. At the end of phacoemulsification and IOL implantation, complete viscoelastic removal should meticulously be attained as retained viscoelastic can hinder graft adhesion (Fig. 10.13).

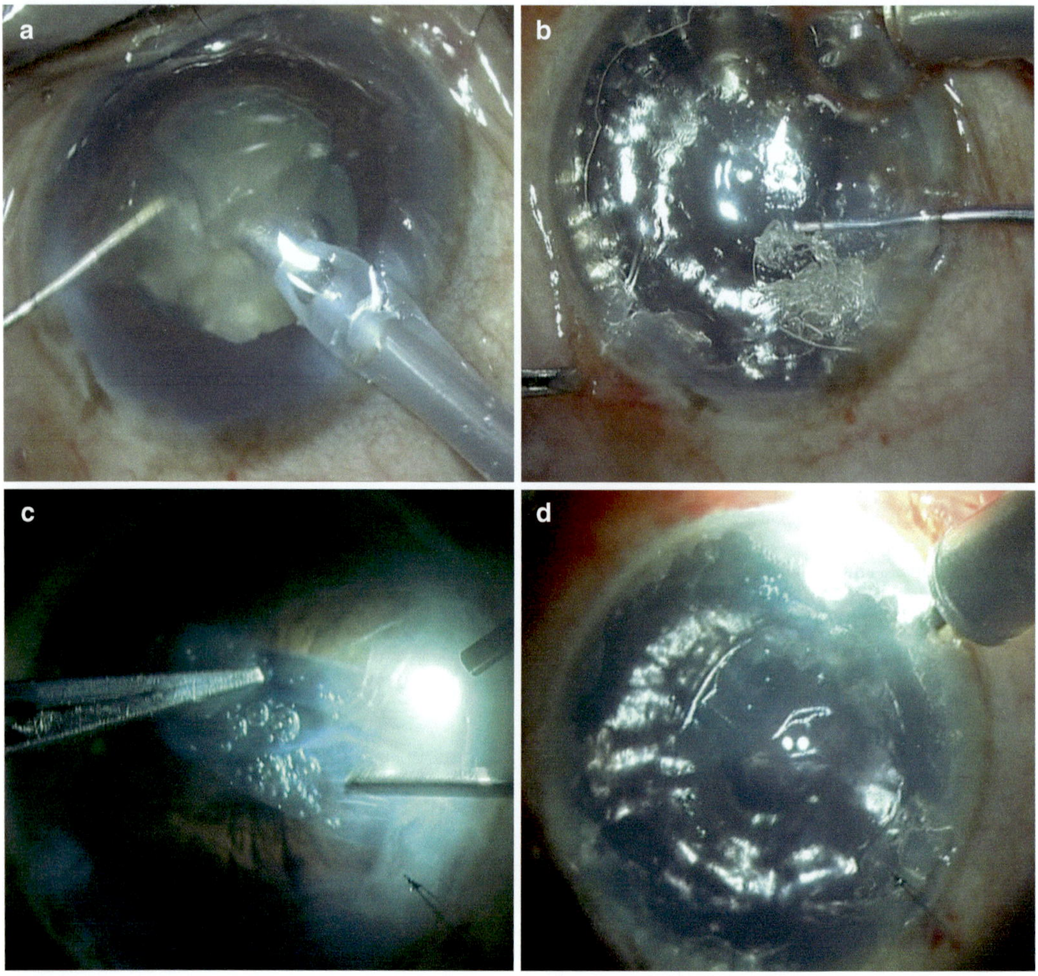


**Fig. 10.13** Fuch's dystrophy with cataract: (**a**) Phacoemulsification performed with PCIOL implantation in the bag; (**b**) Descemetorhexis done using air pump-assisted technique; (**c**) PDEK graft injected and E-PDEK technique used to determine graft orientation and to help unroll the graft; (**d**) Graft floated up, centered, and edge folds removed

Hydrophobic acrylic IOLs are preferred to be implanted in eyes requiring endothelial keratoplasty. Hydrophilic IOLs are preferably avoided if endothelial keratoplasty is planned either in the current or a future sitting in order to avoid the risk of IOL opacification that exists with hydrophilic IOLs. A thin layer of calcium phosphate accumulates beneath the anterior optical surface of hydrophilic IOLs in the central visual area (area spared by pupil/anterior capsulorhexis) following direct and prolonged contact of intracameral air or long-acting gas with the IOL. Opacification risk can also increase in these IOLs with a longer period of high pressure. This results in decreased visual acuity and contrast sensitivity and occurs irrespective of the manufacturer or exact composition of the hydrophilic lens material. Since these are sub-surface opacities, the only treatment possible is IOL exchange.

## 10.15 PDEK in Eyes with Buphthalmos

These eyes have larger diameter corneas and deeper ACs. They therefore have challenges in sizing of graft and unrolling the graft. A PDEK graft can vary in size generally from about 7 to 8.5 mm. The author has rarely got grafts as large as 9.5 mm, but this is not predictable and therefore, if the surgeon is preparing the graft himself/herself, one challenge is getting an appropriately sized graft. If the surgeon is ordering a PDEK graft from the eye bank, he can however ask for a larger sized graft. In contrast, in DMEK, larger sized grafts are possible; however, the greater manipulation that may be required in DMEK grafts as well as the inability to use very young grafts as can be used in PDEK must be considered before choosing between DMEK, PDEK, or DSAEK in these patients. Air tamponade and excessive postoperative IOP rise should be monitored for and avoided in the postoperative period to avoid progressive visual loss. Many of these patients may already have a tube or trabeculectomy and all precautions advised to be taken in such cases apply here as well.

## 10.16 ICE Syndrome

Patients with ICE syndrome have peripheral anterior synechiae (PAS) and iris defects which may need to be attended to. Bleeding while releasing PAS can lead to hyphema, blood clots interfering with free graft movement, a fibrinous atmosphere in the AC, blood in the interface and increased postoperative inflammation or IOP. The author prefers to release PAS under air using the air pump-assisted technique. The pressurized air prevents bleeding into the AC and allows rapid clotting and cessation of bleeding. In addition, pupilloplasty techniques may need to be used to repair iris defects (Fig. 10.14). Any co-existing glaucoma may also need to be attended to medically or surgically (same or two different sittings) [5]. Intra-cameral tPA and enoxaparin have been tried to decrease fibrin formation. However the risk of post-operative hyphema should be balanced against the risk of fibrin formation. More studies are required for estimating the ideal dose to balance this risk to optimal levels [16–18].

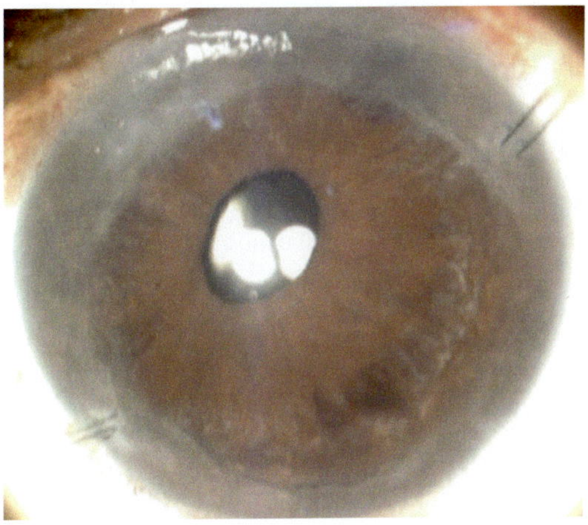

**Fig. 10.14** Postoperative slitlamp image of PDEK done in case of irido-corneal-endothelial syndrome

## 10.17 Combined Surgeries

PDEK can be combined with various surgeries such as phacoemulsification, pupilloplasty, secondary IOL implantation, glaucoma surgeries, anterior vitrectomy, and squint. Many of these cases have been discussed in the preceding sections already (Figs. 10.15, 10.16, and 10.17).

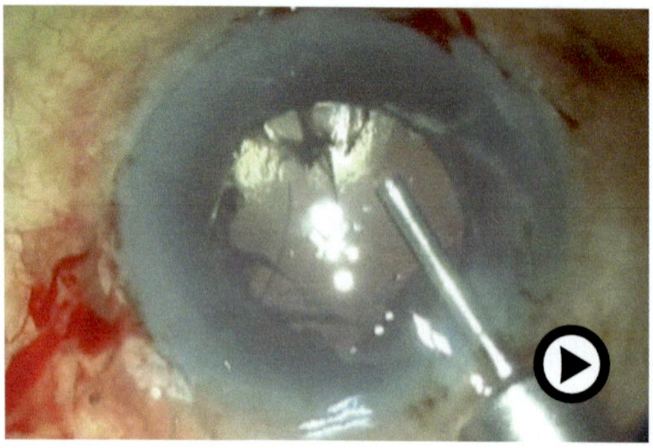

**Fig. 10.15** PDEK + Iris repair (https://doi.org/10.1007/000-dhn)

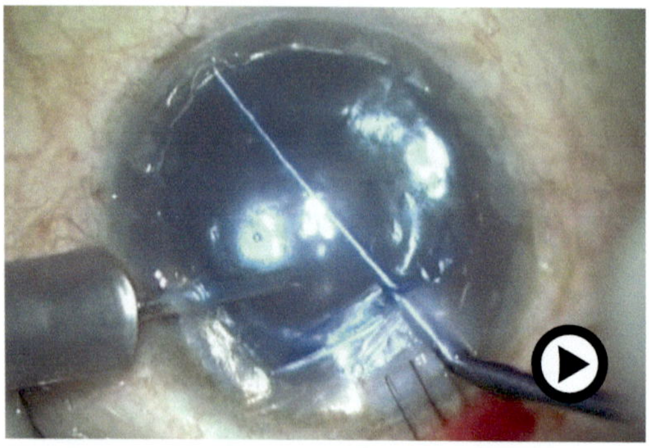

**Fig. 10.16** Phaco with PDEK and HDS (https://doi.org/10.1007/000-dhm)

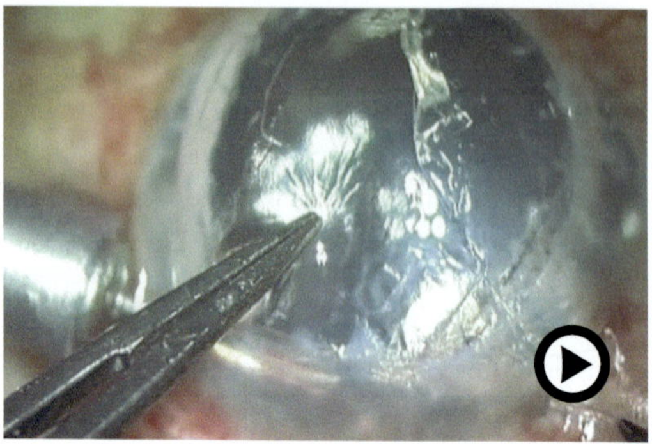

**Fig. 10.17** Phaco with PDEK on failed graft (https://doi.org/10.1007/000-dhp)

## References


1. Agarwal A, Dua HS, Narang P, Kumar DA, Agarwal A, Jacob S, Agarwal A, Gupta A. Pre-Descemet's endothelial keratoplasty (PDEK). Br J Ophthalmol. 2014;98(9):1181–5.
2. Agarwal A, Agarwal A, Narang P, Kumar DA, Jacob S. Pre-Descemet endothelial keratoplasty with infant donor corneas: a prospective analysis. Cornea. 2015;34(8):859–65.
3. Jacob S, Narasimhan S, Agarwal A, Agarwal A, A I S. Air pump-assisted graft centration, graft edge unfolding, and graft uncreasing in young donor graft pre-descemet endothelial keratoplasty. Cornea. 2017;36(8):1009–13.
4. Jacob S. Use of pressurized air infusion for pre-descemet's endothelial keratoplasty (PDEK)—The air pump assisted PDEK technique. Open Ophthalmol J. 2018;12:175–18.
5. Air pump assisted PDEK. Soosan jacob 6 2 min with audio final. https://www.youtube.com/watch?v=onK1R0DG-ow. Accessed 19 Aug 2020.
6. Jacob S, Agarwal A, et al. Endoilluminator-assisted transcorneal illumination for Descemet membrane endothelial keratoplasty: enhanced intraoperative visualization of the graft in corneal decompensation

secondary to pseudophakic bullous keratopathy. J Cataract Refract Surg. 2014;40(8):1332–6.
7. Jacob S, Agarwal A, Kumar DA. Endoilluminator-assisted Descemet membrane endothelial keratoplasty and endoilluminator-assisted pre-Descemet endothelial keratoplasty. Clin Ophthalmol. 2015;9:2123–5.
8. Native means of graft stabilization: host descemetic scaffolding and wound scaffolding to decrease the risk for graft detachment in DMEK and PDEK. J Cataract Refract Surg. 2019;45(8):1059–1063.
9. Jacob S, Agarwal A, Kumar DA, Agarwal A, Agarwal A, Satish K. Modified technique for combining DMEK with glued intrascleral haptic fixation of a posterior chamber IOL as a single-stage procedure. J Refract Surg. 2014;30(7):492–6.
10. Jacob S. PDEK and E PDEK with Glued IOL with post op Soosan Jacob 7.16 min; 2014. https://www.youtube.com/watch?v=2Od4h9OB60M. Accessed 1 Dec 2019.
11. Jacob S. Glued IOL with OCT guided PDEK Soosan Jacob 6 min; 2015. https://www.youtube.com/watch?v=QpDgFkA6fZY&list=PLOLM5nX3h_taUkT5ftFzwE_-JmGx6HeWO&index=5. Accessed 1 Dec 2019.
12. Jacob S. PDEK for PBK and pre descemetic scarring Soosan Jacob 5.2 mins with audio; 2016. https://www.youtube.com/watch?v=ikbuOyHx_wg&list=PLOLM5nX3h_taUkT5ftFzwE_-JmGx6HeWO&index=20. Accessed 1 Dec 2019.
13. Jacob S. E PDEK Glued IOL Soosan Jacob 6 min with Audio; 2014. https://www.youtube.com/watch?v=KIA7HevO8ns&list=PLOLM5nX3h_taUkT5ftFzwE_-JmGx6HeWO&index=14. Accessed 1 Dec 2019.
14. Jacob S. E PDEK with 5 yr old donor graft in failed DSAEK Soosan Jacob 5.23 min; 2015. https://www.youtube.com/watch?v=Udpqmj-c6Ng&list=PLOLM5nX3h_taUkT5ftFzwE_-JmGx6HeWO&index=2. Accessed 1 Dec 2019.
15. Jacob S. E-PDEK with phaco in failed penetrating graft Soosan Jacob 4.01 min; 2014. https://www.youtube.com/watch?v=jZpkxvNNBBE&list=PLOLM5nX3h_taUkT5ftFzwE_-JmGx6HeWO&index=13. Accessed 1 Dec 2019.
16. Mulpuri L, Ouano DP, Riaz KM, et al. Intracameral enoxaparin for Descemet membrane endothelial keratoplasty: a pilot safety study. Cornea. 2024:1–8. (Published Ahead-of-Print).
17. Dastjerdi MH. Letter Regarding: Intracameral Enoxaparin for Descemet Membrane Endothelial Keratoplasty: A Pilot Safety Study. Cornea. 2024. Epub ahead of print.
18. Osaadon P, Belfair N, Lavy I, et al. Intracameral r-tPA for the management of severe fibrinous reactions in TASS after cataract surgery. European Journal of Ophthalmology. 2022;32(1):200–4.

# Host Descemetic Scaffolding

# 11

Soosan Jacob

## 11.1 Introduction

Descemet's membrane endothelial keratoplasty (DMEK) [1–3] and pre-Descemet's membrane endothelial keratoplasty (PDEK) [4, 5] are gaining in popularity secondary to the advantages that they offer over Descemet's Stripping Automated Endothelial Keratoplasty (DSAEK). This includes better corrected and uncorrected visual acuity, less higher order aberrations, better contrast sensitivity, faster recovery, less induction of hypermetropic refractive error, and lesser immune response [6, 7].

Despite this, its uptake by corneal surgeons around the world has been slower due to various reasons—loss of the DMEK or PDEK graft during preparation; difficulty in identifying orientation within the AC, difficult maneuvering within the AC, increased risk of graft detachment, and so on [8–15]. The availability of pre-prepared, pre-marked, pre-stained, pre-loaded grafts; more refined techniques such as the endo-illuminator-assisted DMEK (described by the author) as well as other techniques for enhancing visualization and identifying graft orientation [16] as well as better described techniques for graft unrolling have made wider acceptance of these surgeries possible. However, graft detachment still accounts for a significant proportion of postoperative complications and is a greater problem following combined surgeries such as DMEK/PDEK when combined with phaco, trabeculectomy, or tube shunt and also following surgery in complex eyes such as aphakia, vitrectomized eye, eyes with absent iris, and eyes with glaucoma drainage devices [8–15]. The Jacob's air pump-assisted technique that uses pressurized air infusion facilitates various steps of PDEK as well as increases graft adherence in both DMEK and PDEK [17, 18]. The author has also described another technique called host Descemetic scaffolding that also decreases incidence of graft detachment and may be used in combined surgeries/complex eyes or even in routine cases during the learning curve [19–22]. It may be done in case of both PDEK and DMEK grafts (Fig. 11.1).

Though advantageous, this technique is not a must for every case of DMEK and PDEK. It helps as a supplementary technique but need not be an essential part of the surgical technique. The advantage it offers is scaffolding to the graft and decreased rate of graft detachment. It may there-

**Supplementary Information** The online version contains supplementary material available at https://doi.org/10.1007/978-981-97-3469-6_11. The videos can be accessed individually by clicking the DOI link in the accompanying figure caption or by scanning this link with the SN More Media App.

S. Jacob (✉)
Dr. Agarwal's Refractive and Cornea Foundation, Chennai, India

Dr. Agarwal's Eye Hospital and Eye Research Centre, Chennai, India



S. Jacob (ed.), *Mastering DMEK and PDEK*, https://doi.org/10.1007/978-981-97-3469-6_11

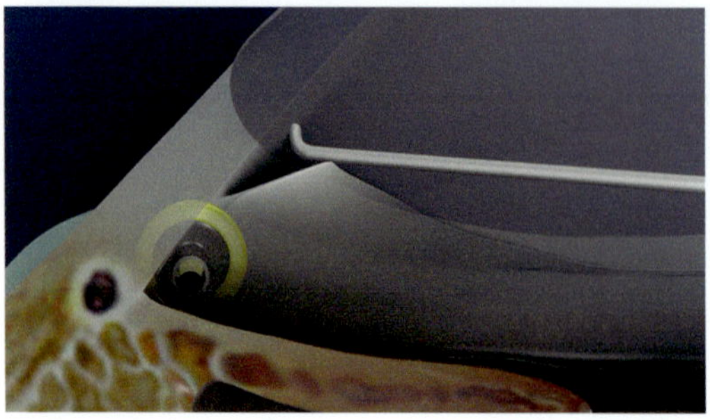

**Fig. 11.1** The host Descemetic scaffolding technique uses a reverse Sinskey hook to pull the host DM out from underneath the graft and release it to lie posterior to the graft, thereby supporting it from the underside

fore be used in complex cases depending on individual surgeon experience and choice of surgical procedures.

## 11.2 Technique

The diameter of the host Descemetorhexis is made about 0.5–1 mm smaller than the graft diameter along both sides of at least one axis. The graft is then injected into the anterior chamber (AC). It is unrolled, centered, and floated up against the host stroma. An anterior chamber maintenance (ACM) connected to pressurized air is then inserted into the AC. This can be done by connecting the ACM to the air pump present in newer phaco machines or using the fluid air exchange system present in posterior vitrectomy systems. The pressurized air holds the graft up against the stroma. During the subsequent maneuvers, it also creates space in the AC, prevents the AC from collapsing while instruments are inserted through the incision and thereby prevents graft-instrument touch and consequent graft damage. For more on the use of the air pump in thin membrane endothelial keratoplasty, see chapter on air pump-assisted TMEK.

Once the graft has been centered and floated up, it lies within the Descemetorhexis all around except along the axis where the Descemetorhexis was made smaller. In the two opposite quadrants along this axis, the graft overlaps the host Descemet's membrane from the posterior aspect. If left as such, this would increase the risk of detachment along these two quadrants. However, the host Descemetic scaffolding technique instead uses a reverse Sinskey hook to pull the host DM out from underneath the graft and release it to now lie posterior to the graft, thereby supporting it from the underside (Fig. 11.1). This is done by placing the reverse Sinskey at the edge of the overlap and pulling it out by following the outline of the graft (thereby preventing any graft touch). Once one edge is caught, the whole extent of host DM overlap can be teased out by moving the tip of the reverse Sinskey just outside the edge of the graft. Thus, the host DM scaffolding can be done successfully without touching the graft itself. Once the host DM is brought to thus lie under the graft, it acts as a scaffold holding the graft up and sandwiching it between itself and the overlying stroma. This scaffold helps prevent graft detachment in the postoperative period and is especially useful in complex cases (Figs. 11.2a–c and 11.3a–d).

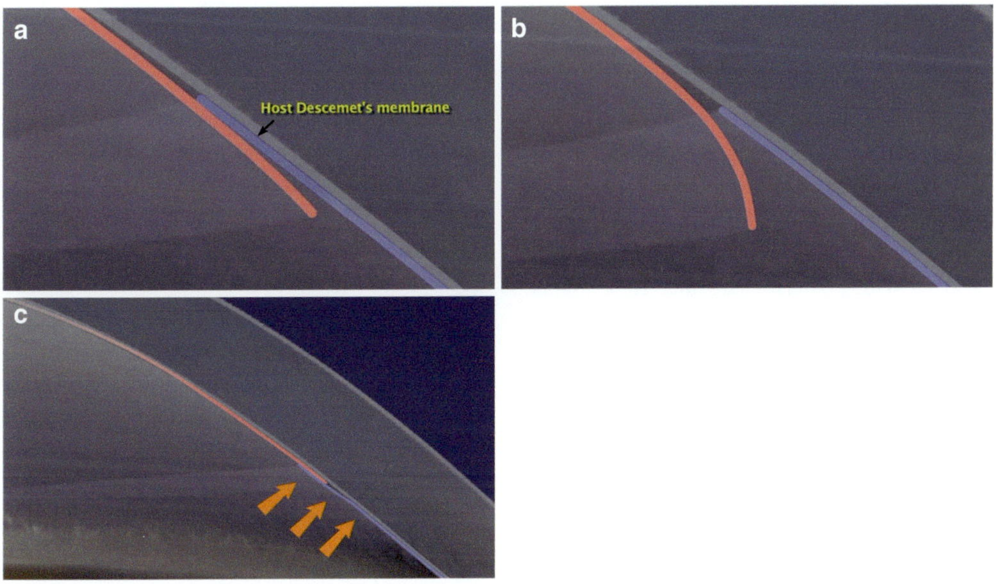


**Fig. 11.2** Relationship between rim of peripheral host Descemet's membrane (DM) and graft: (**a**, **b**) Host DM above graft predisposes to graft detachment; (**c**) Host DM below graft scaffolds graft and holds it in place

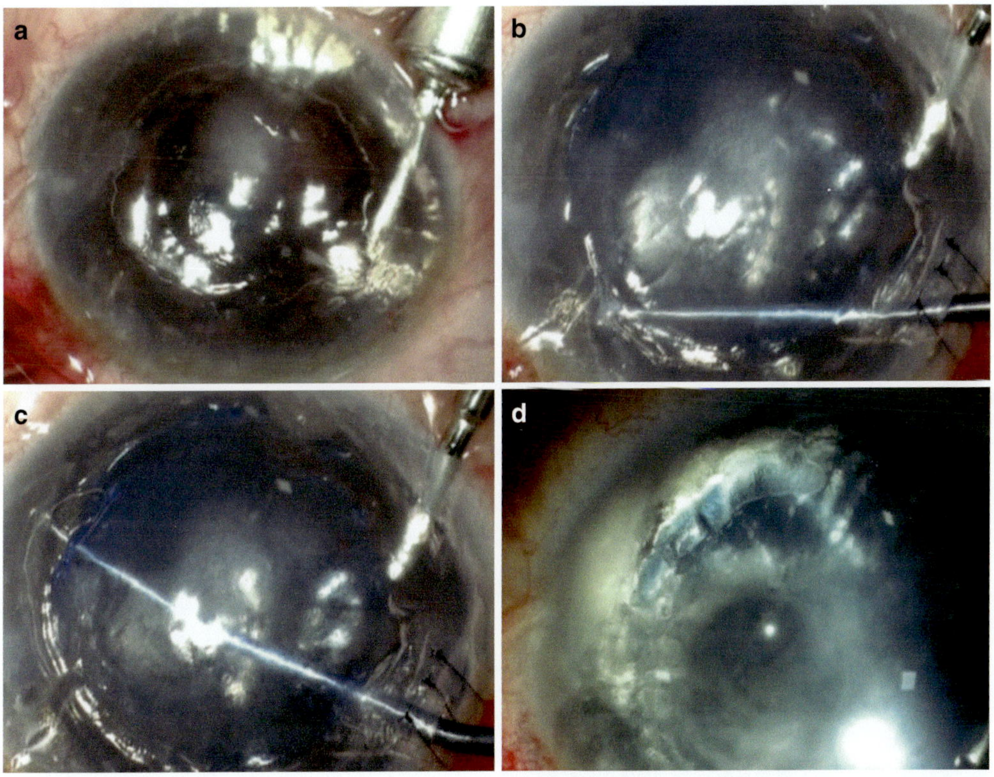


**Fig. 11.3** Host Descemetic Scaffolding: (**a**) Descemetorhexis that is slightly smaller than the size of the graft, in at least some quadrants is made; (**b**) The PDEK graft is injected, unrolled, centered, floated up, and edge folds removed. The graft lies below the Descemetorhexis in some areas; (**c**) The peripheral rim of host Descemet's membrane is teased out from between the graft and the stroma to lie beneath the graft. It thus now scaffolds the graft preventing detachment; (**d**) The overlap of the graft by the host Descemet's membrane from the posterior aspect is seen

## 11.3 Advantage

Immediately postoperatively, air or long-acting gas is used as a tamponade to provide support for the graft. However, in eyes with an incomplete iris; secondary IOL fixation in the form of intrascleral haptic fixation/sutured scleral fixated IOL/iris fixated IOL or ACIOL; vitrectomized eyes; eyes with posterior capsular rent; aphakic eyes and eyes with glaucoma drainage device or trabeculectomy—air/gas may not remain within the AC. It may either migrate posteriorly into the vitreous cavity or may escape through the glaucoma drainage tube. This results in insufficient air support for the graft in the postoperative period resulting in an increased risk of graft detachment. The host Descemetic scaffold is especially useful in such situations to give an additional layer of support for the graft in the absence of air support (Fig. 11.4a–c).

Sometimes, graft edges show a tendency to curl after surgery thereby initiating a detachment from the site. This can be prevented from happening in the quadrants of scaffolding by the host DM holding the graft firmly in place (Fig. 11.5). Host Descemetic scaffolding is also useful in combined surgeries where risk of detachment is higher.

Though host Descemetic scaffolding may be done over a larger extent of the graft, two opposite quadrants is generally enough. No edema or bullae were seen by the author over the area of scaffolding. Ideally, the host should not be stripped close to the graft edge with only a thin

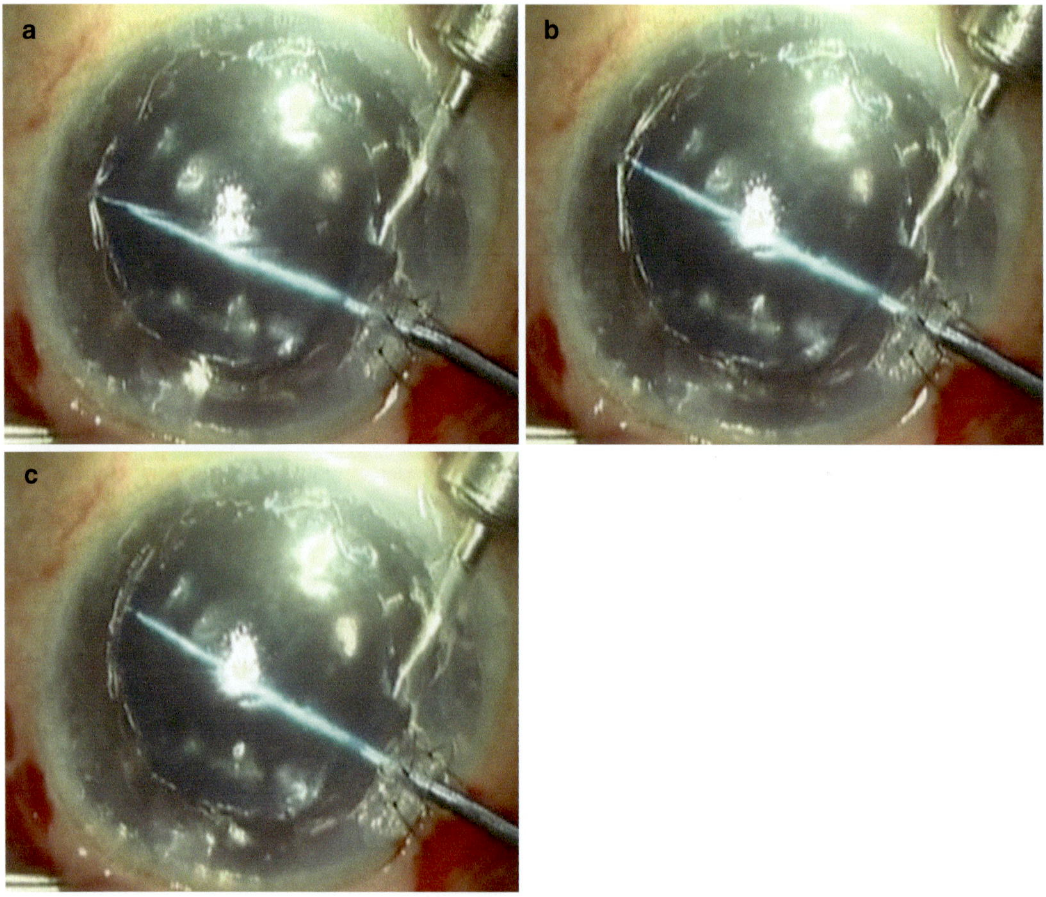


**Fig. 11.4** Host Descemetic Scaffolding: (**a**, **b**) The peripheral rim of host Descemet's membrane is teased out from above the graft to lie beneath it; (**c**) It lies below the graft thus scaffolding the graft and preventing detachment

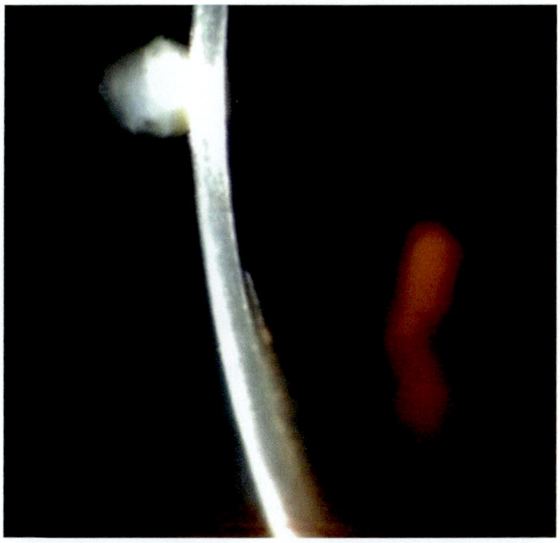

**Fig. 11.5** Slit lamp image showing host Descemetic rim in the inferior corneal periphery

rim of overlap. The host scaffolding rim should cover the graft sufficiently towards the pupil to prevent the graft from slipping out. This is especially important for inferior scaffolding where air bubble support is also less.

## 11.4 Wound Scaffolding

This technique is similar in that its aims to provide a scaffolding to the graft except that wound scaffolding is used in the incision area and host Descemetic scaffolding may be done in the opposite quadrant [19–22]. Wound scaffolding is done by sandwiching part of the peripheral edge of the graft within the wound. This is done in a similar manner to the host Descemetic scaffolding described above. After the graft has been unfolded and floated up, it is centered, peripheral edge folds unfolded and uncreased. The graft edge if overlaps the wound, can be very successfully provided a scaffolding within the wound. This is done by drawing the graft edge into the wound using a reverse Sinskey hook. It is however confined to within 50% of the width of the wound in order to prevent a wick syndrome. If it does cross an extent of 50%, it is folded back within the wound to lie within 50%. This may be used in isolation. If combined with a host Descemetic scaffolding in the opposite quadrant, the graft can get good postoperative support (Figs. 11.6a, b and 11.7a, b).

**Results**: The author has had excellent results with the host Descemetic and wound scaffolding techniques. It is easy to perform with the air pump providing continuous air infusion and preventing the anterior chamber from collapsing. Bilateral or multi-point host Descemetic scaffolding may be done as also a combination of host descemetic scaffolding and wound scaffolding (Fig. 11.8a–c). Postoperatively, the graft attaches well and the overlying cornea shows no signs of edema or bulla formation. The corneal endothelial count is as after regular PDEK or DMEK.

**Other Advantages**: It has advantages of decreasing graft detachment in complex and combined cases as well as during the learning curve. It allows the patient to get all the advantages that DMEK and PDEK offer in comparison to DSAEK (Fig. 11.9). It also avoids the use of other techniques that have been used for decreasing graft detachment such as transcorneal mattress sutures which can damage or even tear the graft and also long-acting gas which has disadvantages of a longer time to visual recovery, greater risk of IOL opacification, and delayed fitness for air travel [23, 24].

**Complications**: A Descemetorhexis larger than the graft size can prevent this procedure from being done. Attempting to perform this procedure without simultaneously also using the air pump-assisted technique can result in graft detachment and graft damage. For wound scaffolding, the graft should be within 50% of the width of the wound. Leaving the graft outside the wound after wound scaffolding can result in a wick syndrome and infection and this should be avoided. Care should be taken to verify that the host DM is under the graft throughout its extent. If the host DM is not brought out from under the graft, this can become an area with an increased risk of detachment.

**Anterior Segment OCT**: This shows the graft margin being scaffolded by the host DM. It also shows the host DM trapped within the wound in case of wound scaffolding. The margins of the

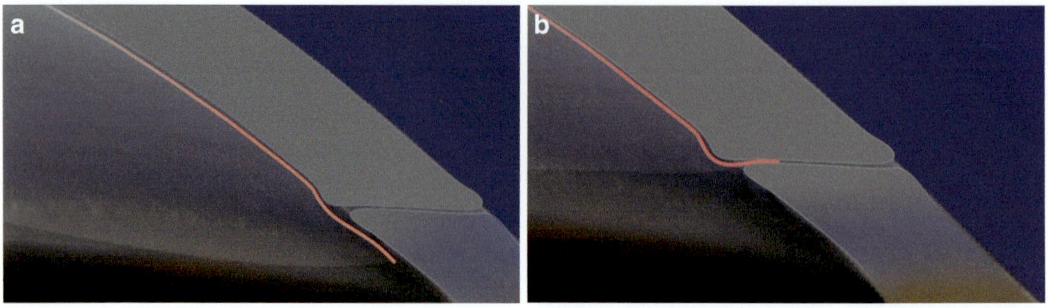


**Fig. 11.6** Wound scaffolding: (**a**) Wound scaffolding is done by sandwiching part of the peripheral edge of the graft within the wound; (**b**) If the graft edge overlaps the wound, it can be very successfully scaffolded within the wound by drawing the graft edge into the wound using a reverse Sinskey hook

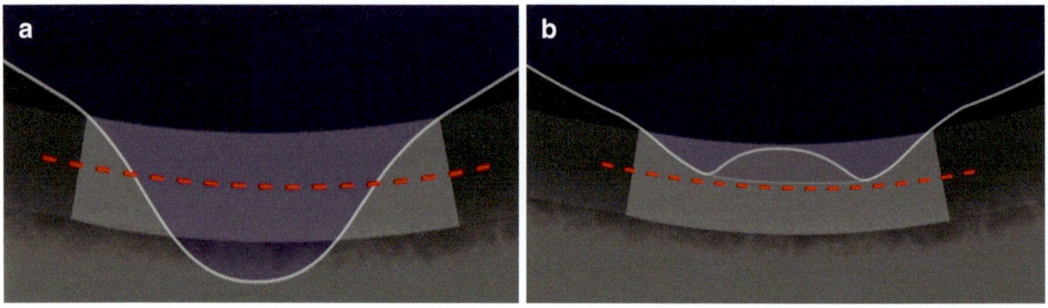


**Fig. 11.7** Wound scaffolding: (**a**) Wound scaffolding is confined to within 50% of the width of the wound in order to prevent a wick syndrome; (**b**) If it does cross an extent of 50%, it is folded back within the wound to lie within 50%

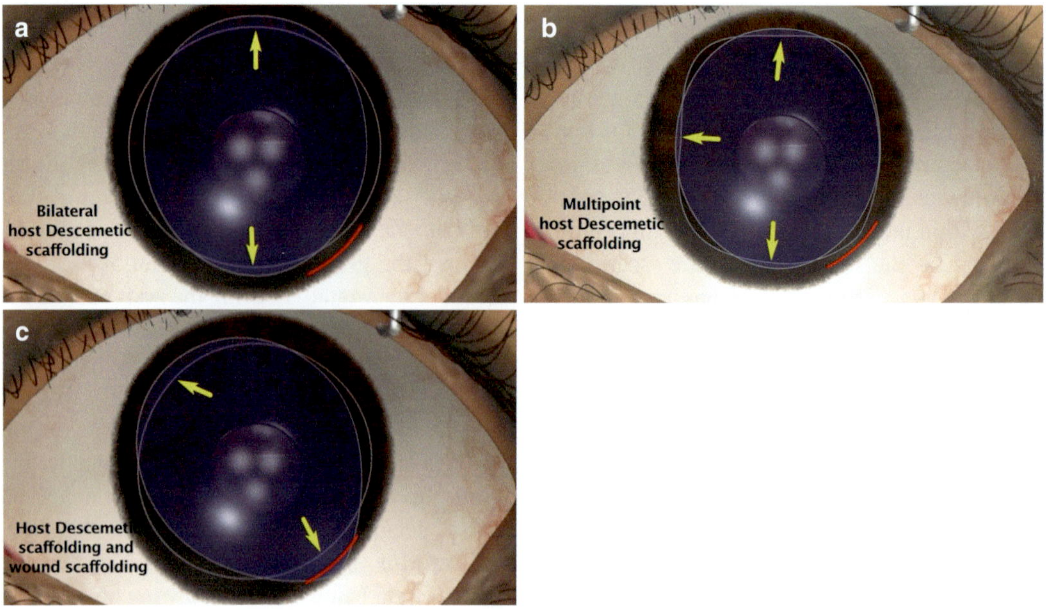


**Fig. 11.8** (**a**, **b**) Bilateral and multi-point host Descemetic scaffolding; (**c**) Combination of host Descemetic with wound scaffolding

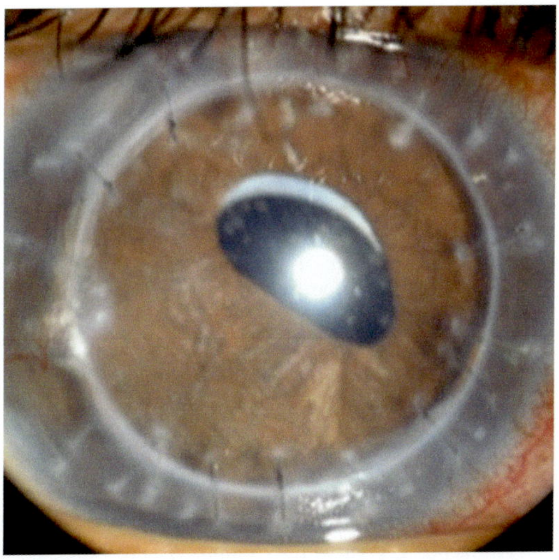

**Fig. 11.9** Postoperative slit lamp image showing PDEK for a failed penetrating keratoplasty using host Descemetic scaffolding technique. A well-attached graft and clear cornea are seen

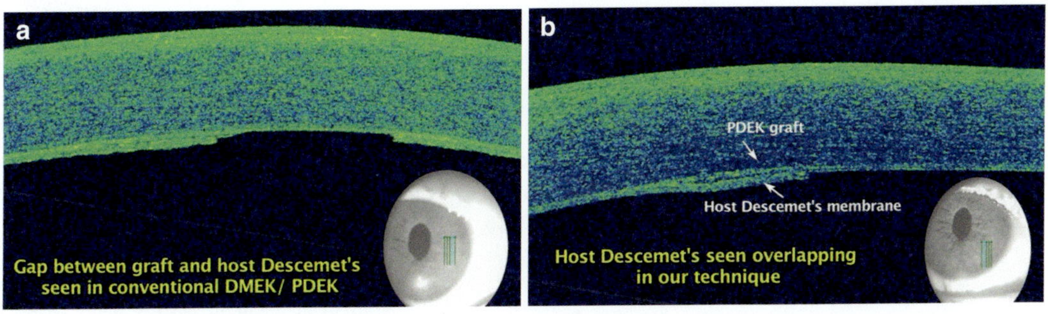


**Fig. 11.10** ASOCT imaging: (**a**) Conventional PDEK is seen with a gap between the graft and the host peripheral rim; (**b**) The peripheral rim of host's Descemet's membrane is seen scaffolding the PDEK graft

host DM may erroneously be interpreted as a graft detachment and care should be given to the site of OCT, direction of the scan as well as the direction of the detached margin in order to differentiate an edge of the host DM from a detached graft (Fig. 11.10a, b).

## 11.5 Conclusion

The host Descemetic and wound scaffolding techniques in concert with the air pump-assisted technique allows good graft adherence and prevents graft detachment postoperatively in both PDEK and DMEK. This may be employed by advanced surgeons, especially in complex cases. The rim of scaffolding should be sufficiently broad and not too thin (Fig. 11.11).

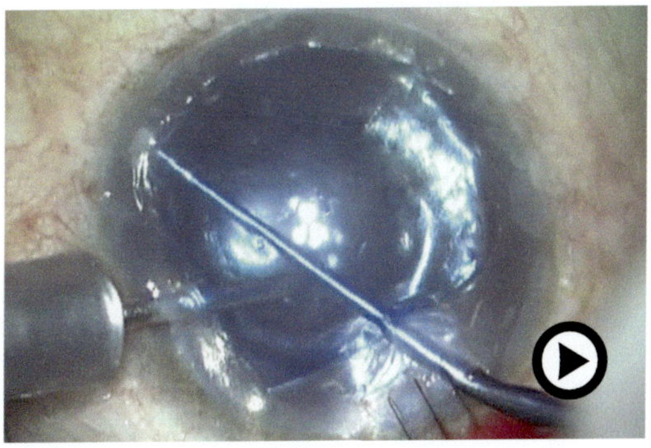

**Fig. 11.11** Host descemetic scaffolding (https://doi.org/10.1007/000-dhq)

## References


1. Melles GR, Ong TS, Ververs B, van der Wees J. Descemet membrane endothelial keratoplasty (DMEK). Cornea. 2006;25:987–90.
2. Price MO, Price FW Jr. Descemet's membrane endothelial keratoplasty surgery: update on the evidence and hurdles to acceptance. Curr Opin Ophthalmol. 2013;24(4):329–35.
3. Kruse FE, Schrehardt US, Tourtas T. Optimizing outcomes with Descemet's membrane endothelial keratoplasty. Curr Opin Ophthalmol. 2014;25(4):325–34.
4. Dua HS, Faraj LA, Said DG, Gray T, Lowe J. Human corneal anatomy redefined: a novel pre-Descemet's layer (Dua's layer). Ophthalmology. 2013;120(9):1778–85.
5. Agarwal A, Dua HS, Narang P, Kumar DA, Agarwal A, Jacob S, Agarwal A, Gupta A. Pre-Descemet's endothelial keratoplasty (PDEK). Br J Ophthalmol. 2014;98(9):1181–5.
6. Maier AK, Gundlach E, Gonnermann J, Klamann MK, Bertelmann E, Rieck PW, Joussen AM, Torun N. Retrospective contralateral study comparing Descemet membrane endothelial keratoplasty with Descemet stripping automated endothelial keratoplasty. Eye (Lond). 2015;29(3):327–32. https://doi.org/10.1038/eye.2014.280. Epub 2014 Nov 21.
7. Goldich Y, Artornsombidth P, Avni-Zauberman N, Perez M, Ulate R, Elbaz U, Rootman DS. Fellow eye comparison of corneal thickness and curvature in descemet membrane endothelial keratoplasty and descemet stripping automated endothelial keratoplasty. Cornea. 2014;33(6):547–50.
8. Liarakos VS, Monnereau C, Dapena I, Melles GRJ. Learning curve of Descemet membrane endothelial keratoplasty (DMEK) worldwide—Multicenter trial on DMEK. Panoptis. 2013;25(2):68–75. http://www.panoptisjournal.gr/images/Panoptis/pdfs/issue2/LEARNING_CURVE.pdf. Accessed 27 Dec 2018.
9. Feng MT, Price MO, Miller JM, Price FW. Air reinjection and endothelial cell density in Descemet membrane endothelial keratoplasty: five-year follow-up. J Cataract Refract Surg. 2014;40:1116–21.
10. Rodríguez-Calvo-De-Mora M, Quilendrino R, Ham L, et al. Clinical outcome of 500 consecutive cases undergoing Descemet's membrane endothelial keratoplasty. Ophthalmology. 2015;122:464–70.
11. Melles GRJ, Ong TS, Ververs B, van der Wees J. Preliminary clinical results of Descemet membrane endothelial keratoplasty. Am J Ophthalmol. 2008;145(2):222–7.
12. Guerra FP, Anshu A, Price MO, Price FW. Endothelial keratoplasty: fellow eyes comparison of Descemet stripping automated endothelial keratoplasty and descemet membrane endothelial keratoplasty. Cornea. 2011;30:1382–6.
13. Guerra FP, Anshu A, Price MO, Giebel AW, Price FW. Descemet's membrane endothelial keratoplasty: prospective study of 1-year visual outcomes, graft survival, and endothelial cell loss. Ophthalmology. 2011;118:2368–73.
14. Price MO, Giebel AW, Fairchild KM, Price FW. Descemet's membrane endothelial keratoplasty. Prospective multicenter study of visual and refractive outcomes and endothelial survival. Ophthalmology. 2009;116:2361–8.
15. Siggel R, Adler W, Stanzel TP, et al. Bilateral descemet membrane endothelial keratoplasty. Cornea. 2016;35:772–7.
16. Jacob S, Agarwal A, Agarwal A, Narasimhan S, Kumar DA, Sivagnanam S. Endoilluminator-assisted transcorneal illumination for Descemet membrane endothelial keratoplasty: enhanced intraoperative visualization of the graft in corneal decompensation secondary to pseudophakic bullous keratopathy. J Cataract Refract Surg. 2014;40(8):1332–6.
17. Jacob S. Use of pressurized air infusion for pre-descemet's endothelial keratoplasty (PDEK)—The air pump assisted PDEK technique. Open Ophthalmol J. 2018;12:175–80.
18. Jacob S, Narasimhan S, Agarwal A, Agarwal A, A I S. Air pump-assisted graft centration, graft edge unfolding, and graft uncreasing in young donor graft pre-Descemet endothelial keratoplasty. Cornea. 2017;36(8):1009–13.
19. Jacob S, Agarwal A, Agarwal A, Agarwal A, et al. Native means of graft stabilization: host descemetic scaffolding and wound scaffolding to decrease the risk for graft detachment in DMEK and PDEK. J Cataract Refract Surg. 2019;45(8):1059–63.
20. Jacob S. Host descemetic scaffold for pre-descemet and descemet membrane endothelial keratoplasty. Presented at the ASCRS_ASOA Annual Meeting, Washington, DC, USA, April 2018.
21. Jacob S. 'Host descemetic scaffolding' technique preserves thin grafts [video]. Ocular Surgery News; 2018. https://www.healio.com/ophthalmology/cornea-external-disease/news/online/%7B9703e028-dce3-4608-9f54-3de9f43a74e1%7D/video-host-descemetic-scaffolding-technique-preserves-thin-grafts. Accessed 29 Apr 2019.
22. Jacob S. Host descemetic scaffolding Soosan Jacob with audio 2 min. https://www.youtube.com/watch?vZ_zHqdKyWYPY. Accessed 29 Apr 2019.
23. Rickmann A, Szurman P, Jung S, Boden KT, Wahl S, Haus A, Boden K, Januschowski K. Impact of 10% SF6 gas compared to 100% air tamponade in Descemet's membrane endothelial keratoplasty. Curr Eye Res. 2018;43(4):482–6.
24. von Marchtaler PV, Weller JM, Kruse FE, Tourtas T. Air versus sulfur hexafluoride gas tamponade in descemet membrane endothelial keratoplasty: a fellow eye comparison. Cornea. 2018;37(1):15–9.

# 12 Complications in DMEK: Prevention and Management

Mohamed Gamal Elghobaier, Marianne O. Price, and Francis W. Price

## 12.1 Introduction

Descemet membrane endothelial keratoplasty (DMEK) is considered the best surgical treatment for endothelial dystrophy and pseudophakic bullous keratopathy (PBK). The diseased host corneal endothelium and Descemet membrane is replaced with corresponding healthy donor tissue through a small incision. DMEK provides better visual and refractive outcomes, faster recovery, and lower risk of immunologic rejection than penetrating keratoplasty (PK) or earlier iterations of endothelial keratoplasty (EK). However, as with any other surgical procedure, complications may occur. Careful case selection and good training can minimize DMEK complications.

**Supplementary Information** The online version contains supplementary material available at https://doi.org/10.1007/978-981-97-3469-6_12. The videos can be accessed individually by clicking the DOI link in the accompanying figure caption or by scanning this link with the SN More Media App.

M. G. Elghobaier · M. O. Price · F. W. Price (✉)
Price Vision Group, Indianapolis, IN, USA
e-mail: marianneprice@cornea.org; francisprice@pricevisiongroup.net

## 12.2 Complications of Donor Tissue Preparation (Video 12.1)

### 12.2.1 Tissue Damage

While isolating the donor endothelium and Descemet membrane, the tissue could be torn or experience endothelial cell loss because of excessive manipulation [1]. Donor factors are important, e.g. age, cause of death, death to preservation time, and previous eye surgery or trauma (Fig. 12.1). Some eye banks utilize a donor risk rating scale that considers diabetes severity and duration [2].

A direct peeling method, such as the Submerged Cornea Using Backgrounds Away (SCUBA) method, is the most widely used method of DMEK graft preparation because it preserves the graft from dryness and decreases the

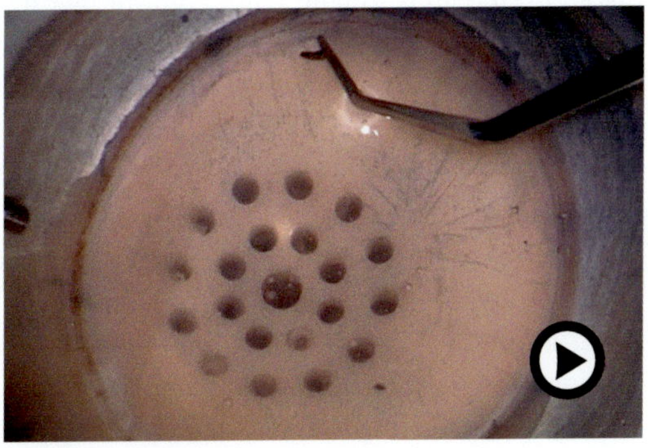

**Video 12.1** Tissue damage (https://doi.org/10.1007/000-dht)


S. Jacob (ed.), *Mastering DMEK and PDEK*, https://doi.org/10.1007/978-981-97-3469-6_12

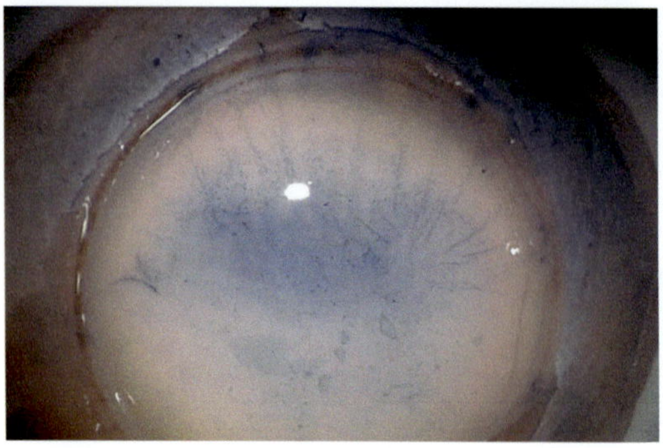

**Fig. 12.1** Radial stress marks due to stress exerted when collecting the donor tissue while the multiple dots are due to cell loss resulting from long death to preservation time

surface tension while detaching it from the stroma [3, 4]. We have described the "smile configuration" which indicates tensile stress and predicts horse shoe tear formation during graft lifting. To solve this problem, the pull point should be switched to another point with less tension [4].

## 12.2.2 Irregular Graft Thickness

SCUBA produces a uniform graft thickness [5] while pneumatic dissection could end up with irregular graft thickness because of inclusion of some pre Descemetic layer or deep stroma or a combination of type 1 and 2 bubbles.

## 12.2.3 Wrong Stamping

Some surgeons prefer to have an orientation mark placed on the graft to help them confirm that the endothelium is facing the anterior chamber after the donor tissue is uncurled in the recipient anterior chamber. An orientation stamp usually takes the shape of an inverted F or S (Fig. 12.2). Both are associated with minimal endothelial cell loss. A human error could happen if a Sinskey hook end is used to stamp a straight F or S letter (instead of being inverted). To prevent this, stamping should be done only by using a stamping instrument. Wrong stamping might result in implanting the graft in a wrong orientation with subsequent early graft failure [1, 6]. A picture of the donor tissue from the endothelial side is included in the donor box and should be reviewed to make sure of the stamp shape.

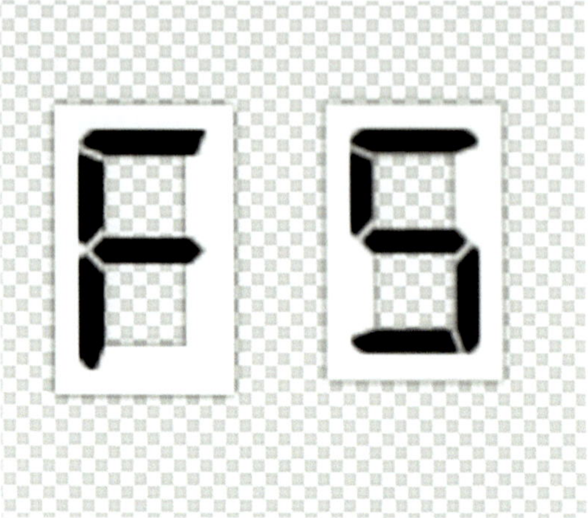

**Fig. 12.2** A comparison between the digital F and S showing that the S has a larger footprint (F is formed by 4 digital units while S is formed by 5 digital units). This is applicable to the S and F stamps of the same size

## 12.2.4 Tissue Loss

Lamellar keratoplasty makes it possible to use the same corneoscleral button to save vision in multiple patients. Punching out the anterior corneal lamella with a 2–3 mm trephine to stamp the DMEK graft sacrifices the anterior lamella. In our practice, we don't stamp the DMEK graft in order to decrease tissue manipulation.

## 12.2.5 Improper Graft Trephination

The most common difficulty with trephination is pushing too hard and causing a full-thickness punch. With PK we are used to pushing hard to make sure we get a complete trephination, whereas with EK, we prefer to just go a little past the Descemet membrane. Small grafts include fewer healthy donor endothelial cells, and we try to avoid grafts less than 7.5 mm in diameter. Large grafts can increase the difficulty of intraoperative manipulation, but can be helpful in eyes where the anterior chamber (AC) will not shallow, such as post vitrectomy or with large corneal diameters [1, 5].

### 12.2.6 Poor Graft Staining

Trypan blue 0.06% (VisionBlue, DORC International, Netherlands) is found to be safe and efficient in staining the DMEK graft. Insufficient staining will result in poor visualization particularly if operating on a hazy cornea [7].

Preloaded DMEK grafts should be stained longer when prepared for shipping overseas. Staining time of the operating room (OR) prepared grafts is usually 60–90 s, while preloaded eye bank grafts should be stained for 2–5 min.

Cost is sometimes a consideration with using a stain, but significant complications may result when non-commercialized stains or non-FDA-approved stains are used, primarily when the wrong stain is actually used like gentian violet.

## 12.3 Problems Related to Tissue Preservatives and Storage

Optisol GS (Bausch & Lomb, Irvine, CA) is the most widely used cold storage solution in the USA [8] although some newer preservatives such as Eusol and Kerasave (Alchimia, Italy) have become available [8, 9]. Using outdated preservatives or preserving tissues above the recommended temperature will lead to tissue damage (Fig. 12.3).

Eye banks have to ship tissues in large containers to utilize more wet ice. Airline delays and mishandling containers should be taken into consideration. Death to surgery time for tissues transported within the USA is usually less than 6 days while it is 8–11 days for tissues shipped overseas. The advantage of using ice is that when ice and water are combined, they produce a constant temperature of 4 °C. If exposed to the warmer environment, the ice melts cooling the container. If exposed to a colder environment, the water freezes warming the container.

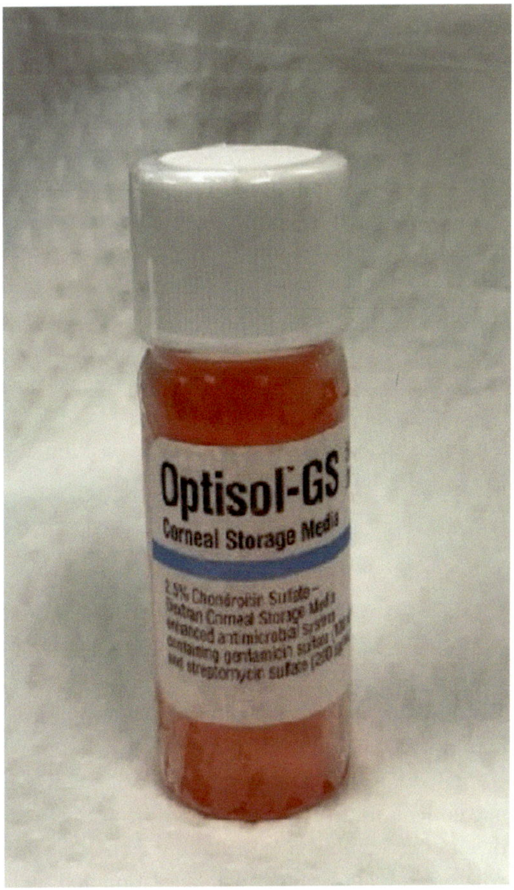


**Fig. 12.3** The most commonly used tissue preservatives in the USA is Optisol GS

## 12.4 Intraoperative Complications

### 12.4.1 Complications Related to Surgical Steps Prior to Graft Insertion

#### 12.4.1.1 Anesthesia-Related Complications

General anesthesia is not preferred because of possible risk of serious complications which might end in death. In our practice, we prefer topical anesthesia with IV sedation as injections with orbital infiltration can result in serious complications such as retrobulbar hemorrhage, optic nerve damage, brainstem anesthesia, or ocular perforation. Subconjunctival anesthesia is usually insufficient while subtenon infiltration is technically more difficult and both could result in ocular perforation or subconjunctival hemorrhage and overall swelling of the conjunctiva.

We use a combination of topical and intracameral 1% lidocaine with topical lidocaine (either 2% with epinephrine or 4% plain) anesthesia and intravenous sedation with monitoring of vital signs. We don't usually recommend intracameral anesthetics for vitrectomized eyes as they might reach the retina and optic nerve making it impossible for the patient to fixate on the microscope light or for the surgeon to determine if the IOP is too high at the end of the case by asking the patient if they can see the light of the microscope.

### 12.4.2 Complications Related to Scleral Retraction Sutures

We start surgery by placing superior and inferior partial thickness scleral bridle sutures. Potential complications include taking a deep bite with the needle leading to scleral perforation, retinal tear or vitreous hemorrhage, or taking a shallow bite which results in conjunctival laceration and ineffective eye stabilization. One needs to carefully avoid vessels to avoid subconjunctival bleeding (Fig. 12.4). The sutures are essentially not only fixating the eye, but allow moving the eye in different directions while the graft is being positioned.

### 12.4.3 Complications Related to Surgical Incisions

Although a scleral tunnel incision is less astigmatic and self-sealing, it is technically more difficult than a corneal incision and usually requires cauterization. Button holing could happen if the tunnel is too shallow or premature entry if the tunnel is too deep. It is more difficult to perform phacoemulsification through a scleral tunnel in combined cases. Other potential problems include iris prolapse, iris trauma, or even iridodialysis.

A corneal incision is easier and quicker and temporal placement is preferred because it causes less surgically induced astigmatism. A corneal incision has to be sutured immediately after graft implantation to prevent graft escape. Corneal sutures can be associated with astigmatism, infection and foreign body sensation, and can be removed after 1–2 weeks.

## 12.5 Complications Related to Host DM Scoring and Removal

Residual DM tags work as a mechanical barrier against graft attachment and can be removed by bimanual I/A [7]. Deep scoring may result in stromal scratches which could impair graft attachment and allow fluid ingress into the interface. Any disrupted posterior

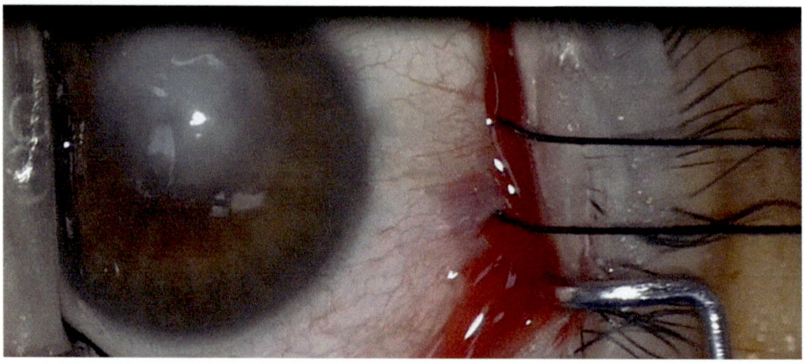

**Fig. 12.4** Conjunctival laceration and subconjunctival hemorrhage secondary to scleral retraction sutures

stromal fibers should be amputated close to the stroma using 23G intraocular scissors. DM in Fuchs patients is easier to strip in comparison with PBK particularly for young patients. In all cases, trypan blue stains loose areas of DM and stroma.

### 12.5.1 Poor Visualization

Visualization is more challenging in patients with dark irides, and dense arcus is particularly a problem when performing the lower iridotomy. Corneal edema is also challenging while extensive stromal scarring is an indication for penetrating keratoplasty (PK) rather than DMEK. Intraoperative hyphema should be well managed because it makes direct visualization difficult and impairs image quality of intraoperative OCT. Intraoperative bleeding can be managed with irrigation, raising the IOP temporarily, localization with either air or viscoelastic, and just waiting for the bleeding to stop while using the above adjunctive measures.

For better visualization, we advise use of trypan blue to densely stain the donor or to highlight the stromal bed and DM tags; using an intraoperative OCT (Fig. 12.5), hand held slit lamp or endoilluminator to confirm orientation [10]; and finally debridement of epithelium. However, we prefer to not debride the epithelium until the donor is in the anterior chamber to minimize the risk of introducing recipient epithelium into the anterior chamber.

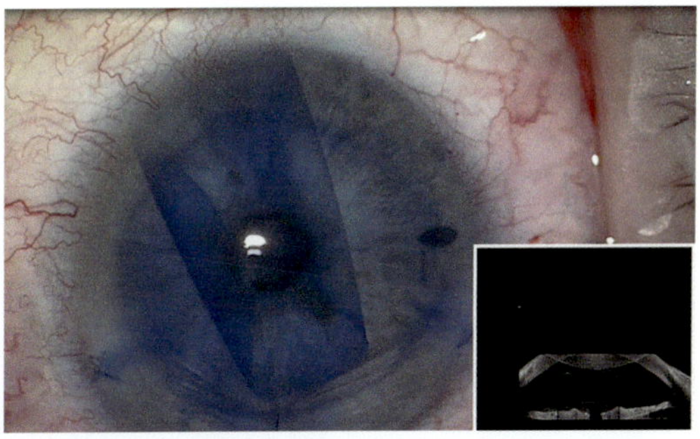

**Fig. 12.5** Intraoperative OCT (iOCT) in the right bottom part of the screen showing the correct graft orientation

When DMEK is combined with phacoemulsification, a capsulorhexis of 5–5.5 mm may be preferred to minimize forward displacement of the IOL during graft manipulation and to minimize IOL touch to the graft [5].

### 12.5.2 Complications Related to the Donor Graft

#### 12.5.2.1 Donor Graft Damage

The donor tissue can be damaged if handled with inappropriate instruments or poor technique. Graft loading into the injector is best done using a no-touch technique. An anterior chamber IOL can traumatize the graft, and it is preferable to exchange it for a posterior chamber IOL with sulcus, iris, or scleral fixation.

#### 12.5.2.2 Donor Graft Loss

The graft can be ejected from the eye just after injection if the AC pressure exceeds ambient pressure (Fig. 12.6). Shallowing of the AC before removing the injector and removing it slowly helps keep the graft in the AC. Injecting the graft off axis in relation to the main incision helps trap it in the AC.

#### 12.5.2.3 Graft Decentration

The graft should be attached centrally or slightly superiorly because the air/gas bubble that promotes graft attachment moves superiorly when the patient is in an erect position. For eyes left phakic, decentering the graft nasally allows more room for a future temporal incision with cataract surgery.

## 12.6 Difficult Unscrolling and Unfolding (Video 12.2)

Different techniques have been suggested according to the graft conformation inside the eye [11].

Delivering DMEK tissue in a trifold configuration with the endothelium inward has also been suggested to reduce surgical trauma to donor endothelial cells and facilitate unfold-

**Fig. 12.6** Partial expulsion of the DMEK graft after implantation in the AC. (**b**) Pulling the graft in using microforceps (**a**)

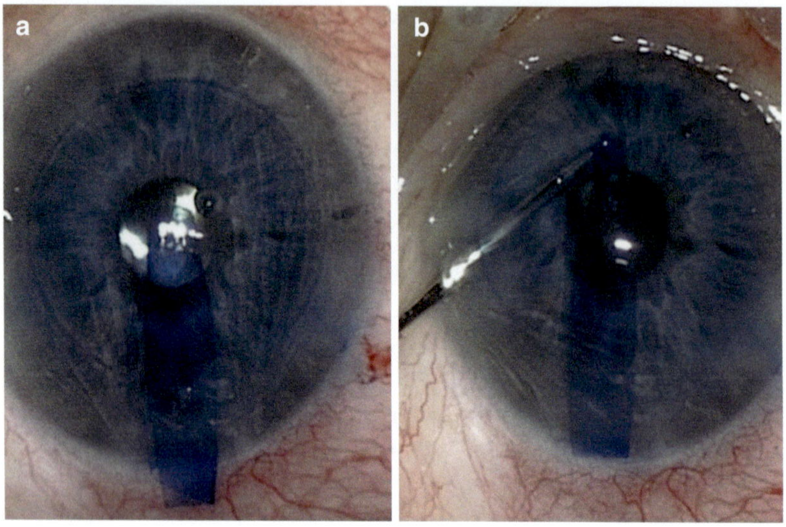

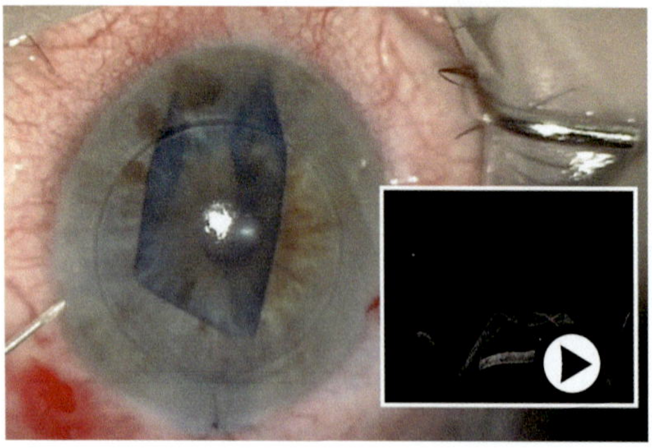

**Video 12.2** Difficult unfolding of DMEK graft (https://doi.org/10.1007/000-dhs)

ing especially using a pull in method so the graft can be held in position while it unfolds [12]. Many surgeons prefer to use grafts from 60- to 70-year-old donors as grafts from younger donors are more difficult to uncurl. If younger donors are used, often a technique of AC shallowing with compression of the donor between the cornea and iris is used to unfold.

A more recent method is Hansen's incisions in which two small incisions are made in the periphery to facilitate an endothelium out graft to curl with a three-sided configuration like a colonial hat (Personal communication Mark Hansen).

## 12.7 Upside Down Graft Implantation

This will lead to graft primary failure and/or graft dislocation (Fig. 12.7). An asymmetric marking or a stamp [13] could be placed on the DM side to aid in determining graft orientation. We prefer to use intraoperative OCT or a hand held slit beam to identify graft orientation [14]. One can also use a cannula to identify whether the scroll of the graft is directed above or below the cannula (Moutsouris sign) [15]. but in our experience, this is difficult in eyes with much edema or poor views through the cornea.

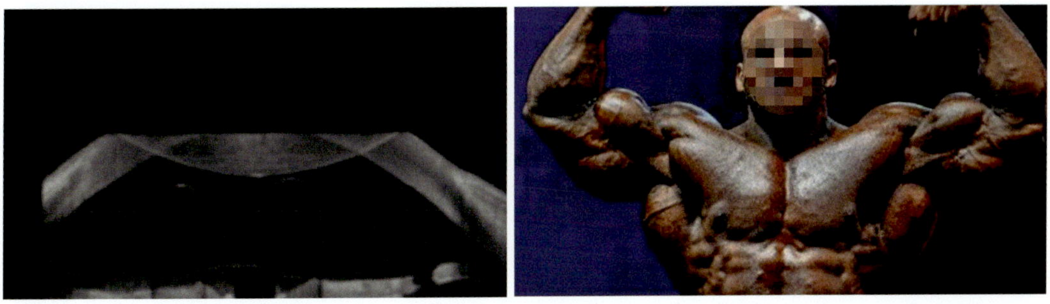

**Fig. 12.7** If you forget the correct graft orientation, remember this body builder's flexed arms (front double biceps pose)

## 12.8 Anterior Segment Complications

### 12.8.1 Hyphema (Video 12.3)

The most common cause of hyphema is performing a peripheral iridectomy (PI). Other causes could include iatrogenic iris trauma especially when operating on a shallow AC, creating a scleral tunnel, IOL explantation or exchange, and spontaneous hyphema (Fig. 12.8 and Video 12.3).

An inferior PI is an important step in DMEK surgery because it reduces the risk for pupillary block glaucoma [5]. Performing the PI in the far periphery places it close to the major vessels of the circulus iridis major increasing the chance of hyphema or causing a localized iridodialysis, while performing it in the mid periphery of the iris will delay clearing of the air tamponade covering the PI and increase the risk of postoperative pupillary block.

We found that the risk of hyphema secondary to PI was not significantly associated with preoperative use of anticoagulants or patient age [16]. The risk of hyphema was higher when DMEK was combined with cataract extraction and IOL implantation. The occurrence of intraoperative hyphema was not associated with poorer postoperative visual acuity or increased endothelial cell loss.

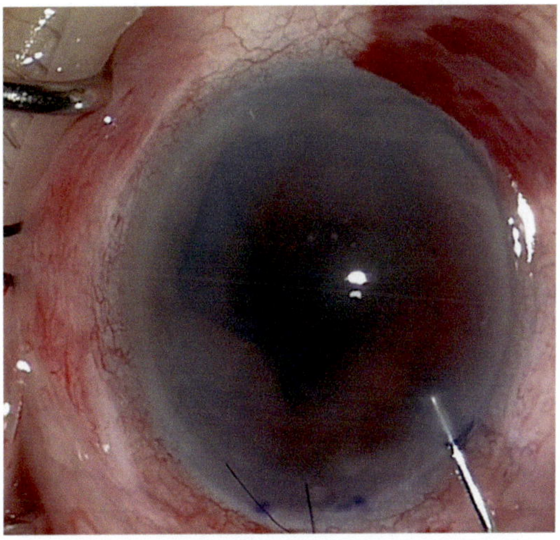

**Fig. 12.8** Intraoperative hyphema; both blood and the graft are inside the eye

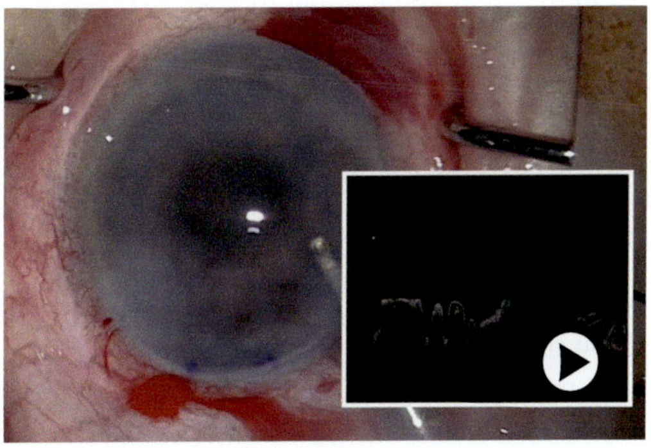

**Video 12.3** Intraoperative hyphema (https://doi.org/10.1007/000-dhr)

The PI could be performed preoperatively using Nd:Yag laser or intraoperatively [17]. Laser PI has its own complications such as postoperative IOP spike, uveitis, hyphema, focal lens opacity, and diplopia.

## 12.9 IOL Subluxation or Decentration

Air tamponade can be complicated with IOL decentration or dislocation either in the AC or in the vitreous cavity. Zonular dialysis due to ocular trauma, pseudoexfoliation, previous ocular surgery, or systemic syndromes, for example, Marfan syndrome is a strong predisposing factor. If zonular dialysis is suspected, bag support, for example, by capsular tension ring (CTR) should be performed before DMEK, with or without reducing the size of the air bubble.

## 12.10 Anterior Chamber Depth/Pressure Fluctuation

Sudden shallowing of the AC can cause graft ejection out of the eye with risk of graft damage or intraocular infection. Sudden deepening of the AC, as when hydrating the wounds at the end of surgery, can decrease air bubble size and detach the graft. Fluctuation in the AC pressure can predispose to rebleeding from a PI.

## 12.11 Collateral Damage to the Eye Structures

Aggressive tapping on the ocular surface could result in corneal abrasion, zonular dialysis, cataract, and ocular bleeding. Often the epithelium has an associated anterior membrane dystrophy or sub-epithelial scar with Fuchs dystrophy or long-standing decompensation.

## 12.12 Intraoperative Floppy Iris Syndrome (IFIS)

Most cases of IFIS are seen when combined with phacoemulsification because of longer surgery time and possible iris manipulation. Iris prolapse will increase time of surgery, predispose to uveitis, intraocular infection, and hyphema. However, constricting the pupil after performing phacoemulsification and before DMEK will manage IFIS efficiently.

## 12.13 Posterior Segment Complications

### 12.13.1 Vitreous Loss

Vitreous loss can happen during DMEK. Aphakia, zonular dehiscence, unnoticed posterior capsular tear (PCT), large capsulotomies without anterior capsule coverage of the optic, or aggressive technique can be predisposing factors.

We prefer pars plana vitrectomy (PPV) over bimanual anterior vitrectomy because it ensures cleaning vitreous from the AC, no enlargement of the PCT, and less chance of retinal traction.

If vitreous loss is noticed after the graft has been injected into the AC, then one has to evaluate the extent of prolapse. One should clean all the incision sites of prolapsed vitreous with cellulose sponges and scissors. If the pupil become round and the vitreous is minimal, then we would reposition the graft and inject air as usual. The air typically pushes the vitreous back into the posterior chamber. If more extensive vitreous is present, then once again clean the incisions of exposed vitreous and suture them closed. Utilizing a pars plana approach, perform a core vitrectomy removing the vitreous in the anterior chamber. Once the vitreous has been pulled out of the AC and the core vitrectomy is complete, then one can restrain the donor as necessary (within the eye) and complete positioning of the donor as planned.

### 12.13.2 Graft Dislocation in the Posterior Segment

We have never had a case of a DMEK donor going into the vitreous cavity. In one case, we injected a donor through the pupil in a pseudophakic patient but retrieved the donor with intraocular forceps. A key here is to make sure one does not have an open conduit to the vitreous cavity and to maintain relatively good overall pressure and formation of the globe so that there is not a large fluid movement to the posterior portions while the graft is in the eye.

In cases of deficient iris/lens diaphragm such as aphakia, aniridia, or large iris defects the air bubble and graft can escape to the posterior segment. A DSEK graft anchored to the cornea with a suture should be considered instead of DMEK [18]. Large iris defects should be sutured. Iris/lens implants should be considered for aniridia. Eyes with artificial irises should have DSEK graft, but keep in mind that for most eyes with an artificial iris, there is a substantial space between the implant and the wall of the eye so a DSEK graft can easily fall back into the posterior portions of the eye, so the graft should be inserted with a pull in technique followed by an immediate injection of air to hold the graft in place and then suture fixation of the graft. If the graft dislocates to the posterior chamber, a PPV would be needed to remove the graft from the vitreous cavity. The graft can damage the retina or predispose to epiretinal membrane formation, retinal traction, or proliferative vitreoretinopathy (PVR) [19]. In case of aphakia, secondary IOL implantation should be performed before DMEK.

### 12.13.3 Retinal Vascular Complications

The ocular perfusion pressure is defined as the ocular arterial pressure minus the IOP, so elevated IOP from air tamponade could cause decreased ocular blood flow. Therefore, we advise testing light perception just after filling the AC with air. If the patient could not see light, the bubble size has to be reduced. This is an advantage of topical anesthesia both at the end of surgery and postoperatively in case of pupillary block.

### 12.13.4 Air and Gas Bubble-Related Complications

#### 12.13.4.1 Wrong Application of Air/Gas Bubble

We prefer to enter the AC with a 30 G needle rather than a cannula in the paracentesis. It is advisable also to inject air near the iris to ensure it is as far from the donor endothelium as possible with slow withdrawal of the needle to prevent air egression. Air escaping behind the iris could lead to pupillary block.

#### 12.13.4.2 Overfilling the AC

This will lead to elevation of the IOP in the early postoperative period with need for partial evacuation. We have recently found that on days with falling barometric pressure, there is an increased chance of air bubbles expanding and blocking the PI.

#### 12.13.4.3 Air/Gas Escape from the AC

In case of bubble escape from the eye, all surgical wounds including the paracentesis have to be sealed tightly by sutures. The bubble could escape to the posterior segment in cases of loss of iris/lens diaphragm and in vitrectomized eyes or to the bleb or filtering device in eyes with prior glaucoma filtration surgery.

#### 12.13.4.4 Injection of Wrong Form of Gas

Gas [20] should be used in the nonexpansile form; 20% for Sulfur Hexafloride (SF6) and 14% for (C3F8). If used by mistake in the expansile form (100%), bubble size will increase leading to serious effects. If discovered in the early postoperative period, gas/air exchange should be performed.

## 12.14 Immediate and Early Postoperative Complications

### 12.14.1 Graft Detachment or Dislocation

Partial graft detachment is the most frequent early postoperative complication, whereas complete graft detachment is relatively rare. Poor graft attachment can be caused by many factors including poor donor graft quality, excessive intraoperative manipulations, and the presence of mechanical barriers, for example, DM tags, interrupted stromal fibers, blood cells, and viscoelastic substance.

There is no fixed rule about when to rebubble or the maximum number of times to rebubble. We prefer early intervention when the detachment affects the visual area because areas that are detached more than 8 weeks become rigid reducing the likelihood of reattachment [21], and long-standing corneal edema will heal by fibrosis which adversely affects vision.

We usually rebubble within the first 1–4 postoperative weeks and prefer to enlarge the residual original air bubble before it has completely dissipated. Our previous study showed that a single rebubble was not associated with endothelial cell loss while two or more were associated with higher endothelial cell loss [22]. The rebubble rate did not differ between preloaded grafts and grafts prepared by the surgeon [23]. Gases, for example, SF6 20% stay in the AC three times longer than air, so these are preferred by some surgeons for rebubble.

### 12.14.2 Loss of Air/Gas Tamponade (Video 12.4)

The patient leaves the OR with an air bubble filling 90% of the AC that disappears within 3–5 days. If the bubble was reduced in size after 60 min of supine position with no eye rubbing, then the patient should return to the OR for rebubble and revision of any leaky wounds.

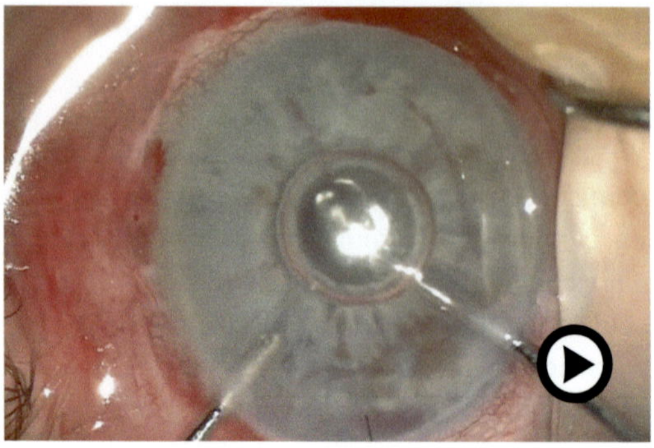

**Video 12.4** Management of air/gas tamponade (https://doi.org/10.1007/000-dhv)

### 12.14.3 Ocular Hypertension (Fig. 12.9)

Increase in IOP can be detected in the early postoperative period and is usually due to pupillary block, angle closure, exacerbation of pre-existing glaucoma [24], hyphema, or it could be surgically induced, for example, inflammation or improper removal of viscoelastics.

Pupillary block is reported to happen in up to 15% of cases [17, 25]; most respond to medical treatment while a minority requires letting some air out. The patient should be examined 1 h after DMEK, and if the IOP is high and the PI is not covered by the air bubble and was plugged with blood clot or was incompletely open, a laser PI should be performed. In case of mechanical forward displacement of the iris, a PI is not effective and reduction of the bubble size is required. If the air bubble was filling less than 80% of the AC, mydriatics will break the pupillary block by moving the pupil edge below the bubble lower margin [5].

### 12.14.4 Early Graft Failure

It is defined as the absence of corneal clearance for a month after surgery. Primary failure may occur in spite of complete attachment of the DMEK graft in the early postoperative period. In some cases, this may be from poor quality tissue or difficulties during surgery. But often no cause

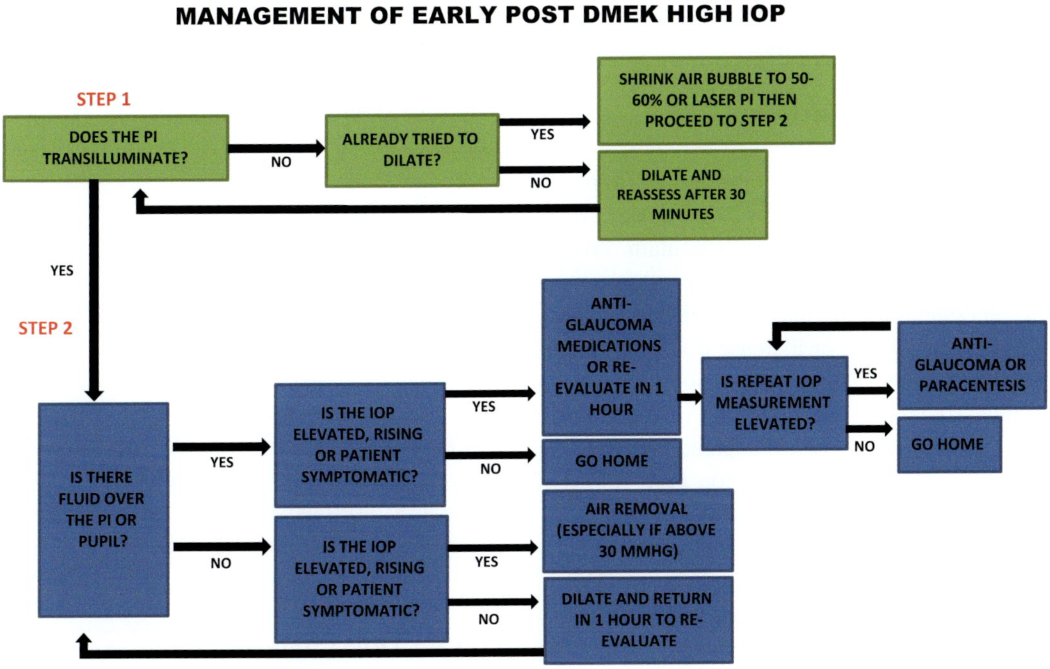


**Fig. 12.9** Post-DMEK hyphema

can be found. Graft detachment is another cause of primary failure if the graft cannot be attached after repeated reinjections of air [26, 27].

Replacement of a failed graft within 1–2 months rehabilitates patients promptly and precludes stromal fibrotic changes that could impair visual outcomes [28].

### 12.14.5 Optical Failure

Unsatisfactory visual outcomes can be caused by graft abnormalities within the pupillary area including folds, irregular central corneal thickness or opacity in the interface, or retained fragments of host DM. Surgical intervention should be considered to correct the optical problems even if the graft is attached [29].

### 12.14.6 Hyphema

Rebleeding from a PI can occur in the early postoperative period, but is rare. Usually, it is mild and responds to bed rest and conservative treatment, but if extensive, it might lead to increased IOP or blood staining if the IOP is not controlled.

### 12.14.7 Postoperative Inflammation

Inflammation in the early postoperative period can be infectious or non-infectious. Eye banks have strict rules about accepting donor tissues to reduce the risk of transmitting infection. Also many surgical centers culture the donor rim and preservative solution.

Several cases of Candida infection after DMEK have been reported. Treatment consisted of topical, oral, intracameral, and/or intravitreal antifungals and partial or total graft removal [30]. Sterile inflammation (postoperative uveitis) can happen in case of excessive manipulation to the iris, for example, IFIS, pupilloplasty, in prolonged and complex cases or because of toxic/allergic reaction to an intraoperative consumable. Fibrin formation in the AC might lead to graft detachment.

## 12.15 Late Postoperative Complications

### 12.15.1 Graft Rejection

DMEK has a significantly lower risk of immunologic rejection than DSEK or PK because DMEK is less antigenic as it doesn't contain stroma. Rejection can be recognized by the classic signs of endothelial rejection (Khodadoust line), keratic precipitates, or increase in corneal thickness [31]. Often it is asymptomatic [32, 33], so regular follow-ups are important to detect early changes. Patients who stop taking steroid eye drops have more risk to develop graft rejection [33]. Less potent steroids (fluorometholone 0.1% or Loteprednol etabonate 0.5%) are sufficient after the first month or two to prevent DMEK rejection and significantly less likely to cause steroid-associated ocular hypertension than more potent steroids such as prednisolone acetate 1% [32, 34].

### 12.15.2 Glaucoma

Steroid-induced glaucoma is the most common cause of late onset IOP elevation. If it happens, IOP can be controlled by antiglaucoma treatment, and tapering strong steroids, or switching to less potent steroids [32, 34]. Surgical intervention is required if IOP cannot be controlled medically. Glaucoma is not the only side effect of long-term topical steroid therapy as it may also cause cataract, increase susceptibility to infection and dry eye and other minor symptoms, for example, stinging and itching.

### 12.15.3 Late Graft Failure

Endothelial decompensation in the absence of documented rejection is the leading cause of late DMEK failure, and prior glaucoma surgery is the main risk factor. In eyes without prior glaucoma surgery, the cumulative probability of 5-year graft survival was 95% [35]. The endothelial cell loss after DMEK is typically 30–34% after 6 months, followed by approximately 9% decrease per year [36, 37]. Failed DMEK is typically treated with DMEK regraft with excellent outcomes.

### 12.15.4 Refractive Changes

On average, DMEK is associated with a small mean hyperopic shift (+0.33 D), but the individual change can range from −2.00 to +4.00 diopters. Also cylinder and keratometric power can change to some extent after DMEK somewhat reducing the precision of preoperative IOL calculations [38]. Refractive stability after DMEK is obtained within 1–3 months [39].

### 12.15.5 Lens Changes

As with any intraocular surgery, DMEK can accelerate crystalline lens changes, particularly in older patients, so we often combine DMEK with cataract surgery in patients over 50 years old. Younger patients can be left phakic. When performing DMEK in phakic eyes, we prefer slight nasal decentration of the graft for easier temporal incision in a future phacoemulsification, and we protect the crystalline lens by constricting the pupil and scoring DM under cohesive viscoelastic. Phacoemulsification can be performed safely after DMEK with minimal endothelial cell loss using a dual viscoelastic technique [40].

IOL calcification has been described and may be associated with metabolic reaction leading to deposition of calcium in the presence of air, pressure effect leading to dehydration of hydrophilic IOLs [41], or inflammatory reaction. The pattern of calcification is superficial in the anterior area of the IOL and in the pupillary area. Management is by IOL exchange.

Pupil abnormalities and posterior synechia such as minor peaking up can happen and were noted more with SF6 tamponade [42]. Possible causes include prolonged high IOP leading to sphincter muscle ischemia and prolonged mydriasis leading to firm contact between the back of the iris and the anterior capsule.

#### 12.15.6 Interface Deposits

The interface should be examined carefully because it could be the site of accumulation of cells in case of epithelial ingrowth or infiltrates in case of infectious keratitis. Other deposits could include blood, viscoelastic substance, metallic particles, pseudoexfoliation material, etc.

#### 12.15.7 Infection

Late onset infection should be considered and patients should be seen routinely to pick up early signs of infection as these patients are on long-term steroid therapy. *Candida glabrata* was the most common organism in tissue culture of the donor rim [43]. Oral, intracameral, and intrastromal antifungals should be prescribed for cases of ocular infection. We have found that 1.6% of donor cultures were positive for fungal contamination [44] PPV should be done if the infection spread to the posterior segment.

#### 12.15.8 Posterior Segment Complications

The rate of developing CME in triple DMEK surgery was not significantly different than in DMEK alone. Topical anti-inflammatory treatment is usually sufficient but some cases might need intravitreal injections [45].

Other posterior segment complications include suprachoroidal hemorrhage, retinal detachment, and retinal vascular occlusion.

### 12.16 Conclusions

Proper case selection, surgical training, and awareness of ways to prevent and treat complications are keys to successful DMEK surgery.

## References


1. Ćirković A, Schlötzer-Schrehardt U, Weller JM, Kruse FE, Tourtas T. Clinical and ultrastructural characteristics of graft failure in DMEK: 1-year results after repeat DMEK. Cornea. 2015;34:11–7.
2. Williams RS, Mayko ZM, Friend DJ, Straiko MD, Clay RD, Stoeger CG. Descemet membrane endothelial keratoplasty (DMEK) tissue preparation: a donor diabetes mellitus categorical risk stratification scale for assessing tissue suitability and reducing tissue loss. Cornea. 2016;35(7):927–31.
3. Giebel AW, Price FW. Descemet's membrane endothelial keratoplasty (DMEK): the bare minimum. In: Price FW, Price MO, editors. DSEK: all you need to know about endothelial Keratoplasty. Thorofare: Slack; 2008. p. 119–46.
4. Tenkman LR, Price FW, Price MO. Descemet membrane endothelial keratoplasty donor preparation: navigating challenges and improving efficiency. Cornea. 2014;33:319–25.
5. McKee Y, Price FW. DMEK. The digital manual of ophthalmic surgery & theory. 2014;1(1).
6. Debellemanière G, Guilbert E, Courtin R, Panthier C, Sabatier P, Gatinel D, Ali S. Impact of surgical learning curve in Descemet membrane endothelial keratoplasty on visual acuity gain. Cornea. 2017;36:1–6.
7. Zeidenweber DA, Tran KD, Sales CS, Wehrer SW, Straiko MD, Terry MA. Prestained and preloaded DMEK grafts: an evaluation of tissue quality and stain retention. Cornea. 2017;36(11):1402–7.
8. Pham C, Hellier CE, Vo MD, Szczotka-Flynn OD, Benetz MA, Ann B, Lass MD. Donor endothelial specular image quality in Optisol GS and Life4°C. Int J Eye Banking. 2013;1(2):1–8.
9. Koo EH, Goodman CF, Vanner EE, Tothova JD, Fout E, Buras W. Eusol-C as corneal cold storage solution: early clinical outcomes of keratoplasty. Cornea. 2022;41:e26–e28.
10. Jacob S, Agarwal A, Kumar DA. Endoilluminator-assisted Descemet membrane endothelial keratoplasty and endoilluminator-assisted pre-Descemet endothelial keratoplasty. Clin Ophthalmol. 2015;9:2123.
11. Veldman PB. www.patientready.org. Accessed 11 Oct 2024.
12. Busin M, Leon P, Scorcia V, Ponzin D. Contact lens-assisted pull-through technique for delivery of tri-folded (endothelium in) DMEK grafts minimizes surgical time and cell loss. Ophthalmology. 2016;123(3):476–83.
13. Veldman PB, Dye PK, Holiman JD, Mayko ZM, Sáles CS, Straiko MD, Stoeger CG, Terry MA. Stamping an S on DMEK donor tissue to prevent upside-down grafts: laboratory validation and detailed preparation technique description. Cornea. 2015;34(9):1175–8.
14. Burkhart ZN, Feng MT, Price MO, Price FW. Handheld slit beam techniques to facilitate DMEK and DALK. Cornea. 2013;32(5):722–4.

15. Dirisamer M, Ham L, Dapena I, Moutsouris K, Droutsas K, van Dijk K, Frank LE, Oellerich S, Melles GR. Efficacy of Descemet membrane endothelial keratoplasty: clinical outcome of 200 consecutive cases after a learning curve of 25 cases. Arch Ophthalmol. 2011;129(11):1435–43.
16. Crews JW, Price MO, Lautert J, Feng MT, Price FW Jr. Intraoperative hyphema in Descemet membrane endothelial keratoplasty alone or combined with phacoemulsification. J Cataract Refract Surg. 2018;44(2):198–201.
17. Gorovoy MS. DMEK complications. Cornea. 2014;33(1):101–4.
18. Price MO, Price FW Jr, Trespalacios R. Endothelial keratoplasty technique for aniridic aphakic eyes. J Cataract Refract Surg. 2007;33(3):376–9.
19. Vasquez-Perez A, Brennan N, Ayoub T, Allan B, Larkin DF, da Cruz L. Descemet membrane endothelial keratoplasty (DMEK) graft dislocation into the vitreous cavity. Cornea. 2019;38(2):173–6.
20. Marques RE, Guerra PS, Sousa DC, Ferreira NP, Gonçalves AI, Quintas AM, Rodrigues W. Sulfur hexafluoride 20% versus air 100% for anterior chamber tamponade in DMEK: a meta-analysis. Cornea. 2018;37(6):691–7.
21. Müller TM, Verdijk RM, Lavy I, Bruinsma M, Parker J, Binder PS, et al. Histopathologic features of Descemet membrane endothelial keratoplasty graft remnants, folds, and detachments. Ophthalmology. 2016;123:2489–97.
22. Feng MT, Srinivas SP, Miller JM, Price FW. Air reinjection and endothelial cell density in Descemet membrane endothelial keratoplasty: five-year follow-up. J Cataract Refract Surg. 2014;40:1116–21.
23. Regnier M, Auxenfans C, Maucort-Boulch D, Marty A-S, Damour O, Burillon C, et al. Eye bank prepared versus surgeon cut endothelial graft tissue for descemet membrane endothelial keratoplasty: an observational study. Medicine (Baltimore). 2017;96:e6885.
24. Naveiras M, Dirisamer M, Parker J, Ham L, van Dijk K, Dapena I, et al. Causes of glaucoma after descemet membrane endothelial keratoplasty. Am J Ophthalmol. 2012;153:958–966.e1.
25. Maier A-KB, Wolf T, Gundlach E, Klamann MKJ, Gonnermann J, Bertelmann E, et al. Intraocular pressure elevation and post-DMEK glaucoma following descemet membrane endothelial keratoplasty. Graefes Arch Clin Exp Ophthalmol. 2014;252:1947–54.
26. Cirkovic A, Schlötzer-Schrehardt U, Weller JM, Kruse FE, Tourtas T. Clinical and ultrastructural characteristics of graft failure in DMEK: 1-year results after repeat DMEK. Cornea. 2015;34(1):11–7.
27. Heinzelmann S, Böhringer D, Eberwein P, Reinhard T, Maier P. Graft dislocation and graft failure following descemet membrane endothelial keratoplasty (DMEK) using precut tissue: a retrospective cohort study. Graefes Arch Clin Exp Ophthalmol. 2017;255(1):127–33.
28. Price MO, Feng MT, McKee Y, Price FW Jr. Repeat Descemet membrane endothelial keratoplasty: secondary grafts with early intervention are comparable with fellow-eye primary grafts. Ophthalmology. 2015;122(8):1639–44.
29. Baydoun L, Melles GR. Refining the terminology of graft failure in reports on endothelial keratoplasty outcomes. JAMA Ophthalmol. 2016;134(2):125–6.
30. Thompson M, Carli D. First reported case of donor related candida endophthalmitis after descemet membrane endothelial keratoplasty. Open Ophthalmol J. 2017;11:117–21.
31. Baydoun L, Livny E, Ham L, Bruinsma M, Melles GRJ. 360-degree Scheimpflug imaging to predict allograft rejection after Descemet membrane endothelial keratoplasty. Cornea. 2016;35:1385–90.
32. Price MO, Price FW Jr, Kruse FE, Bachmann BO, Tourtas T. Randomized comparison of topical prednisolone acetate 1% versus fluorometholone 0.1% in the first year after Descemet membrane endothelial keratoplasty. Cornea. 2014;33:880–6.
33. Price MO, Scanameo A, Feng MT, Price FW. Descemet's membrane endothelial keratoplasty: risk of immunologic rejection episodes after discontinuing topical corticosteroids. Ophthalmology. 2016;123:1232–6.
34. Price MO, Feng MT, Scanameo A, Price FW. Loteprednol Etabonate 0.5% gel vs. prednisolone acetate 1% solution after descemet membrane endothelial keratoplasty: prospective randomized trial. Cornea. 2015;34:853–8.
35. Schlögl A, Tourtas T, Kruse FE, Weller JM. Long-term clinical outcome after descemet membrane endothelial keratoplasty. Am J Ophthalmol. 2016;169:218–26.
36. Parker J, Dirisamer M, Naveiras M, Ham L, Van der Wees J, Melles GR. Endothelial cell density after descemet membrane endothelial keratoplasty: 1-to 4-year follow-up. Am J Ophthalmol. 2011;151(6):1107.
37. Price MO, Giebel AW, Fairchild KM, Price FW Jr. Descemet's membrane endothelial keratoplasty: prospective multicenter study of visual and refractive outcomes and endothelial survival. Ophthalmology. 2009;116(12):2361–8.
38. Schoenberg ED, Price FW Jr, Miller J, McKee Y, Price MO. Refractive outcomes of Descemet membrane endothelial keratoplasty triple procedures (combined with cataract surgery). J Cataract Refract Surg. 2015;41(6):1182–9.
39. van Dijk K, Ham L, Tse WH, Liarakos VS, Quilendrino R, Yeh RY, Melles GR. Near complete visual recovery and refractive stability in modern corneal transplantation: descemet membrane endothelial keratoplasty (DMEK). Contact Lens Anterior Eye. 2013;36(1):13–21.
40. Burkhart ZN, Feng MT, Price FW, Price MO. One-year outcomes in eyes remaining phakic after Descemet membrane endothelial keratoplasty. J Cataract Refract Surg. 2014;40:430–4.
41. MacLean KD, Apel A, Wilson J, Werner L. Calcification of hydrophilic acrylic intraocular lenses associated with intracameral air injec-

tion following DMEK. J Cataract Refract Surg. 2015;41:1310–4.
42. Arnalich-Montiel F, Pérez-Sarriegui A, Lauzirika G, Porrua L, Hernández-Verdejo JL. Pupillary abnormalities in descemet membrane endothelial keratoplasty after nearly full tamponade. Cornea. 2017;36:290–4.
43. Tu EY, Majmudar PA. Adjuvant stromal amphotericin B injection for late-onset DMEK infection. Cornea. 2017;36(12):1556–8.
44. Doshi H, Pabon S, Price MO, Feng MT, Price FW Jr. Overview of systemic Candida infections in hospital settings and report of Candida after DMEK successfully treated with antifungals and partial graft excision. Cornea. 2018;37(8):1071–4.
45. Heinzelmann S, Maier P, Böhringer D, Hüther S, Eberwein P, Reinhard T. Cystoid macular oedema following Descemet membrane endothelial keratoplasty. Br J Ophthalmol. 2015;99:98–102.

# Postoperative Handling and Management of Graft Detachments

13

Lamis Baydoun, Silke Oellerich, and Gerrit R. J. Melles

## 13.1 Introduction

Endothelial keratoplasty (EK), in particular Descemet membrane endothelial keratoplasty (DMEK), has revolutionized modern endothelial keratoplasty procedures with its unprecedented clinical outcomes and lower complication rates [1–9]. With the introduction of EK, however, graft detachment has emerged as a new complication. It is the most common complication after DMEK and "feared" by novel surgeons especially when adopting the DMEK technique [2, 10–15]. Higher detachment rates are noted for DMEK, while techniques that utilize thicker endothelial grafts, such as (Ultrathin-) Descemet membrane (automated) endothelial keratoplasty (DS(A)EK) or Pre-Descemet's endothelial keratoplasty (PDEK) report lower detachment rates [5, 16–18]. Main uncertainties in dealing with DMEK detachments are: (1) how to avoid them, (2) which ones to treat, and (3) when is the best timing for treatment?

Technique standardization, a continuous increase in surgical experience and the use of non-expansible intracameral gas tamponades (such as SF6) to support graft adhesion, contributed to a significant decrease in detachment rates within the past years [2, 19–25]. Although most detachments are benign, this common complication requires special attention as its treatment, i.e., repeat complete intracameral air (or gas) injection (the so-called re-bubbling) may induce endothelial cell damage that may subsequently influence graft function and threaten graft longevity. The focus of this chapter will be on the management of DMEK graft detachments.

L. Baydoun (✉)
Department of Ophthalmology, University Hospital Münster, Münster, Germany

ELZA Institute, Zurich/Dietikon, Switzerland

Netherlands Institute for Innovative Ocular Surgery, Rotterdam, The Netherlands
e-mail: dr.lamisbaydoun@gmail.com

S. Oellerich
Netherlands Institute for Innovative Ocular Surgery, Rotterdam, The Netherlands

G. R. J. Melles
Netherlands Institute for Innovative Ocular Surgery, Rotterdam, The Netherlands

Melles Cornea Clinic Rotterdam, Rotterdam, The Netherlands

NIIOS-USA, San Diego, CA, USA

## 13.2 What Is a Graft Detachment?

Graft detachment, also named dehiscence or dislocation, is a lack of adherence between the endothelial graft and the recipient posterior cornea. Depending on the kind of endothelial transplant, there is a (partial) lack of adherence between the donor Descemet membrane (DM) and recipient stroma in DMEK, between the donor stroma and recipient stroma in DS(A)EK and the pre-Descemet stromal layer and the


S. Jacob (ed.), *Mastering DMEK and PDEK*, https://doi.org/10.1007/978-981-97-3469-6_13

recipient stroma in PDEK. The space between the detached graft and the recipient stroma is filled with aqueous humor. Classifying the extension and configuration of detachments aids in determining which detachments may require treatment and which do not.

## 13.3 Classifying Graft Detachments

### 13.3.1 Detachment Extension

A graft detachment can either be complete or partial. *Complete detachments* occur less frequently. The graft is usually floating flat (unfolded from limbus to limbus) or folded as a (partial) roll in the anterior chamber. Complete detachments are typically visually significant because of the diffuse corneal edema owing to the inability of the endothelial cells to deswell the cornea when not properly positioned against the recipient stroma.

*Partial detachments* occur more frequently. These can range from edge detachments to those that extend to ≤1/3 of the graft surface area (also classified as minor detachments) or to >1/3 of the graft surface area (also classified as major detachments) (Fig. 13.1) [26]. Minor detachments usually do not impair visual acuity and are therefore considered benign unless they involve the visual axis. Major detachments, on the other hand, often involve the optical zone and hereby affect visual performance. Although initially edematous, the cornea overlying a partial detachment may often (entirely) clear within weeks or months due to the endothelial cells re-populating the "naked" posterior stroma. In eyes with major detachments, these corneas are prone to decompensate later again (Fig. 13.2) [27–30].

### 13.3.2 Detachment Configuration

Assessing the detachment configuration [31] helps in deciding for necessity and timing of treatment which will be addressed later in this chapter. The following configurations can be observed (Figs. 13.1 and 13.3):

1. Graft roll is free-floating in the anterior chamber (Fig. 13.3a).
2. Flat detachment that follows the corneal curvature but does not adhere to the recipient stroma (Fig. 13.3b).
3. A wavy graft detachment over several quadrants that shows areas with partial attachment (Fig. 13.3c).
4. Deep detachment protruding into the recipient anterior chamber with or without adherence to surrounding ocular structures such as the iris (Fig. 13.3d).
5. Inward folds that typically produce larger graft detachments than the area of the fold (Fig. 13.3e).
6. Flat or deep detachment with the graft edges curling up towards the iris indicating an upside-down orientation of the graft.

However, not all detachment configurations necessarily require treatment. While some grafts are attached immediately after surgery, others may initially be partially detached or detach partially from the recipient stroma during the deswelling process of the cornea within the first week after DMEK (Fig. 13.4) [26]. These initial partial detachments often re-attach spontaneously (Fig. 13.5) or corneal clearance can occur within the first postoperative weeks despite persistent detachment (Fig. 13.2) [25, 27–30]. A detachment may therefore also be considered as

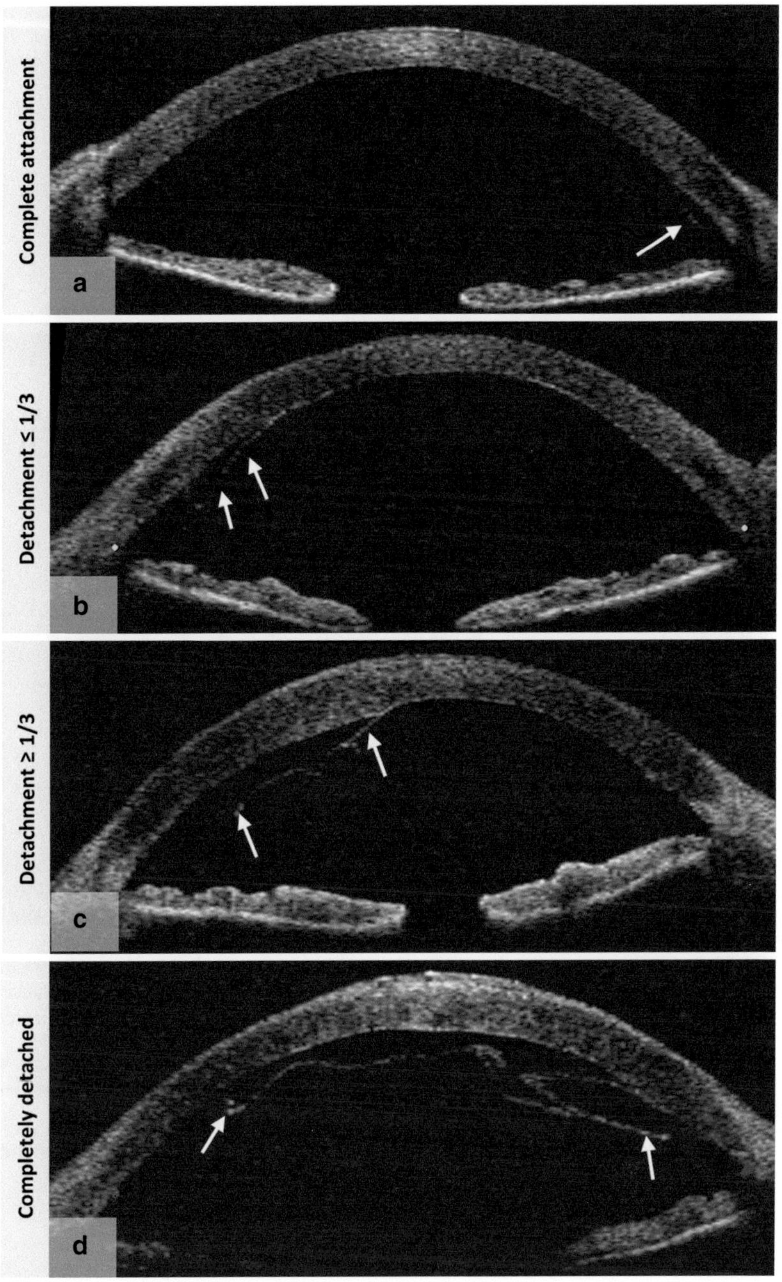


**Fig. 13.1** AS-OCT images displaying the graft adherence status after Descemet membrane endothelial keratoplasty (DMEK). (**a**) Complete attachment. (**b**) Minor detachment: Descemet graft detachment over ≤1/3 of the graft surface area, not affecting the visual axis. (**c**) Major detachment: detachment >1/3 of the graft surface area. (D) subtotal or total graft detachment. (Modified figure from reference [26])

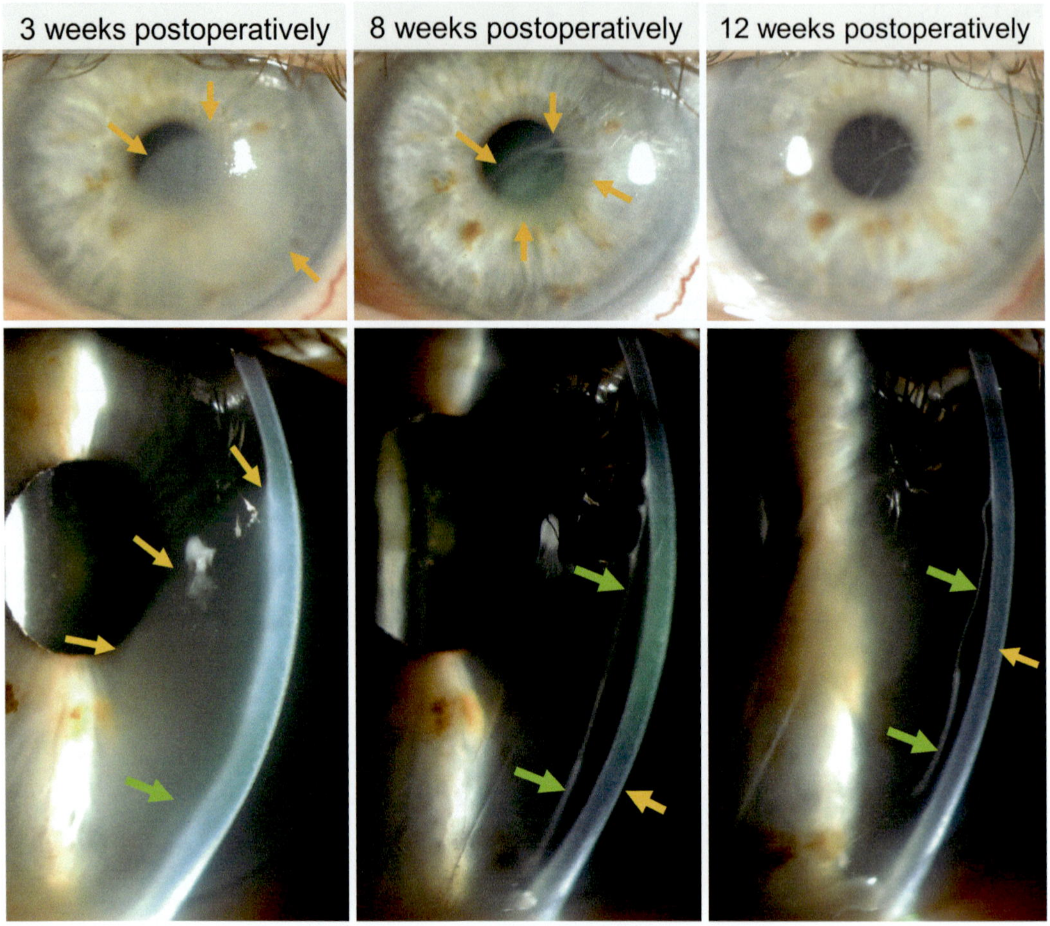


**Fig. 13.2** Slit-lamp photographs of a transplanted cornea with a major graft detachment three (Left), eight (Middle), and 12 weeks (Right) after Descemet membrane endothelial keratoplasty. Note that the edema (orange arrows) overlying the Descemet detachment (green arrows) resolves with time, and that stromal thinning with concomitant corneal clearance progresses from the periphery towards the corneal center (Modified figure from reference [27])

part of a wound healing process rather than a complication per se. In contrast, detachments that persist or enlarge, without showing a tendency of re-attachment or corneal clearance, may require intervention. Or is it possible to prevent graft detachments?

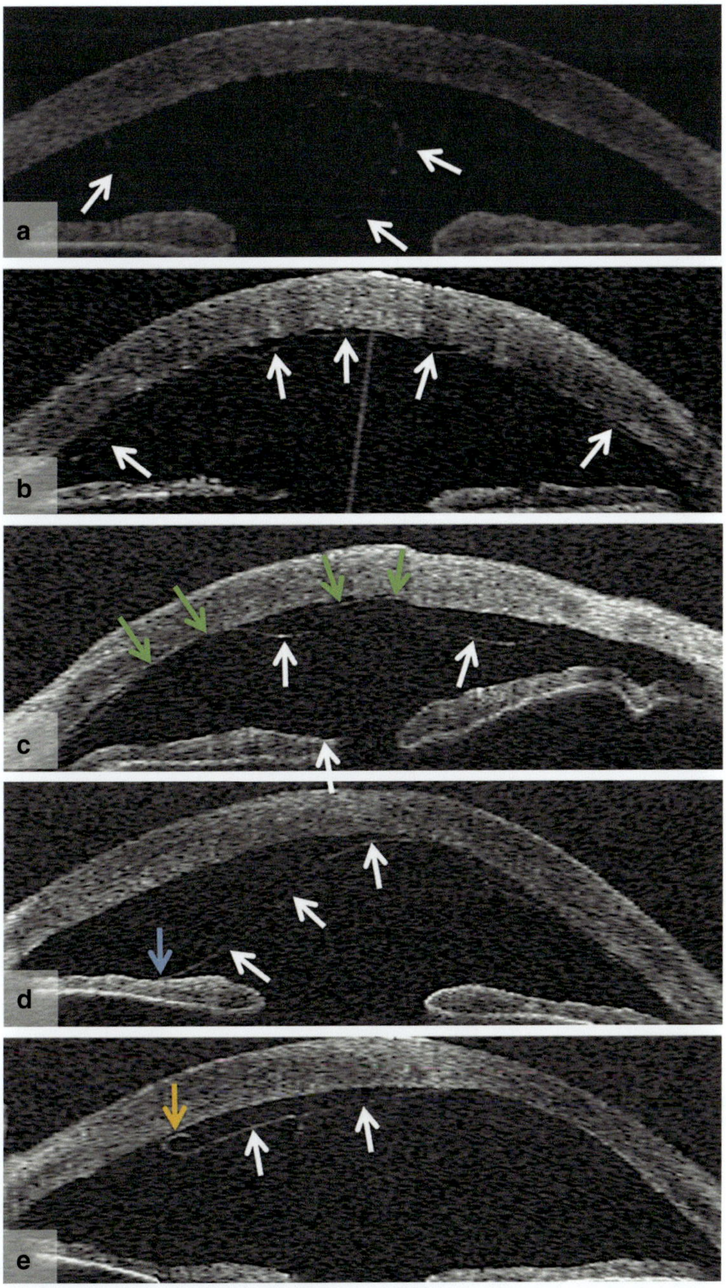


**Fig. 13.3** AS-OCT images showing five forms of DMEK graft detachment (white arrows) configurations. (**a**) With a free-floating roll in the anterior chamber. (**b**) With a flat detachment that follows the corneal curvature but without any apparent tendency for the graft to adhere, spontaneous re-attachment may be awaited because the graft may be a "slow responder" that does not benefit from immediate re-bubbling. Such grafts may be re-bubbled from 2 to 4 weeks after surgery when endothelial function may have been restored. Note that such a graft configuration (well positioned but just slightly detached) may also be indicative of an upside-down position of the graft. (**c**) With a wavy detachment over several quadrants that shows areas with partial attachment (green arrows) may be re-bubbled rather quickly because the detachment is too large to expect spontaneous re-attachment, i.e., detachment may persist owing to physical separation rather than lack of endothelial functionality. (**d**) Detachments protruding far into the anterior chamber may be eligible for early re-bubbling because the tissue often adheres to surrounding ocular structures such as the iris (blue arrow). (**e**) Inward folds (orange arrow) typically produce a somewhat larger graft detachment that may spontaneously re-attach over time, but sometimes requires re-bubbling. (Modified figure from reference [31])

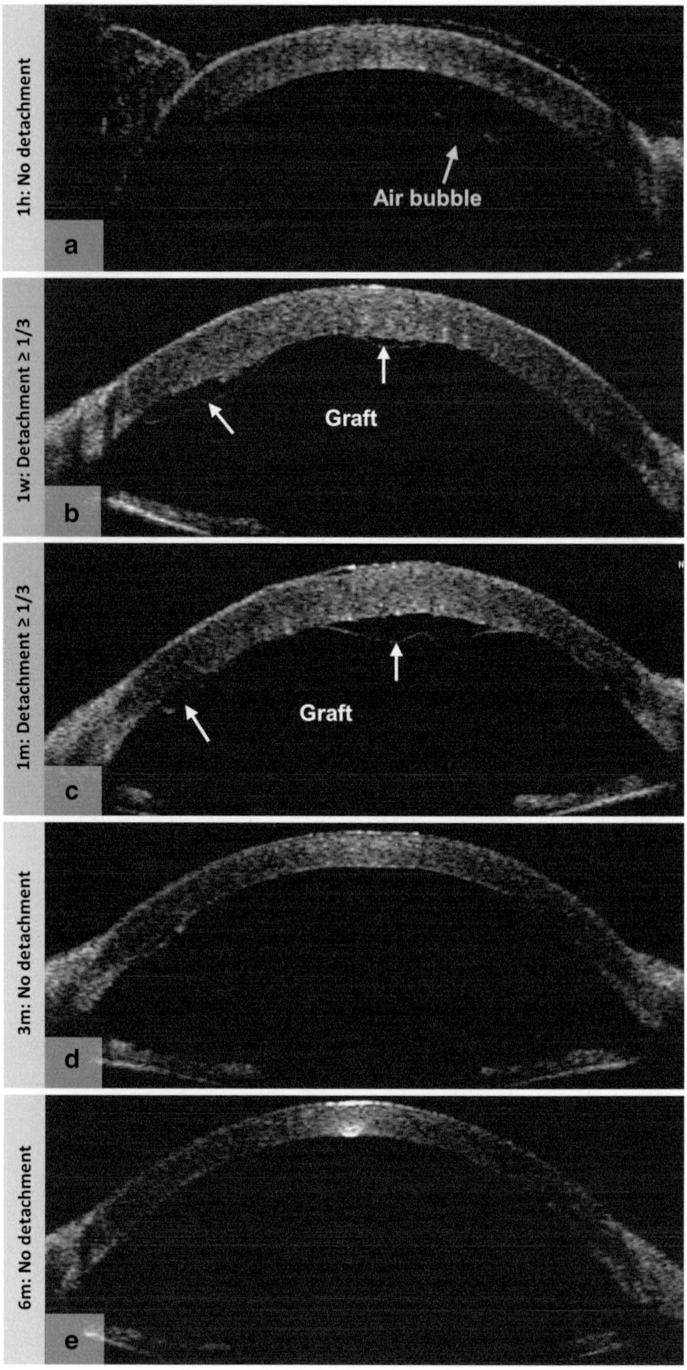


**Fig. 13.4** AS-OCT images of a cornea at 1 h to 6 months after Descemet membrane endothelial keratoplasty (DMEK). (**a**) On the 1-h. AS-OCT, complete adherence of the Descemet graft is seen, (**b**) followed by a minor partial detachment (white arrows) at 1 week and (**c**) 1 month and (**d**, **e**) re-attachment at 3 and 6 months postoperatively. (Taken from reference [26])

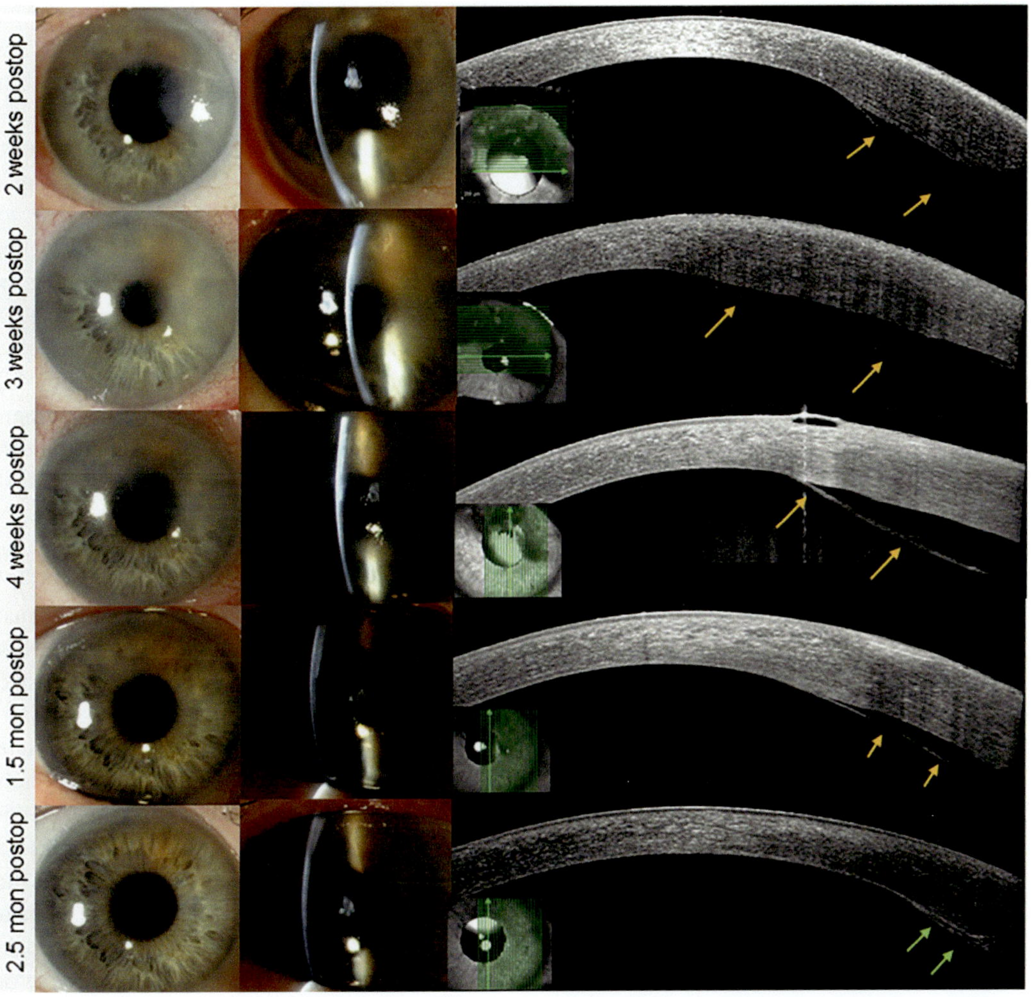


**Fig. 13.5** Slit-lamp (left) and OCT images (right) of a right eye at different follow-up points from 2 weeks (upper row) until 2.5 months (lower row) after Descemet Membrane Endothelial Keratoplasty. The initially detached graft (orange arrows) and corneal edema extends from two to three weeks postoperatively. The initially detached Descemet graft (orange arrows) re-attached spontaneously to the recipient posterior stroma, with major resolution of the stromal edema (green arrows)

## 13.4 Intervention or Prevention: Why Does the Graft Detach and How to Avoid it?

Already the famous Dutch scholar, Desiderius Erasmus (1466–1536) from Rotterdam, "posted" the quote "prevention is better than cure," which implies that managing diseases or complications starts with preventing them from happening in the first place. In other words, postoperative management of graft detachments starts with prevention. Hence, being aware of the origin and sources of graft detachments will help avoiding or at least reducing detachment rates. In the past years, growing surgical experience, and for some surgeons, the use of intracameral gas tamponades could lower the incidence of graft separation significantly [2, 19–25]. Still, every surgeon will encounter detached grafts, especially during the learning curve. Most detachments originate from avoidable mistakes performed preoperatively, intraoperatively, and postoperatively. Knowing the following facts can and will reduce this undesired DMEK-complication more quickly and will help avoiding it continuously.

### 13.4.1 Preoperative Precautions

1. Damage to the endothelial cells during graft preparation may cause graft areas that are devoid of endothelial cells. These areas may be more prone to detach.

   *Tip*: Minimize graft manipulation and direct damage and trephine a graft area that remained mostly unaffected [32–36].
2. Grafts with tears or hanging fragments result from challenging preparation. Such grafts often behave differently in the anterior chamber and may therefore be unpredictable and more difficult to unfold leaving residual graft folds that may detach more easily.

   *Tip*: Remove torn graft edges early during preparation to avoid "hanging" graft pieces that will be difficult to handle in the anterior chamber [35].
3. Avoid grafts that are (relatively) too large for proper intracameral graft fit because the graft will inevitably fold (e.g., in phakic eyes, or eyes with anterior synechia) or detach if covering an irregular stromal hump (e.g., in posterior surface irregularities or in failed penetrating grafts).

   *Tip*: Measure the area of the aimed graft position and chose trephination size accordingly [37].

### 13.4.2 Intraoperative Precautions

1. Avoid left-behind host DM remnants and remove a lamellar splitting of the DM (the so-called double layer) that is found in about 10% of eyes with Fuchs endothelial corneal dystrophy.

   *Tip*: Perform a thorough descemetorhexis, preferably under air to improve visualization of the DM. The "double layer" can often be removed more easily with a scraper instead of a reversed Sinskey hook. If the tissue does not go off easily, you may already be digging into the corneal stroma. Note that stromal surface damage and irregularities may be another source for improper graft adherence [37–42].
2. Guarantee correct graft orientation before complete unfolding to not mistakenly lift the graft when positioned upside-down.

   *Tip*: Hence, make sure the graft scrolls are facing up towards the corneal stroma (Fig. 13.6) and the endothelium faces the iris. To confirm correct graft orientation, one can check the "Moutsouris sign" (i.e., placing a cannula underneath the graft folds, if the tip of the cannula turns blue the graft is correctly oriented, if not the graft is lying upside-down) [43, 44]. Other surgeons manage this key step by marking the graft asymmetrically, stamping an "S" and/or "F" on the DM or by using an intraoperative Optical Coherence Tomography (OCT) [45–49].
3. Prominent posterior stromal surface irregularities as observed in the area of the corneal tunnel incision or in a penetrating graft may induce a graft detachment.

   *Tip*: Adjust the graft size and decenter the graft away from bulking stromal areas [37].
4. Peripheral graft curls/"inward folds" may spring off the posterior corneal surface often producing a larger detachment than the area of the curl itself.

   *Tip*: Assure complete graft unfolding at the end of the surgery and confirm that the peripheral graft border is round and has no straight lines. The latter may indicate an inward fold. By repeated tapping on the outer corneal surface (the so-called bubble-bumping maneuver) over the area of the graft curl while the anterior chamber is filled with a movable air bubble, the air and fluid movement may open and completely unfold the graft [43, 44].
5. During air/fluid exchange or air/gas reduction from the anterior chamber, the DMEK graft may accidently detach either by an abrupt collapse of the anterior chamber, by directly injecting fluid near the graft edge, or by mechanically detaching it with the cannula.

   *Tip*: Perform this step carefully by aspirating the air slowly and refilling the chamber before it collapses. Do not inject the fluid towards the graft but rather downwards or to the sides of the paracentesis. Choose a paracentesis that is not covered by the DMEK graft.
6. At the end of the surgery, good pressurization is a key step to promote graft adhesion [43].

   *Tip:* Ensure good pressurization before the air bubble time, but also after the air/fluid exchange or tamponade reduction.

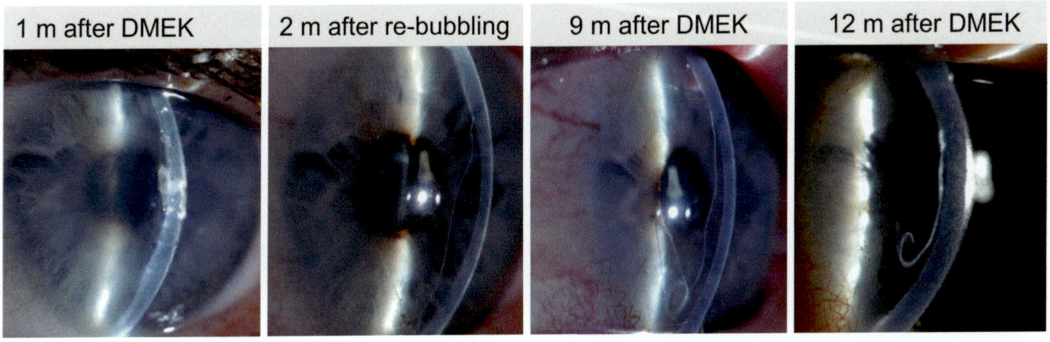


**Fig. 13.6** Slit-lamp images of an eye 1 and up to 12 months after DMEK. At 1 month postoperatively the cornea shows diffuse corneal edema. Two months after re-bubbling the cornea has cleared significantly but the graft is still detached. In the slit-lamp images at 9 and 12 months postoperatively the wrong graft orientation becomes obvious (graft is curling towards the iris instead of towards the corneal stroma

### 13.4.3 Postoperative Precautions

1. The patient is recommended to maintain a supine position for 1–2 days to support graft adhesion. Anterior chamber air is majorly resorbed within this time [43, 44].

   *Tip*: Stress this importance to the patient and make it "his/her part of a successful surgery."
2. Eye rubbing may cause graft displacement.

   *Tip*: Instruct the patient not to rub the eye.

Besides the above-mentioned points, the use of intraocular viscoelastics during DMEK was associated with graft detachments [50]. In contrast, a larger air bubble size at the termination of surgery may result in a lower detachment risk after DMEK [51, 52]. One may consider to cut the air tamponade time in uncomplicated Fuchs dystrophy eyes from 60 to 45 or 30 min since this did not result in more DMEK detachments [53]. An association of detachments and the use of DMEK grafts prepared from younger donors could not be confirmed consistently [54, 55]. Further, a technique modification in which the host DM or the incision were used for graft scaffolding has been recently suggested to reduce the risk of DMEK and PDEK detachments. An air pump-assisted technique has also been described to decrease graft detachment [56, 57].

## 13.5 Detached or Not Detached: Assessing the Graft Adherence Status

### 13.5.1 Slit-Lamp

Graft detachments can usually be diagnosed at the slit-lamp. In areas of failed corneal clearance and persistent corneal thickening and edema, a detached graft is often the underlying cause and can be seen in longitudinal section as a white line or structure at the posterior corneal surface protruding into the anterior chamber. Sometimes, the detachment is better visible when scanning it in longitudinal section while the patient is looking to the right or left.

Remember, that a detachment will not always catch your eye naturally, you need to search for it by examining the entire posterior cornea from limbus to limbus with the slit-light.

### 13.5.2 Anterior Segment Optical Coherence Tomography

Although most detachments can be seen at the slit-lamp, the Anterior Segment Optical Coherence Tomography (AS-OCT) has become indispensable in the management of post-EK eyes since it can record the dehiscence early and hereby document its evolution over time.

In eyes where the cornea is entirely swollen and cloudy it can be difficult to visualize the graft attachment status at the slit-lamp due to enhanced corneal reflection from the edema. In those cases, the AS-OCT has become essential to distinguish between an eye with a graft detachment and an eye with an attached graft but delayed endothelial cell function that is slowing corneal clearance (Fig. 13.7) [58]. Delayed corneal clearance is rare, but important to identify because re-bubbling such an eye could cause additional damage to the endothelial cell layer which could prolong corneal clearance even more. Hence, a detached graft may require repeat intracameral air injection if no clearance follows in the coming weeks and eyes with delayed cell function require patience by the patient and the surgeon [30, 58]. If the latter condition extends, for example, more than a month without showing any clearance, one may proceed with repeat keratoplasty to restore vision.

*Tip*

When evaluating graft dehiscence, pay attention to the orientation of the detached scroll at the graft edges. If the DM scroll is facing towards the corneal stroma, the graft is correctly oriented. If the orientation of the DM scroll is facing the iris, i.e., the endothelial side is facing the recipient stroma and not the anterior chamber, this indicates that the graft was positioned upside-down. Remember to always rule out an upside-down graft at the slit-lamp and/or the AS-OCT before indicating a repeat tamponade of the anterior chamber.

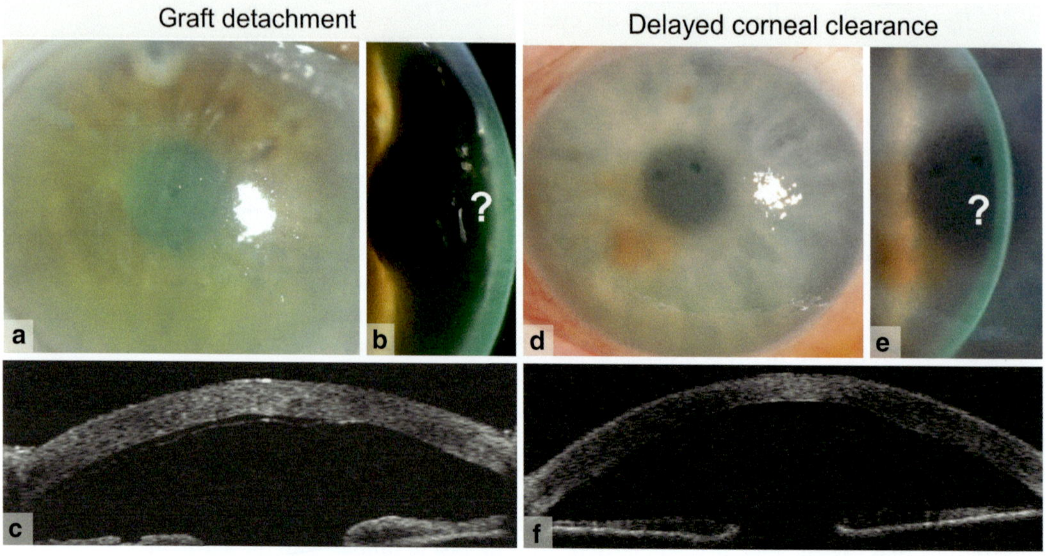


**Fig. 13.7** The figure displays slit-lamp (upper row) and AS-OCT images (lower row) of two eyes with diffuse corneal edema after DMEK. In patient 1 (left column), AS-OCT reveals that graft detachment is the reason for the corneal edema. If persistent, this patient may benefit from re-bubbling. In patient 2 (right column), the graft is completely attached, which may result from a delayed functioning of the transplanted endothelial cells. Await cornea clearance at least 4 weeks after DMEK. If no tendency of corneal clearance is visible, one may consider to proceed with repeat DMEK due to primary graft failure (Modified from Reference [58])

### 13.5.3 The Graft Is Detached: Re-Bubble or Not?

If a graft is detached, a repeat intracameral tamponade of air/gas or the so-called re-bubbling is widely accepted as the treatment of choice for visually significant graft detachments. Yet, there is no common guideline on the ideal indication and timing; hence, the number of re-bubblings reported from different groups ranges between 2.4 and 82% with a mean rate of 28.8% [59]. This diversity results from discrepancies in surgical experience but also from the subjective preferences of each surgeon that is based on the experience with spontaneous resolution of detachments or corneal clearance and outcomes after re-bubbling [10, 11, 15, 26–28, 31, 59–62].

While surgeons may agree that complete and large/major detachments, as well as grafts positioned upside-down, virtually always require re-intervention, the opinions differ when it comes to minor detachments (Fig. 13.8). For the latter, the decision whether to re-bubble or not, depends on the location, configuration, and the extent of the detachment [63].

## 13.6 Complete and Major Detachments

Every novel DMEK surgeon will face complete detachments during their learning curve. With increasing surgical experience these detachments fortunately become very rare as do partial major detachments (>1/3 of the graft surface area). Still, the latter will occur randomly, sometimes without any clear reason.

Complete detachments will not resolve spontaneously and will remain floating flat or as a roll in the host anterior chamber. If great cell damage is expected from the previous DMEK surgery, those grafts may need to be exchanged. However, if the previous surgery was smooth, re-unfolding and/or re-attaching the graft by a re-bubbling procedure may be preferred.

Note that complete and major detachments can also result from an upside-down positioning of the graft. Consider graft exchange or, to save the tissue, graft "flipping" or repositioning was described as a successful treatment option [60, 61].

Concerning major detachments, those corneas may show some corneal clearance tendency, but

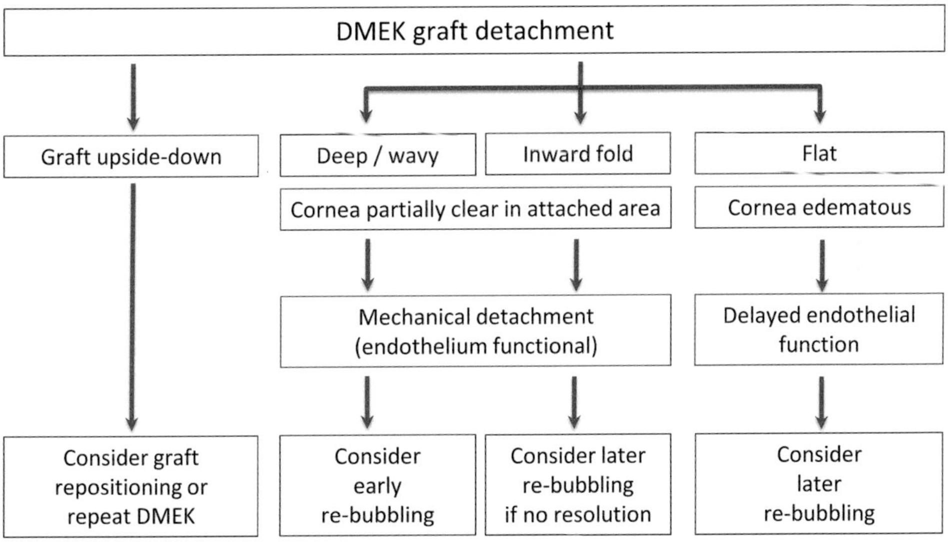


**Fig. 13.8** Decision tree for earlier and later re-bubbling depending on the graft detachment configuration and signs of functional endothelium (Modified from Reference [31])

this can take a couple of months and/or be incomplete. Because long-standing corneal edema has shown to cause fibrotic changes that can affect visual outcomes and because there is evidence that these eyes are at higher risk of decompensating sooner, one may consider timely re-bubbling [64–66].

Another reason for re-bubbling these eyes early is that these detachments often protrude far into the host anterior chamber adhering to surrounding ocular tissue, such as the iris. Hence, these detachments will not re-attach naturally and may therefore need early mechanical separation by re-injecting a tamponade beneath the detached graft to enhance corneal deswelling. The same applies to large detachments that origin from inward folds that will not always spontaneously unfold to allow graft re-attachment. Long-standing untreated detachments become stiff and immobile from fibrotic transformation and persist or shrink to peripheral graft folds [26, 30, 31, 63, 67].

## 13.7 Minor Detachments

In contrast to major graft detachments, minor detachments (≤1/3 of the graft surface area) are often asymptomatic. They frequently resolve by spontaneous re-attachment (Figs. 13.4 and 13.5) or show quick spontaneous clearance of the cornea overlying the persistent detachment. Subsequently, these eyes still obtain excellent visual acuity. Therefore, some surgeons are hesitant to rush into a re-bubbling that may induce endothelial cell damage [19, 31, 63]. On the other hand, if not treated and the edema does not subside, poorer visual outcomes due to fibrotic changes and scarring of the cornea may result [62, 65, 66]. Hence, the dilemma is: await natural resolution or re-injecting air/gas to accelerate graft attachment, corneal clearance, and visual recovery and prevent graft and corneal fibrosis which may also serve a better "cosmetic" result? [62, 65, 67] The answer would be easier if we could foresee which grafts will remain attached and which ones would progress in detaching.

*To predict whether a detachment may persist or extend,* the combined assessment of the postoperative AS-OCT at 1 h and 1 week has been suggested (Fig. 13.9): [26]

1. If the graft was completely attached at 1 week postoperatively, then this graft will remain stable and will most likely not detach anymore.
2. In case a detachment was found at 1 week postoperatively, the AS-OCT scan made at 1 h after surgery may be evaluated, and if this exam:
   (a) also shows the same or a smaller detachment, then spontaneous re-attachment is unlikely.
   (b) shows no detachment, then spontaneously re-attachment is likely, as the detachment at 1 week can be interpreted as a kind of healing process during corneal deswelling.

In clinics, the 1-day postoperative AS-OCT is more commonly performed than the 1-h AS-OCT. As a "rule of thumb," one could use the following strategy if a detachment is found at the 1-week follow-up: Unless the graft is progressing to a major detachment which would justify timely re-bubbling, the patient could be re-scheduled for shorter follow-up visits until 4–6 weeks after DMEK to see if corneal clearance and visual acuity are progressing and the detachment is regressing. The evolution of the detachment, the deturgescence of the cornea, and vision within these first 4–6 weeks will help taking the decision without putting the patient at an additional risk since re-bubbling procedures within this time frame have shown to still be successful though in case of later re-bubbling procedures beyond 4–6 weeks those grafts may become too rigid to allow complete unfolding. When in doubt or shorter follow-up visits cannot be scheduled for logistic reasons, one could proceed with early re-bubbling. Also, patients that possibly complain from ocular discomfort that could relate to the epithelial edema could benefit from earlier repeat tamponade injection. In general, it is also helpful to ask about the patient's impression because if satisfied and subjectively improving one could better postpone the intervention.

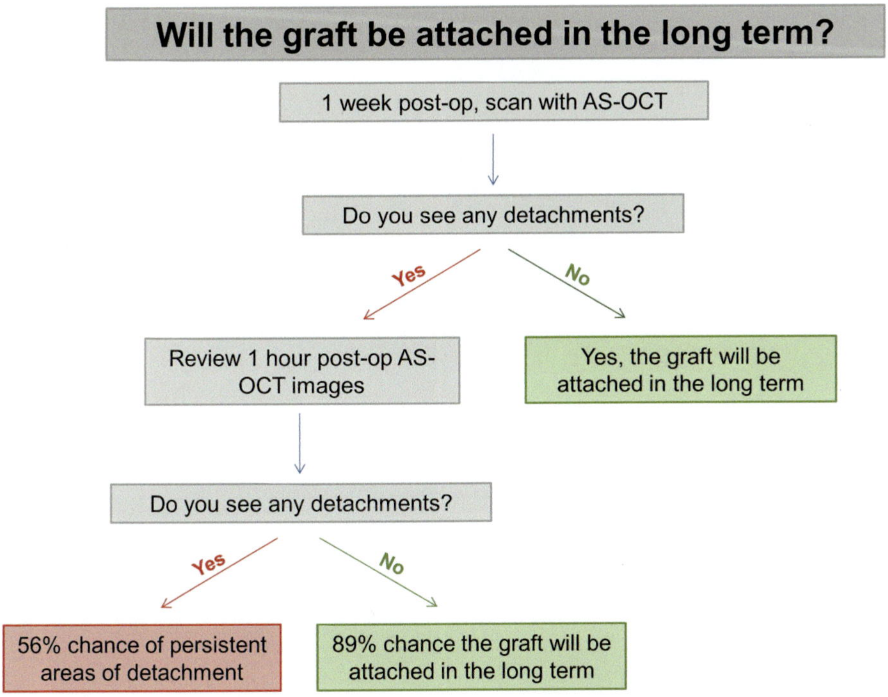


**Fig. 13.9** Prediction tree for estimating a graft's chances of being attached in the long term (taken from Reference [68])

Given that the graft is properly oriented, in our present experience, a single re-bubbling has proven to be sufficient to achieve graft adherence and remarkably quick resolution of the corneal edema already on day 1 after the re-bubbling. Only in very rare cases, also a second DMEK re-bubbling may be necessary. This concerns complex eyes with excessive corneal edema, eyes with DMEK under penetrating grafts (especially with posterior surface irregularities), and those that are difficult to pressurize, such as hypotonic eyes (aphakic eyes or eyes with glaucoma shunts). Patients with such comorbidities may be already prepared before DMEK that an early re-bubbling is more often required than in standard Fuchs endothelial dystrophy eyes and, thus may be considered as part of the primary surgery [69, 70].

## 13.8 The Re-bubbling Procedure

Repeat air injections can be performed under retrobulbar anesthesia, but topical and intracameral anesthesia may also be sufficient. Then, a previously performed paracentesis during DMEK can be re-opened or a new paracentesis can be created with a surgical knife through which a 30-gauge cannula is introduced to inject the air/gas underneath the graft. Subsequently, the tamponade is slightly enlarged and with repeated taps on the outer corneal surface a fluid wave is created to open residual mobile graft folds (the so-called bubble-bumping). If the graft has become rigid from fibrosis already (usually 1–2 months after DMEK), this maneuver may be less effective because of fibrotic changes of the donor tissue not allowing complete graft unfolding. In such cases, these rigid graft folds may be sandwiched between the corneal stroma and the tamponade by further enlarging the tamponade (Fig. 13.10) to pressurize the eye for about 30–60 min (in selected cases if applicable longer). Next, an air–liquid exchange follows to reduce the air bubble [63].

At first glance, the re-bubbling procedure does not appear surgically very demanding since it requires "only" a paracentesis through which the tamponade is injected and enlarged. However,

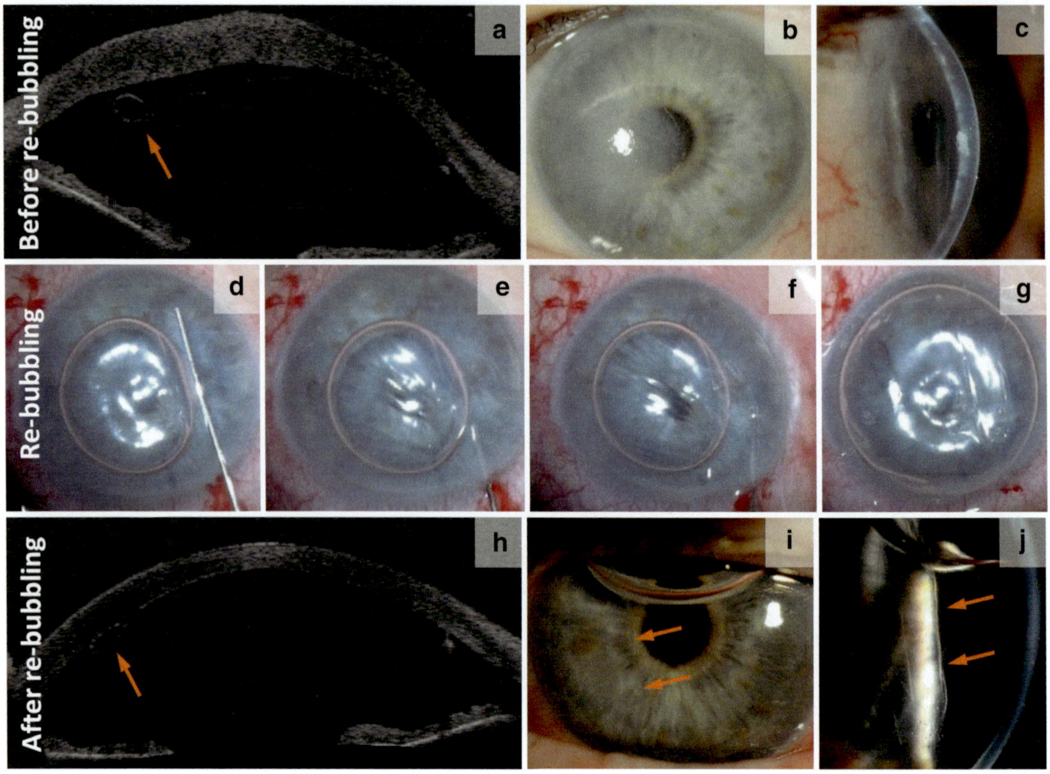


**Fig. 13.10** AS-OCT and intraoperative images of re-bubbling in an eye with a persistent graft fold. An attempt was made to unfold a peripheral scroll with persistent localized corneal edema 11 weeks after DMEK (**a**–**c**). During re-bubbling (**d**–**g**), unfolding was unsuccessful with indirect manipulation from the outer corneal surface (**d**) or direct cannula manipulation (**e** and **f**). Hence, the fold was sandwiched between the air bubble and stroma by a complete air tamponade (**g**). AS-OCT (**h**) and slit-lamp images (**i** and **j**) 1 day after re-bubbling. Note graft attachment and fast corneal clearing despite peripheral persistent fold (orange arrows) while the best-corrected visual acuity improved from 20/50 (0.4) to 20/20 (1.0). (Taken from Reference [63])

this seemingly easy procedure was reported to have been unsuccessful in some cases, was required repeatedly (up to four times) in the same patient or resulted in enlargement of a pre-existing detachment or new separation of attached graft areas, suggesting an additional technical complexity despite its apparent simplicity [5, 31, 60, 63].

Recently, we described two distinctly different approaches for effective re-bubbling (Figs. 13.11 and 13.12) [63]: First, with the "attached area approach," the air cannula is introduced into the anterior chamber in an area where the graft is attached (away from the detachment). This area often allows better visualization of the intraocular structures because this part of the cornea is already clear. On the other hand, this area holds the risk of a novel iatrogenic detachment of the graft by surgical manipulation. Second, with the "detached area approach" the air cannula is introduced into the anterior chamber in the area where the graft is already detached. The risk of a novel detachment may be lower; however, there is a higher chance of extending the detachment by inadvertently injecting air or fluid into the interface because of the poorer visualization caused by stromal edema obscuring the detached graft edge (Fig. 13.13). Hence, when deciding for the air injection, it is helpful to assess the following:

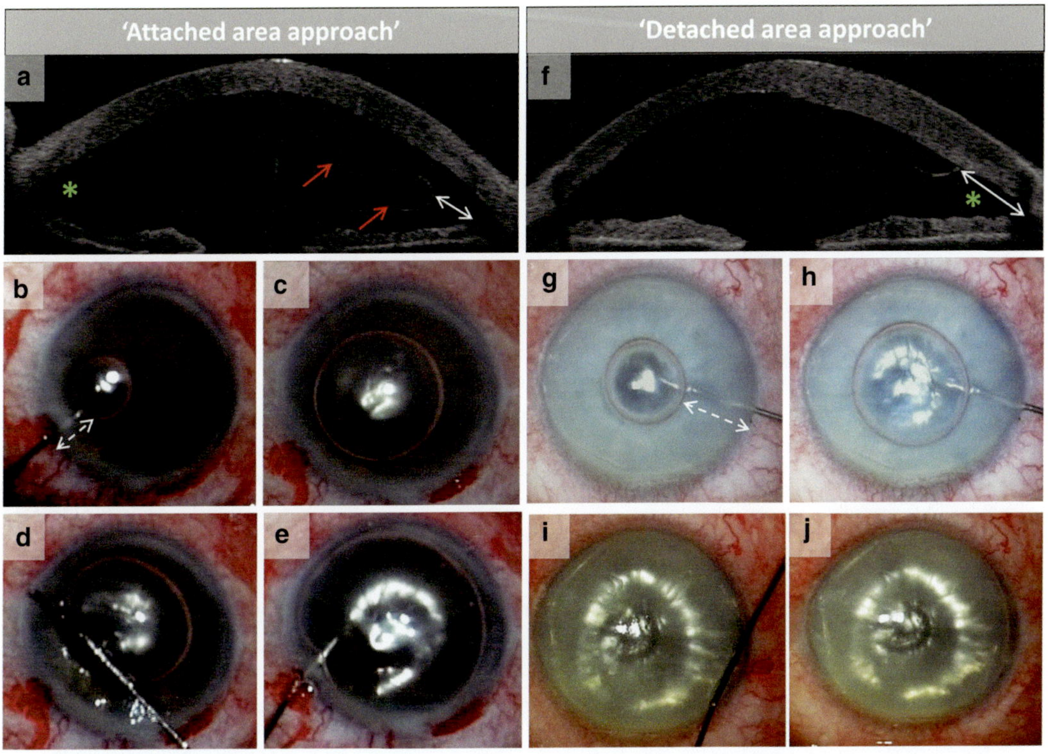


**Fig. 13.11** AS-OCT and intraoperative images of two eyes showing two different rebubbling approaches according to preoperative graft configuration. Images of rebubbling procedures using the attached area approach (**a–e**) and detached area approach (**f–j**). (**a**) The attached area approach may be safer (opposite to the detachment; green asterisk) in the event of a deep detachment (red arrows) in which there is limited space for the air cannula to pass underneath the detached graft (white arrow). Note that with this approach, the air may be injected at the entry site (**b**), after which the air bubble can be enlarged and "rolled" towards the detachment (**c** and **d**), before the anterior chamber is completely filled with air (**e**). The detached area approach (**f–j**) may be chosen when the detached graft edge is located more centrally (green asterisk, white arrow; **f**) so that the air cannula can be positioned underneath the detachment to inject the air (**g**), and filling the anterior chamber (**h**). Peripheral inward curls may be managed by bubble-bumping maneuvers (**i**) before the anterior chamber is completely filled with air (**j**) (Taken from Reference [63])

1. The visibility of the graft edges on both AS-OCT and biomicroscopy
2. The depth of the detachment, that is, the extension of the graft into the anterior chamber (graft–stroma distance)
3. The graft proximity to the limbus, that is, the space available for a surgical entry peripheral to the graft (graft–limbus distance)

Hence, to avoid further enlargement of a detachment, re-bubbling through the attached graft area may be favored with deep detachments when the graft edge reaches the peripheral cornea or when the cornea is very edematous and obscures graft visibility. On the other hand, re-bubbling through the detached graft area may be favored when the detachment is flat and the scroll is located more centrally, leaving room between the graft and iris for the air cannula to dive underneath the detachment. With the detached area approach, avoid injecting the air immediately at the entry site since the air may find the interface and result in an enlargement of the detachment. Both techniques can be suc-

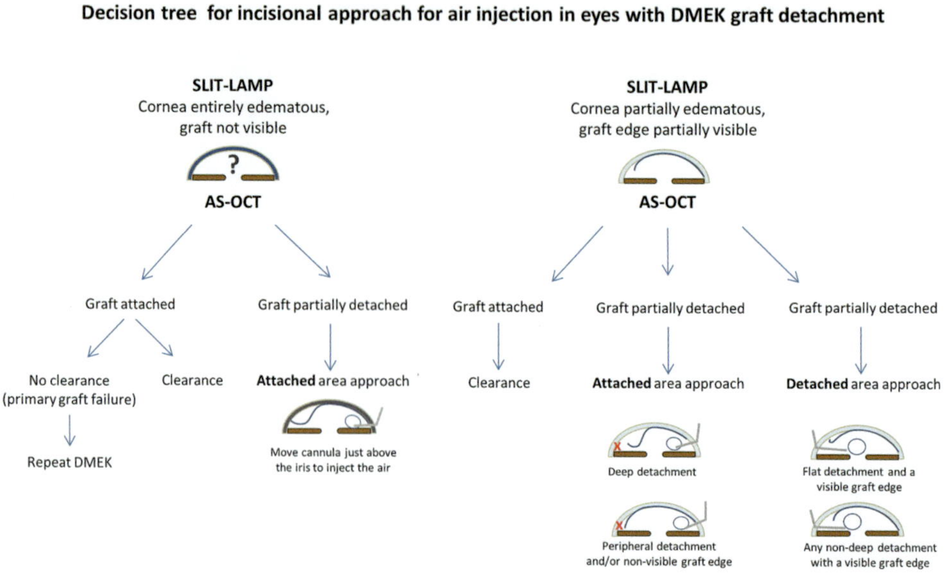


**Fig. 13.12** Decision tree for incisional approach for air injection in eyes with DMEK graft detachment (Taken from Reference [63])

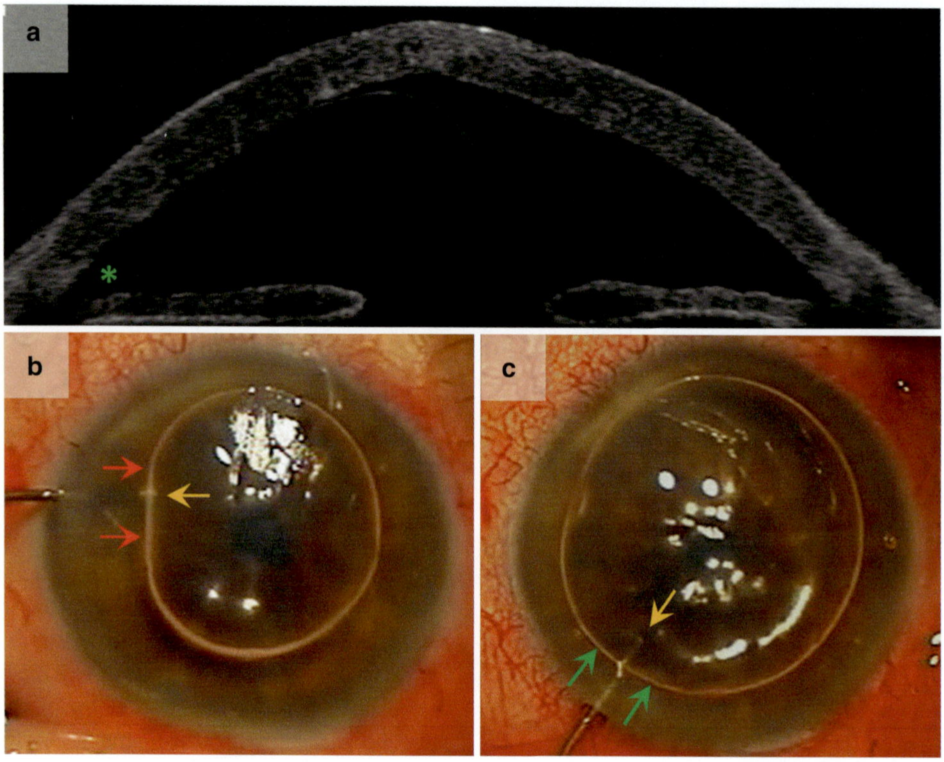


**Fig. 13.13** AS-OCT and intraoperative images of iatrogenically induced detachment at an attached area approach re-bubbling. Preoperative AS-OCT image (**a**) shows the graft configuration and attached area approach for re-bubbling (green asterisk). Intraoperative images (**b** and **c**) show how the graft is detaching with the introduction of the cannula into the anterior chamber. Note how the air bubble is deformed by the graft detachment (red arrows) while the cannula remains outside the air bubble (yellow arrow) (**b**). Enlargement of the air bubble from a new supero-temporal side-port (green arrows) with the tip of the cannula reaching within the air bubble (**c**) is performed to re-attach the graft across the cornea (Taken from Reference [63])

cessful without repeat staining of the graft with trypan blue and without performing venting incisions.

Pressurize the eye well at the end of the surgery. Except for very rare cases, a single re-bubbling is usually enough to achieve good graft adherence. For eyes with diffuse corneal edema, an intraoperative OCT may be useful to avoid re-bubbling complications.

### 13.8.1 Tips for a Successful Re-bubbling

1. Do not rush into a re-bubbling. You have time, unless the graft is majorly or completely detached.
2. Rule out an upside-down graft by checking the graft scrolls at the slit-lamp, AS-OCT or in possible surgical videos.
3. Novel minor detachments at 1 week postoperatively may be temporary and part of a healing process if the graft was previously attached at the first day after surgery, therefore consider not to re-bubble since they may resolve spontaneously.
4. Once the decision has been made to re-operate, plan your re-bubbling properly to avoid complications.
5. In selected cases (e.g., phakics), consider checking before re-bubbling if your iridotomy is still patent.
6. Remember to pressurize the eye well at the end of the re-bubbling.

## 13.9 Conclusion

Graft detachment remains a main complication after DMEK, but numbers are continuously decreasing. Knowing reasons for graft detachment is the primary approach to prevent them and reduce its numbers. Fortunately, many detachments can be temporary, and most detachments are benign, as they are typically small, and asymptomatic because they are located outside of the visual axis. If treatment is required, re-bubbling can be performed successfully in most cases with good visual outcomes although there is still no consensus on the best timing. A graft detachment is not an emergency, so assess the evolution during closer follow-up visits before rushing into a re-bubbling.

**Financial Disclosure** Dr. Baydoun is a consultant for DORC International/Dutch Ophthalmic USA.

## References

1. Baydoun L, Dapena I, Melles G. Evolution of posterior lamellar keratoplasty: PK—DLEK—DSEK/DSAEK—DMEK—DMET. In: Cursiefen C, Jun AS, editors. Current treatment options for Fuchs endothelial dystrophy. Berlin: Springer; 2016. p. 73–85.
2. Rodríguez-Calvo-de-Mora M, Quilendrino R, Ham L, et al. Clinical outcome of 500 consecutive cases undergoing descemet's membrane endothelial keratoplasty. Ophthalmology. 2015;122:464–70.
3. Peraza-Nieves J, Baydoun L, Dapena I, et al. Two-year clinical outcome of 500 consecutive cases undergoing descemet membrane endothelial keratoplasty. Cornea. 2017;36(6):655–60.
4. Baydoun L, Ham L, Borderie V, et al. Endothelial survival after descemet membrane endothelial keratoplasty: effect of surgical indication and graft adherence status. JAMA Ophthalmol. 2015;133:1277–85.
5. Tourtas T, Laaser K, Bachmann B, et al. Descemet membrane endothelial keratoplasty versus descemet stripping automated endothelial keratoplasty. Am J Ophthalmol. 2012;153:1082–90.
6. Guerra F, Anshu A, Price M, et al. Endothelial keratoplasty: fellow eyes comparison of descemet stripping automated endothelial keratoplasty and descemet membrane endothelial keratoplasty. Cornea. 2011;30:1382–6.
7. Schlögl A, Tourtas T, Kruse FE, et al. Long-term clinical outcome after descemet membrane endothelial keratoplasty. Am J Ophthalmol. 2016;169:218–26.
8. Ham L, Dapena I, Liarakos VS, et al. Mid-term results of descemet membrane endothelial keratoplasty (DMEK): 4 to 7 years clinical outcome. Am J Ophthalmol. 2016;171:113–21.
9. Price FW Jr, Feng MT, Price MO. Evolution of endothelial keratoplasty: where are we headed? Cornea. 2015;34:41–7.
10. Dirisamer M, Van Dijk K, Dapena I, et al. Prevention and management of graft detachment in descemet membrane endothelial keratoplasty. Arch Ophthalmol. 2012;130:280–29.
11. Monnereau C, Quilendrino R, Dapena I, et al. Multicenter study of descemet membrane endothelial keratoplasty: first case series of 18 surgeons. JAMA Ophthalmol. 2014;132:1192–8.

12. Price MO, Giebel AW, Fairchild KM, et al. Descemet's membrane endothelial keratoplasty: prospective multicenter study of visual and refractive outcomes and endothelial survival. Ophthalmology. 2009;116:2361–8.
13. Hamzaoglu EC, Straiko MD, Mayko ZM, et al. The first 100 eyes of standardized descemet stripping automated endothelial keratoplasty versus standardized descemet membrane endothelial keratoplasty. Ophthalmology. 2015;122:2193–9.
14. Cursiefen C. Descemet membrane endothelial keratoplasty: the taming of the shrew. JAMA Ophthalmol. 2013;131:88–9.
15. Dapena I, Ham L, Droutsas K, et al. Learning curve in descemet's membrane endothelial keratoplasty: first series of 135 consecutive cases. Ophthalmology. 2011;118:2147–54.
16. Busin M, Madi S, Santorum P, Scorcia V, Beltz J. Ultrathin descemet's stripping automated endothelial keratoplasty with the microkeratome double-pass technique: two-year outcomes. Ophthalmology. 2013;120(6):1186–94.
17. Agarwal A, Dua HS, Narang P, Kumar DA, Agarwal A, Jacob S, Agarwal A, Gupta A. Pre-descemet's endothelial keratoplasty (PDEK). Br J Ophthalmol. 2014;98(9):1181–5.
18. Price MO, Price FW Jr. Descemet's stripping with endothelial keratoplasty: comparative outcomes with microkeratome-dissected and manually dissected donor tissue. Ophthalmology. 2006;113(11):1936–42.
19. Feng MT, Price MO, Miller JM, et al. Air reinjection and endothelial cell density in descemet membrane endothelial keratoplasty: five-year follow-up. J Cataract Refract Surg. 2014;40:1116–21.
20. Güell JL, Morral M, Gris O, Elies D, Manero F. Comparison of sulfur hexafluoride 20% versus air tamponade in descemet membrane endothelial keratoplasty. Ophthalmology. 2015;122:1757–64.
21. Botsford B, Vedana G, Cope L, Yiu SC, Jun AS. Comparison of 20% sulfur hexafluoride with air for intraocular tamponade in descemet membrane endothelial keratoplasty (DMEK). Arq Bras Oftalmol. 2016;79:299–302.
22. Schaub F, Enders P, Snijders K, Schrittenlocher S, Siebelmann S, Heindl LM, et al. One-year outcome after descemet membrane endothelial keratoplasty (DMEK) comparing sulfur hexafluoride (SF 6) 20% versus 100% air for anterior chamber tamponade. Br J Ophthalmol. 2017;101:902–8.
23. Oellerich S, Baydoun L, Peraza-Nieves J, Ilyas A, Frank L, Binder PS, Melles GRJ. Multicenter study of 6-month clinical outcomes after descemet membrane endothelial keratoplasty. Cornea. 2017;36(12):1467–76.
24. Siebelmann S, Lopez Ramos S, Scholz P, Matthaei M, Schrittenlocher S, Heindl LM, Bachmann B, Cursiefen C. Graft detachment pattern after descemet membrane endothelial keratoplasty comparing air versus 20% SF6 tamponade. Cornea. 2018;37(7):834–9.
25. Terry MA, Straiko MD, Veldman PB, Talajic JC, VanZyl C, Sales CS, Mayko ZM. Standardized DMEK technique: reducing complications using prestripped tissue, novel glass injector, and sulfur hexafluoride (SF6) gas. Cornea. 2015;34:845–52.
26. Yeh RY, Quilendrino R, Musa FU, Liarakos VS, Dapena I, Melles GR. Predictive value of optical coherence tomography in graft attachment after descemet's membrane endothelial keratoplasty. Ophthalmology. 2013;120(2):240–5.
27. Dirisamer M, Dapena I, Ham L, van Dijk K, Oganes O, Frank LE, van der Wees J, Melles GR. Patterns of corneal endothelialization and corneal clearance after descemet membrane endothelial keratoplasty for fuchs endothelial dystrophy. Am J Ophthalmol. 2011;152(4):543–555.e1.
28. Dirisamer M, Yeh RY, van Dijk K, Ham L, Dapena I, Melles GR. Recipient endothelium may relate to corneal clearance in descemet membrane endothelial transfer. Am J Ophthalmol. 2012;154(2):290–296.e1.
29. Birbal RS, Parker J, Dirisamer M, Janićijević A, Baydoun L, Dapena I, Melles GRJ. Descemet membrane endothelial transfer: ultimate outcome. Cornea. 2018;37(2):141–4.
30. Dirisamer M, van Dijk K, Dapena I, Ham L, Oganes O, Frank LE, Melles GR. Prevention and management of graft detachment in descemet membrane endothelial keratoplasty. Arch Ophthalmol. 2012;130(3):280–91.
31. Gerber-Hollbach N, Baydoun L, López EF, Frank LE, Dapena I, Liarakos VS, Schaal SC, Ham L, Oellerich S, Melles GRJ. Clinical outcome of rebubbling for graft detachment after descemet membrane endothelial keratoplasty. Cornea. 2017;36(7):771–6.
32. Groeneveld-van Beek EA, Lie JT, Van der Wees J, et al. Standardized "no-touch" donor tissue preparation for DALK and DMEK: harvesting undamaged anterior and posterior donor transplants from the same donor cornea. Acta Ophthalmol. 2013;91:145–50.
33. Lie JT, Birbal R, Ham L, et al. Donor tissue preparation for descemet membrane endothelial keratoplasty. J Cataract Refract Surg. 2008;34:1578–83.
34. Kruse FE, Laaser K, Cursiefen C, Heindl LM, Schlötzer-Schrehardt U, Riss S, Bachmann BO. A stepwise approach to donor preparation and insertion increases safety and outcome of descemet membrane endothelial keratoplasty. Cornea. 2011;30(5):580–7.
35. Livny E, Groeneveld-van Beek EA, Lie JT, Mangundap KM, Bruinsma M, Birbal RS, van der Wees J, Melles GRJ. Minimizing graft preparation failure in descemet membrane endothelial keratoplasty. Cornea. 2017;36(12):1452–7.
36. Ćirković A, Schlötzer-Schrehardt U, Weller JM, Kruse FE, Tourtas T. Clinical and ultrastructural characteristics of graft failure in DMEK: 1-year results after repeat DMEK. Cornea. 2015;34: 11–7.

37. Quilendrino R, Rodriguez-Calvo de Mora M, Baydoun L, Ham L, van Dijk K, Dapena I, Oellerich S, Melles GRJ. Prevention and management of descemet membrane endothelial keratoplasty complications. Cornea. 2017;36(9):1089–95.
38. Laaser K, Bachmann BO, Horn FK, Schlötzer-Schrehardt U, Cursiefen C, Kruse FE. Donor tissue culture conditions and outcome after descemet membrane endothelial keratoplasty. Am J Ophthalmol. 2011;151:1007–18.
39. Weller JM, Schlötzer-Schrehardt U, Kruse FE, et al. Splitting of the recipient's descemet membrane in descemet membrane endothelial keratoplasty—ultrastructure and clinical relevance. Am J Ophthalmol. 2016;172:1–6.
40. Müller TM, Verdijk RM, Lavy I, et al. Histopathologic features of descemet membrane endothelial keratoplasty graft remnants, folds, and detachments. Ophthalmology. 2016;123:2489–97.
41. Dapena I, Ham L, Moutsouris K, et al. Incidence of recipient Descemet membrane remnants at the donor-to-stromal interface after descemetorhexis in endothelial keratoplasty. Br J Ophthalmol. 2010;94:1689–90.
42. Brockmann T, Brockmann C, Maier A-K, et al. Clinicopathology of graft detachment after descemet's membrane endothelial keratoplasty. Acta Ophthalmol. 2014;92:e556–61.
43. Dapena I, Moutsouris K, Droutsas K, et al. Standardized 'no touch' technique for descemet's membrane endothelial keratoplasty (DMEK). Arch Ophthalmol. 2011;129:88–94.
44. Liarakos VS, Dapena I, Ham L, et al. Intraocular graft unfolding techniques in descemet membrane endothelial keratoplasty. JAMA Ophthalmol. 2013;131:29–35.
45. Bachmann BO, Laaser K, Cursiefen C, et al. A method to confirm correct orientation of descemet membrane during descemet membrane endothelial keratoplasty. Am J Ophthalmol. 2010;149:922.
46. Bhogal M, Maurino V, Allan BD. Use of a single peripheral triangular mark to ensure correct graft orientation in descemet membrane endothelial keratoplasty. J Cataract Refract Surg. 2015;41:2022–4.
47. Veldman PB, Dye PK, Holiman JD, et al. The S-stamp in descemet membrane endothelial keratoplasty safely eliminates upside-down graft implantation. Ophthalmology. 2016;123:161–4.
48. Newman LR, Tran KD, Odell K, Dye PK, Galloway J, Sales CS, Straiko MD, Terry MA. Minimizing endothelial cell loss caused by orientation stamps on preloaded descemet membrane endothelial keratoplasty grafts. Cornea. 2019;38(2):233–7.
49. Saad A, Guilbert E, Grise-Dulac A, et al. Intraoperative OCT-assisted DMEK: 14 consecutive cases. Cornea. 2015;34:802–7.
50. Chaurasia S, Price FW Jr, Gunderson L, Price MO. Descemet's membrane endothelial keratoplasty: clinical results of single versus triple procedures (combined with cataract surgery). Ophthalmology. 2014;121(2):454–8.
51. Leon P, Parekh M, Nahum Y, et al. Factors associated with early graft detachment in primary descemet membrane endothelial keratoplasty. Am J Ophthalmol. 2018;187:117–24.
52. Ćirković A, Beck C, Weller JM, Kruse FE, Tourtas T. Anterior chamber air bubble to achieve graft attachment after DMEK: is bigger always better? Cornea. 2016;35:482–5.
53. Santander-García D, Peraza-Nieves J, Müller TM, Gerber-Hollbach N, Baydoun L, Liarakos VS, Dapena I, Oellerich S, Van Dijk K, Melles GRJ. Influence of intraoperative air tamponade time on graft adherence in descemet membrane endothelial keratoplasty. Cornea. 2019;38(2):166–72.
54. Rodríguez-Calvo-de-Mora M, Groeneveld-Van Beek EA, Frank LE, et al. Association between graft storage time and donor age with endothelial cell density and graft adherence after descemet membrane endothelial keratoplasty. JAMA Ophthalmol. 2016;134:91–4.
55. Sales CS, Terry MA, Veldman PB, Mayko ZM, Straiko MD. Relationship between tissue unscrolling time and endothelial cell loss. Cornea. 2016;35:471–6.
56. Jacob S. Use of pressurized air infusion for pre descemet's endothelial keratoplasty (PDEK)—the air pump assisted PDEK technique. Open Ophthalmol J. 2018;12:175–18.
57. Jacob S, Narasimhan S, Agarwal A, Agarwal A, A I S. Air pump-assisted graft centration, graft edge unfolding, and graft uncreasing in young donor graft pre-descemet endothelial keratoplasty. Cornea. 2017;36(8):1009–13.
58. Moutsouris K, Dapena I, Ham L, Balachandran C, Oellerich S, Melles GR. Optical coherence tomography, Scheimpflug imaging, and slit-lamp biomicroscopy in the early detection of graft detachment after descemet membrane endothelial keratoplasty. Cornea. 2011;30(12):1369–75.
59. Deng SX, Lee WB, Hammersmith KM, Kuo AN, Li JY, Shen JF, Weikert MP, Shtein RM. Descemet membrane endothelial keratoplasty: safety and outcomes: a report by the American Academy of Ophthalmology. Ophthalmology. 2018;125(2):295–310.
60. Price MO, Giebel AW, Fairchild KM, Price FW Jr. Descemet's membrane endothelial keratoplasty: prospective multicenter study of visual and refractive outcomes and endothelial survival. Ophthalmology. 2009;116:2361–8.
61. Dragnea DC, Nobacht S, Gericke A, Parker J, Oellerich S, Ham L, Melles GRJ. Postoperative repositioning of inverted descemet membrane endothelial keratoplasty grafts. Cornea. 2019;38(2):162–5.
62. Price FW Jr, Price MO. To intervene or not to intervene: that is the question. Ophthalmology. 2015;122(1):6–7.
63. Fernández López E, Baydoun L, Gerber-Hollbach N, Dapena I, Liarakos VS, Ham L, et al. Rebubbling

techniques for graft detachment after descemet membrane endothelial keratoplasty. Cornea. 2016;35:759–64.
64. Ham L, Dapena I, Liarakos VS, Baydoun L, van Dijk K, Ilyas A, Oellerich S, Melles GR. Midterm results of descemet membrane endothelial keratoplasty: 4 to 7 years clinical outcome. Am J Ophthalmol. 2016;171:113–21.
65. Baydoun L, van Dijk K, Dapena I, Musa FU, Liarakos VS, Ham L, Melles GR. Repeat descemet membrane endothelial keratoplasty after complicated primary descemet membrane endothelial keratoplasty. Ophthalmology. 2015;122: 8–16.
66. Van Dijk K, Parker J, Liarakos VS, Ham L, Frank LE, Melles GRJ. Incidence of irregular astigmatism eligible for contact lens fitting after descemet membrane endothelial keratoplasty. J Cataract Refract Surg. 2013;39:1036–46.
67. Müller TM, Verdijk RM, Lavy I, Bruinsma M, Parker J, Binder PS, Melles GR. Histopathologic features of descemet membrane endothelial keratoplasty graft remnants, folds, and detachments. Ophthalmology. 2016;123(12):2489–97.
68. Melles & Dapena. How to get started with Standardized 'no-touch' DMEK. Netherlands Institue for Innovative Ocular Surgery 2014.
69. Birbal RS, Baydoun L, Ham L, et al. Effect of surgical indication and preoperative lens status on descemet membrane endothelial keratoplasty outcomes. Am J Ophthalmol. 2020;212:79. [Epub ahead of print].
70. Parker J, Quilendrino R, Yeh R-Y, Naveiras M, Dirisamer M. DMEK complications. In: Melles and Dapena, editors. How to get started with DMEK. 2014.

# Complications in PDEK 14

Soosan Jacob

## 14.1 Complications in Harvesting Graft

The PDEK graft is created by injecting air into a corneo-scleral button in order to try and obtain a type 1 Big Bubble (BB). The Type 1 BB was first described by Harminder Dua [1–8] and it corresponds to a cleavage plane being formed between the pre-Descemet's layer (PDL), Descemet's membrane (DM), and endothelium on one side and the stroma on the other side. Complications can occur while preparing the PDEK graft [9–11].

## 14.2 No Big Bubble

Sometimes, injection of air into the corneo-scleral graft results in only emphysema and not the development of a BB. In this case, the needle is connected to a 1 mL syringe filled with Trypan blue stained BSS and advanced to a central, superficial plane. Injection of the BSS often yields a Type 1 BB, which can then be gently enlarged further with BSS or Trypan blue in the same manner. The advantage of using Trypan blue is that it allows better visibility of the graft and also stains the graft at the same time (Fig. 14.1).

S. Jacob (✉)
Dr. Agarwal's Refractive and Cornea Foundation, Chennai, India

Dr. Agarwal's Eye Hospital and Eye Research Centre, Chennai, India



S. Jacob (ed.), *Mastering DMEK and PDEK*, https://doi.org/10.1007/978-981-97-3469-6_14

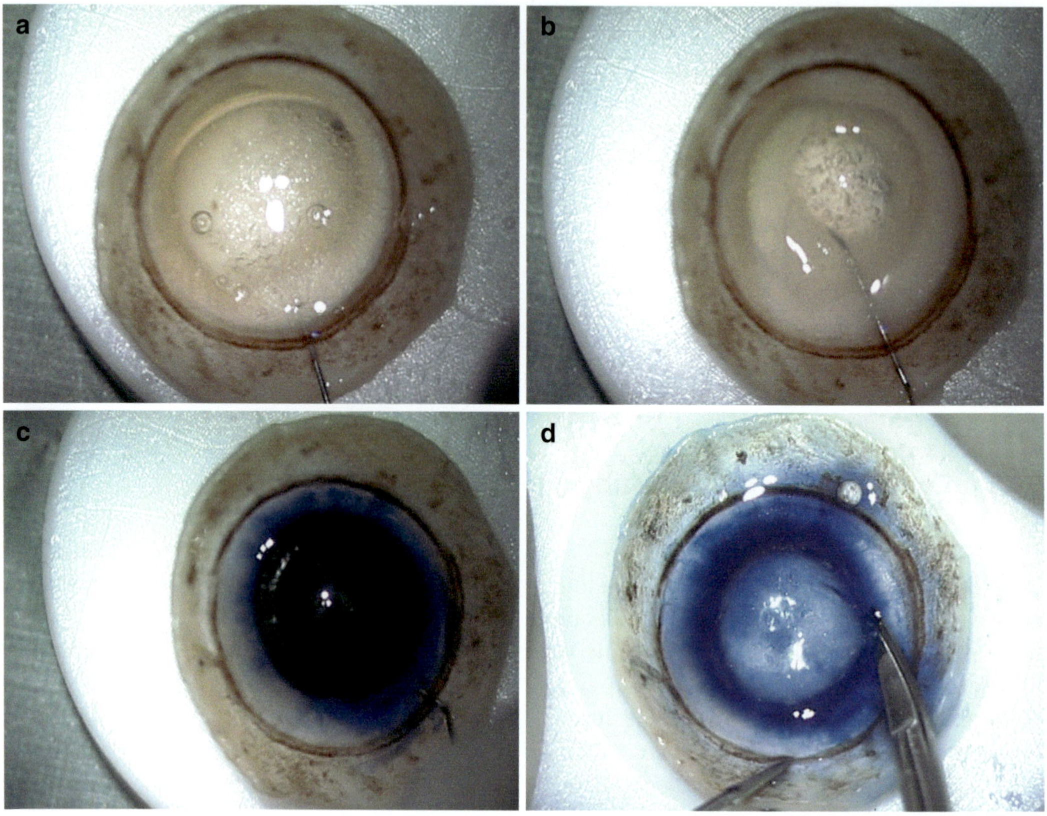


**Fig. 14.1** (**a**) Only tissue emphysema and no bubble after injecting air; (**b**) Big bubble initiated with storage medium; (**c**) Big bubble enlarged with Trypan blue; (**d**) Big bubble cut with Vannas scissors

## 14.3 Small Big Bubble

If the initial BB from air injection is small, it can be enlarged by slowly further injecting air. Alternately, the needle can be connected to a 1 mL syringe filled with BSS or Trypan blue and advanced to enter the BB. Injecting the fluid into the BB results in a slow, controlled expansion to the desired size. Use of Trypan blue has the advantage of both staining the bubble and allowing more accurate measurement of the size of the bubble with a caliper. Note: The caliper is only held above the BB and not touching it while measuring in order to avoid endothelial cell loss. The actual graft size obtained is usually larger than estimated with the caliper because of the dome shape of the graft. An estimated size of 7.5 mm while dome shaped often results in a graft of about 8 mm which is generally sufficient in most cases. However, larger dome-shaped BBs are also frequently obtained resulting in graft sizes of up to 8.5–9 mm (Fig. 14.2).

If despite all efforts a small Type 1 BB is formed, a larger hybrid PDEK-DMEK graft may be harvested by deflating the Type 1 BB, scoring the DM along three sides, peeling it towards the center up to the margin of the Type 1 BB, then using a trephine of the desired size to cut the graft in a manner so that the entire PDEK graft together with part of the DM on the sides is harvested. This graft has advantage of a bigger size but needs to be handled with greater care as there are areas where only the DM is there. In such areas, it may therefore behave like a DMEK graft in terms of difficulty in graft handling.

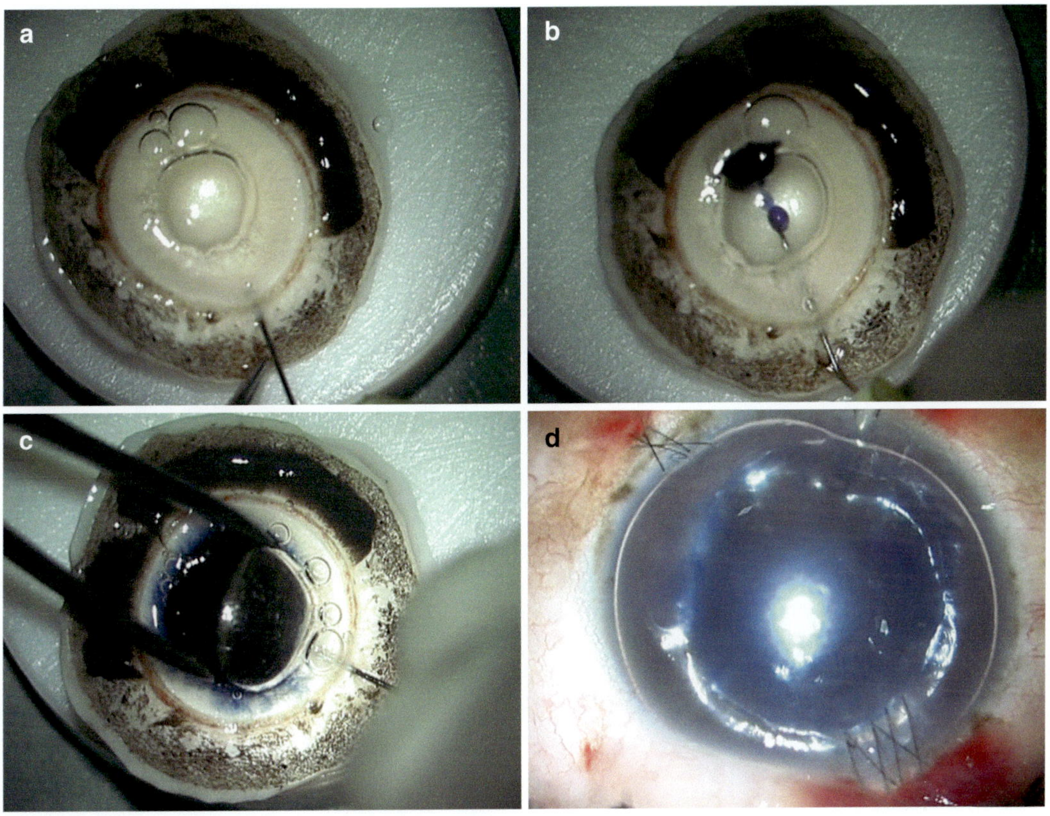


**Fig. 14.2** (**a**) Small big bubble; (**b**) Needle advanced into BB; (**c**) BB enlarged with Trypan blue to 7.5 mm; (**d**) The graft measures 8 mm in the unscrolled floated position

## 14.4 Type Two Big Bubble

A type 2 BB may form instead of a Type 1 if the air passes into a plane between the Descemet's membrane and the pre-Descemet's layer. A Type 2 BB corresponds to a DMEK graft. Its formation can be prevented to some extent by the Soper technique where the DM is scored on the periphery of the corneal rim in order to allow any air that goes into the type 2 bubble plane to just escape through the breaks in the DM instead of lifting up the DM. It can also be avoided by using the PDEK clamp [9]. The author's personal technique is to put small punctures on the endothelial side around the edge of the graft and within the limbus in order to still allow air to escape, thus avoiding a DMEK graft while also avoiding the DM from being dragged a may potentially happen with the Soper technique.

**Proceed as DMEK:** If despite all precautions, a Type 2 BB is formed, the bubble is expanded gently with either air or Trypan blue. Once it is of adequate size, the bubble is opened at the edge with a 15-degree blade and the fluid aspirated. It is then cut with the desired size trephine. Alternately if stamping is desired, it can be cut with the Vannas along the periphery leaving a hinge, following which it is reflected carefully, stamped (following the usual procedure), laid back and trephined (Fig. 14.3).

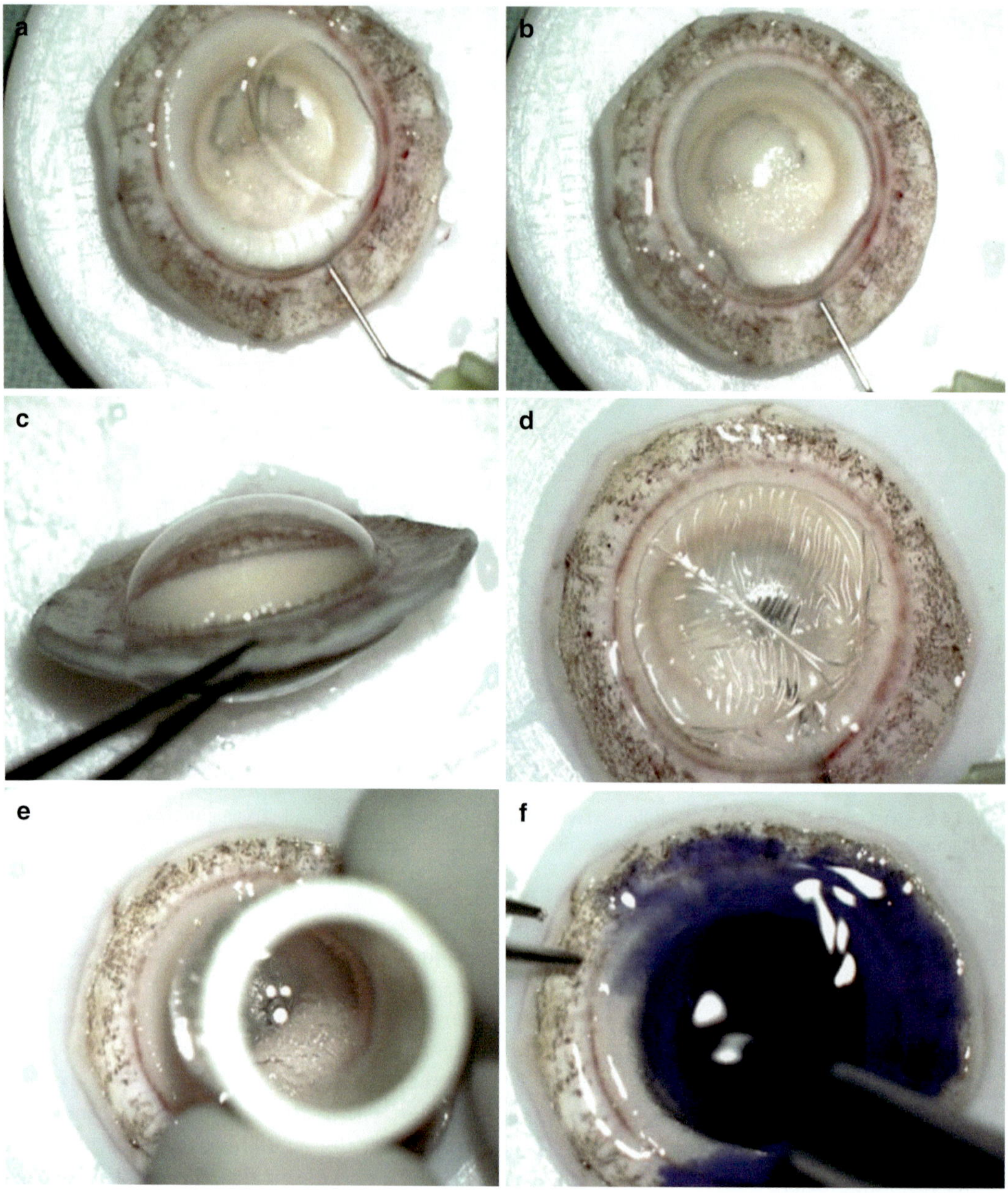


**Fig. 14.3** (**a**) Type 2 BB being formed; (**b**) Type 2 BB expanded; (**c**) Type 2 BB seen fully expanded; (**d**) Bubble is opened and cut along the edge; (**e**) The graft is punched to get a DMEK graft; (**f**) The graft is stained with Trypan blue

## 14.5 Type Three Big Bubble

**Proceed as PDEK:** If the Type 2 is small and only at the extreme periphery and has just started to be formed, the wall of the Type 2 bubble is cut open at the edge with a 15-degree blade Air leakage is avoided by using a blunt instrument like the closed arms of a McPherson forceps to separate the Type 2 from the Type 1 by pressing down on the Type 2 in the periphery and air or Trypan blue is gently injected to preferentially expand the Type 1 BB. Once it is of adequate size, it is cut with Vannas scissors, taking care to include the separated DM in the

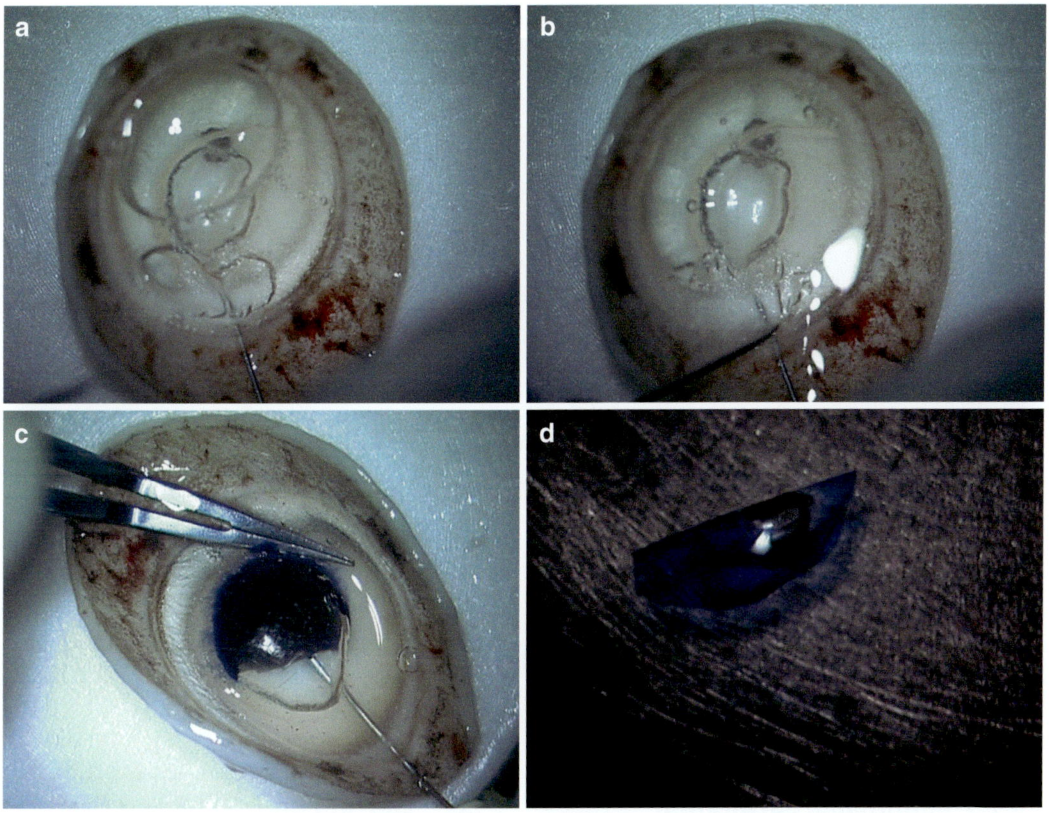


**Fig. 14.4** (**a**) Type 3 BB; (**b**) Entry made into wall of Type 2 BB to allow trapped air to escape and to prevent further enlargement of Type 2 BB; (**c**) Type 1 BB enlarged; (**d**) PDEK graft with split layers at one edge obtained

periphery. The surgery is then continued as PDEK (Fig. 14.4).

**Proceed as DMEK:** If the Type 2 BB is large, the bubble is further expanded gently with either air or Trypan blue. Once it is of adequate size, the bubble is opened at the edge with a 15-degree blade and fluid or air aspirated from within the bubble. It is then spread out and cut with the desired size trephine. Alternately if stamping is desired, it can be cut with the Vannas along the periphery leaving a hinge, following which it is reflected, stamped (following the usual procedure), laid back, and trephined.

## 14.6 Burst Bubble

Excessive air pressure can lead to a bursting of the bubble, both Types 1 and 2. In the event that the bubble bursts from the side, the graft can still be used. However, if it has burst from the center, it has to be discarded (Fig. 14.5).

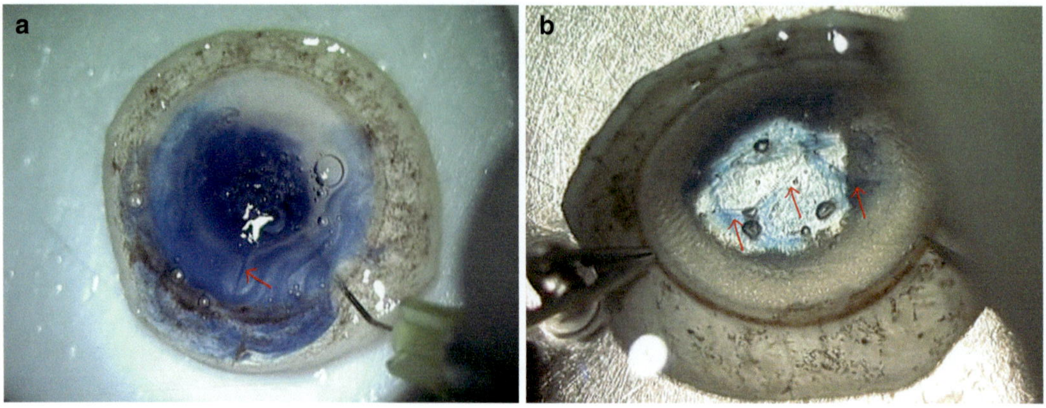


**Fig. 14.5** (**a**) BB burst at the edge can still be harvested and used; (**b**) BB burst through the center cannot be used

## 14.7 Needle Perforation

### 14.7.1 Epithelial Perforation

In this case, it is easy to just withdraw the needle, reinsert at a more superficial plane, and reinject.

### 14.7.2 Endothelial Perforation

With a perforation to the periphery, the needle is withdrawn and then reinserted from the opposite side and bubble creation proceeded with. The previous perforation generally does not interfere with bubble creation.

With perforation at the center, bubble creation can become challenging since any air or fluid injected will keep leaking out through the endothelial perforation. In this case, a DMEK or DSAEK may be proceeded with. An alternative is to use viscoelastic for bubble creation, taking care once the graft is created and cut that the viscoelastic is washed off so as to prevent it from interfering with graft adhesion. Endothelial perforation can be prevented by not advancing the graft too far into the cornea before injecting air. A peripheral location of the needle is sufficient to create the BB.

## 14.8 Getting an Exact Sized Graft

This is important, especially in very small eyes or while doing PDEK for a failed penetrating keratoplasty. In this case, after expanding the bubble with Trypan blue, the dye is aspirated out again, thus collapsing the bubble completely. A trephine of the desired dimension is then used to make a partial thickness cut on the graft making sure to remain within the stained edges. The graft is then gently lifted up and placed in storage medium. In case of any uncut edge, it can be cut with a Vannas scissor (Fig. 14.6).

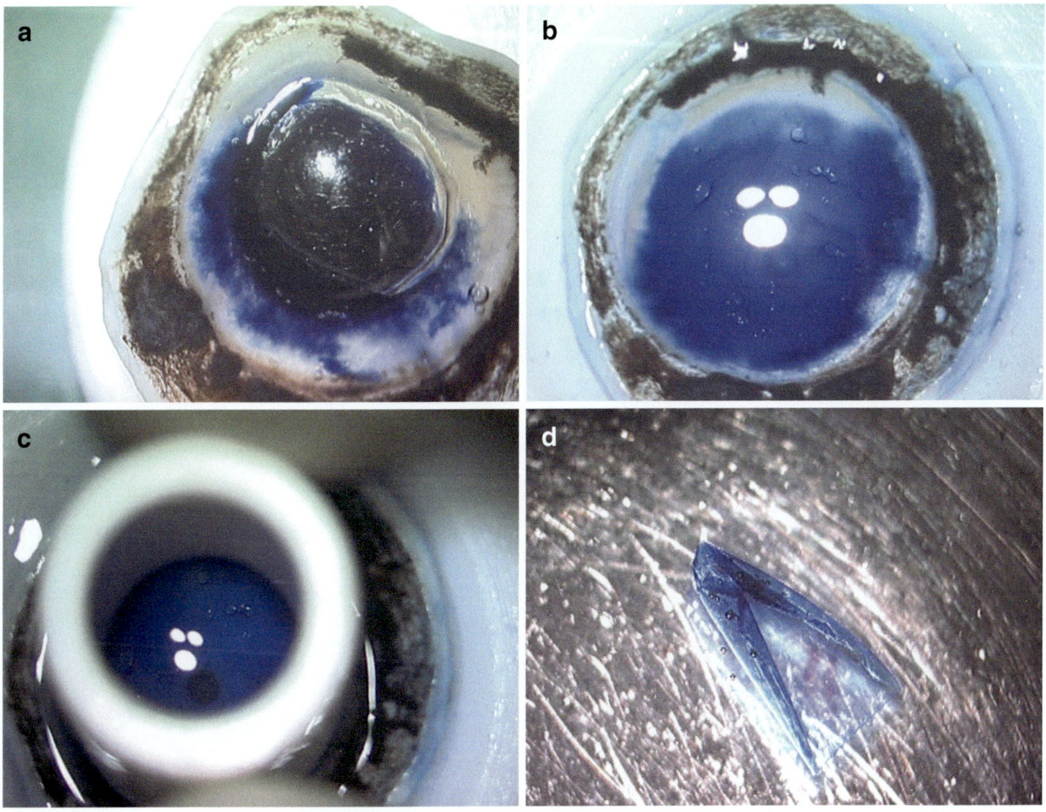

**Fig. 14.6** (**a**) BB created; (**b**) BB aspirated and collapsed; (**c**) Partial thickness trephination. The graft is peeled partially and stamped with irreversible letter; (**d**) Exactly sized PDEK graft harvested. The stamped mark is seen

## 14.9 Intra- and Postoperative Complications

Many of the intra- and postoperative complications are common with that of DMEK and these can be referred to in the DMEK chapter. The PDEK graft being tough and resistant to tear, the following few complications can occur which can however be handled differently from a DMEK graft:

## 14.10 Difficulty in Unscrolling

This can be handled in a similar manner to DMEK. However, complete graft unfolding is not a must in PDEK and extreme edge folds are acceptable. These edge folds can be opened using the air pump-assisted PDEK technique described by the author (SJ) (Fig. 14.7) [10, 11].

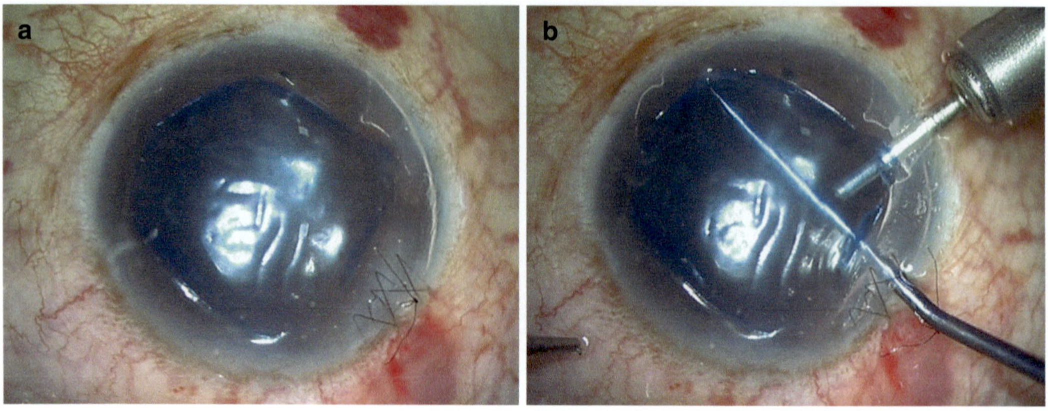


**Fig. 14.7** (**a**) Edge folds seen; (**b**) Edge folds being opened using air pump-assisted PDEK

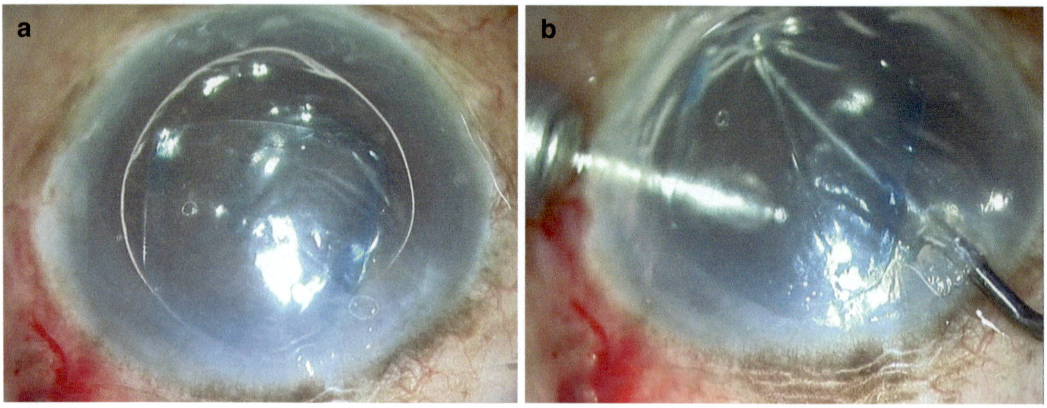


**Fig. 14.8** (**a**) Graft floated up is decentered; (**b**) Decentered graft is recentered using air pump-assisted technique described by the author, SJ

## 14.11 Difficulty in Centering

This too can be handled in a similar manner to DMEK. Again, complete centration prior to floating is not a must in PDEK and a decentered graft can easily be opened and centered using the air pump-assisted PDEK technique (Fig. 14.8) [10, 11].

## 14.12 Creases in the Graft

Graft can easily be uncreased by using a reverse Sinskey and pulling the graft in opposite directions to uncrease it (Fig. 14.9) [10, 11].

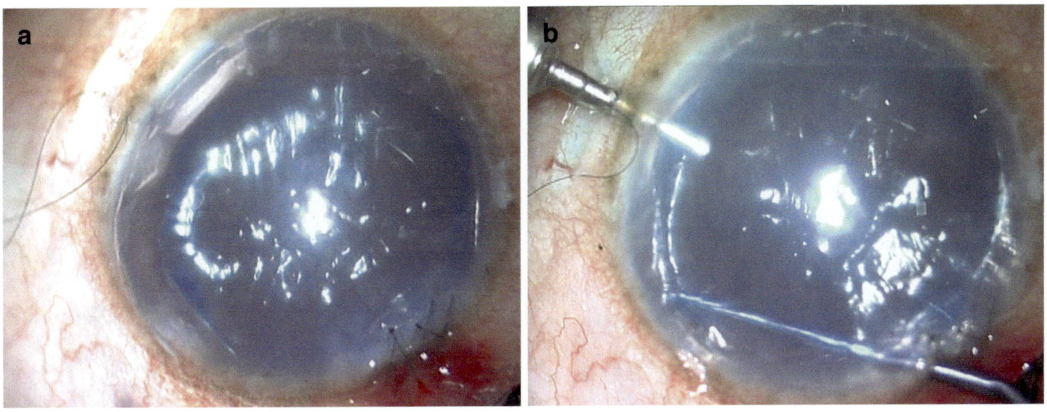


**Fig. 14.9** (**a**) Creases seen in the graft; (**b**) Graft is uncreased using air pump-assisted technique

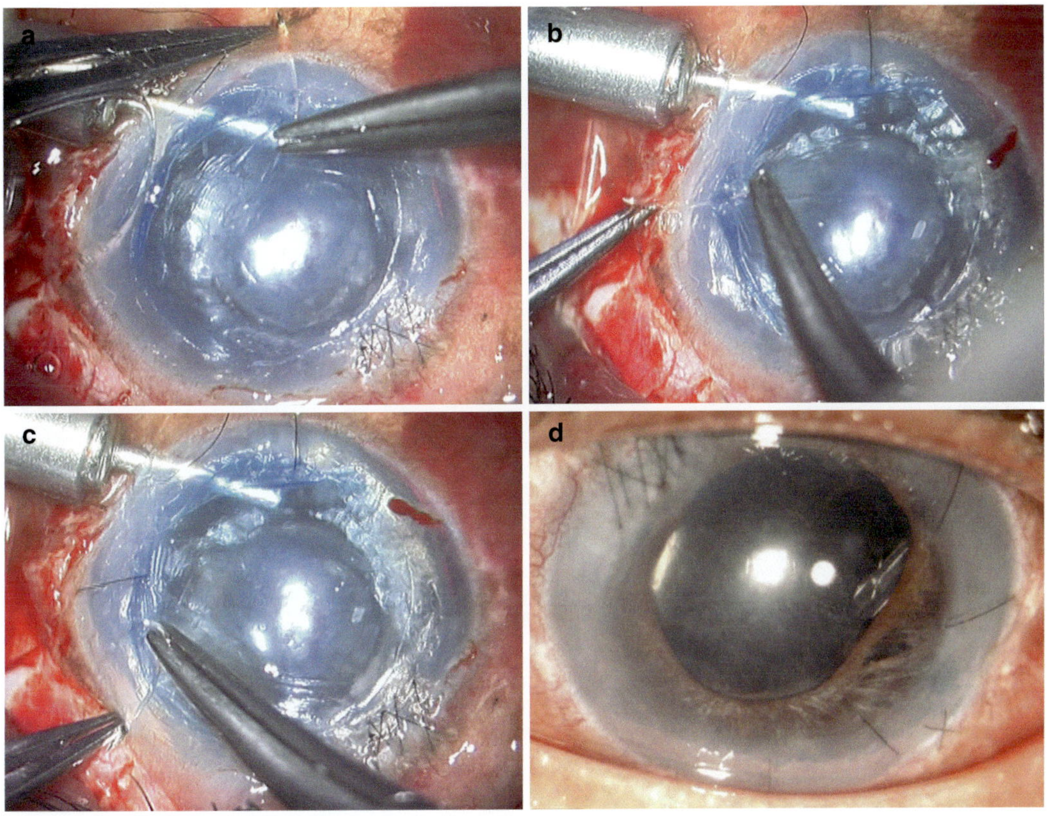


**Fig. 14.10** (**a–c**) Suture being passed through the graft with air pump on and a taut AC; (**d**) Suture tied down decreases postoperative graft detachment

## 14.13 Graft Detachment

The risk of graft detachment is decreased by using the pressurized air infusion from the air-pump assisted technique. In addition, trans-graft sutures may also be applied through areas in the graft which need greater support (e.g., inferior graft) or situations where air tamponade may not be sufficient (e.g., vitrectomized eyes or incomplete iris diaphragm, etc). This is done either with needle pass from endothelium to epithelium direction or with pressurized air infusion and a taut AC, from the epithelial to endothelial direction using a new, sharp needle (Fig. 14.10).

## References


1. Dua HS, Faraj LA, Said DG, Gray T, Lowe J. Human corneal anatomy redefined: a novel pre-Descemet's layer (Dua's layer). Ophthalmology. 2013;120(9):1778–85.
2. Agarwal A, Dua HS, Narang P, Kumar DA, Agarwal A, Jacob S, Agarwal A, Gupta A. Pre-Descemet's endothelial keratoplasty (PDEK). Br J Ophthalmol. 2014;98(9):1181–5.
3. Jacob S. Understanding the PDEK bubble Soosan Jacob with audio 3 3 min. https://www.youtube.com/watch?v=M4n4bCxApAc. Accessed 6 March 2021.
4. Jacob S. My top 10 tips for PDEK BB Soosan Jacob 5 16 min. https://www.youtube.com/watch?v=GMQM7ZINExc. Accessed 6 March 2021.
5. Jacob S. Endothelial keratoplasty playlist. https://www.youtube.com/playlist?list=PLOLM5nX3h_taUkT5ftFzwE_-JmGx6HeWO
6. Agarwal A, Agarwal A, Narang P, Kumar DA, Jacob S. Pre-Descemet endothelial keratoplasty with infant donor corneas: A prospective analysis. Cornea. 2015;34(8):859–65.
7. Sharma N, Devi C, Agarwal R, Bafna RK, Agarwal A. I-PDEK: microscope-integrated OCT-assisted pre-Descemet endothelial keratoplasty. J Cataract Refract Surg. 2021;47(12):e44–8.
8. Moshirfar M, Thomson AC, Ronquillo Y. Corneal endothelial transplantation. In: StatPearls [Internet]. Treasure Island, FL: StatPearls Publishing; 2022.
9. Dua HS, Said DG. Pre-Descemets endothelial keratoplasty: the PDEK clamp for successful PDEK. Eye (Lond). 2017;31(7):1106–10. https://doi.org/10.1038/eye.2017.10.
10. Jacob S. Use of pressurized air infusion for pre Descemet's endothelial keratoplasty (PDEK)—the air pump assisted PDEK technique. Open Ophthalmol J. 2018;12:175–80.
11. Jacob S, Narasimhan S, Agarwal A, Agarwal A, A I S. Air pump-assisted graft centration, graft edge unfolding, and graft uncreasing in young donor graft pre-Descemet endothelial keratoplasty. Cornea. 2017;36(8):1009–13.

# New Frontiers of Corneal Endothelial Regeneration: Descemet Membrane Endothelial Transfer, Descemet Stripping Only, Hemi-DMEK, Quarter-DMEK, and Cultured Corneal Endothelial Cells

15

Philip W. Dockery, Jack S. Parker, and Gerrit R. J. Melles

## 15.1 Introduction

Descemet membrane endothelial keratoplasty (DMEK) has revolutionized surgery to replace diseased or decimated corneal endothelial cells in patients with corneal endothelial dysfunction, including Fuchs endothelial dystrophy (FED) and bullous keratopathy (BK) [1]. However, DMEK is often regarded technically challenging, and postoperatively chronic topical steroid use and long-term clinical follow-up are required [2]. Furthermore, in many areas of the world, corneal tissue remains scarce [3–5]. Less invasive or less technically challenging procedures are under development to improve upon DMEK outcomes.

**Supplementary Information** The online version contains supplementary material available at https://doi.org/10.1007/978-981-97-3469-6_15. The videos can be accessed individually by clicking the DOI link in the accompanying figure caption or by scanning this link with the SN More Media App.

P. W. Dockery
Parker Cornea, Birmingham, AL, USA

J. S. Parker (✉)
Parker Cornea, Birmingham, AL, USA

Netherlands Institute for Innovative Ocular Surgery–USA (NIIOS–USA), San Diego, CA, USA

G. R. J. Melles
Netherlands Institute for Innovative Ocular Surgery–USA (NIIOS–USA), San Diego, CA, USA

Netherlands Institute for Innovative Ocular Surgery (NIIOS), Rotterdam, The Netherlands

Melles Cornea Clinic, Rotterdam, The Netherlands

## 15.2 Descemet Membrane Endothelial Transfer

### 15.2.1 Corneal Clearance with Imperfect Endothelial Keratoplasties

In the early years of endothelial keratoplasty, it was believed that dysfunctional endothelial cells must be replaced with an attached graft to restore corneal clarity [6]. In 2009, Balachandran et al. [7] challenged this notion with a report of two cases of partial DMEK graft detachment with eventual corneal clearance in patients with FED (Fig. 15.1). In the years following, similar reports were shared in patients with FED whose Descemet stripping (automated) endothelial keratoplasty (DS(A)EK) or DMEK grafts detached [8, 9]. In a 2011 population of patients with FED, Dirisamer et al. [10] demonstrated that corneas with partially detached grafts generally cleared, even if the graft was placed (inadvertently)


S. Jacob (ed.), *Mastering DMEK and PDEK*, https://doi.org/10.1007/978-981-97-3469-6_15

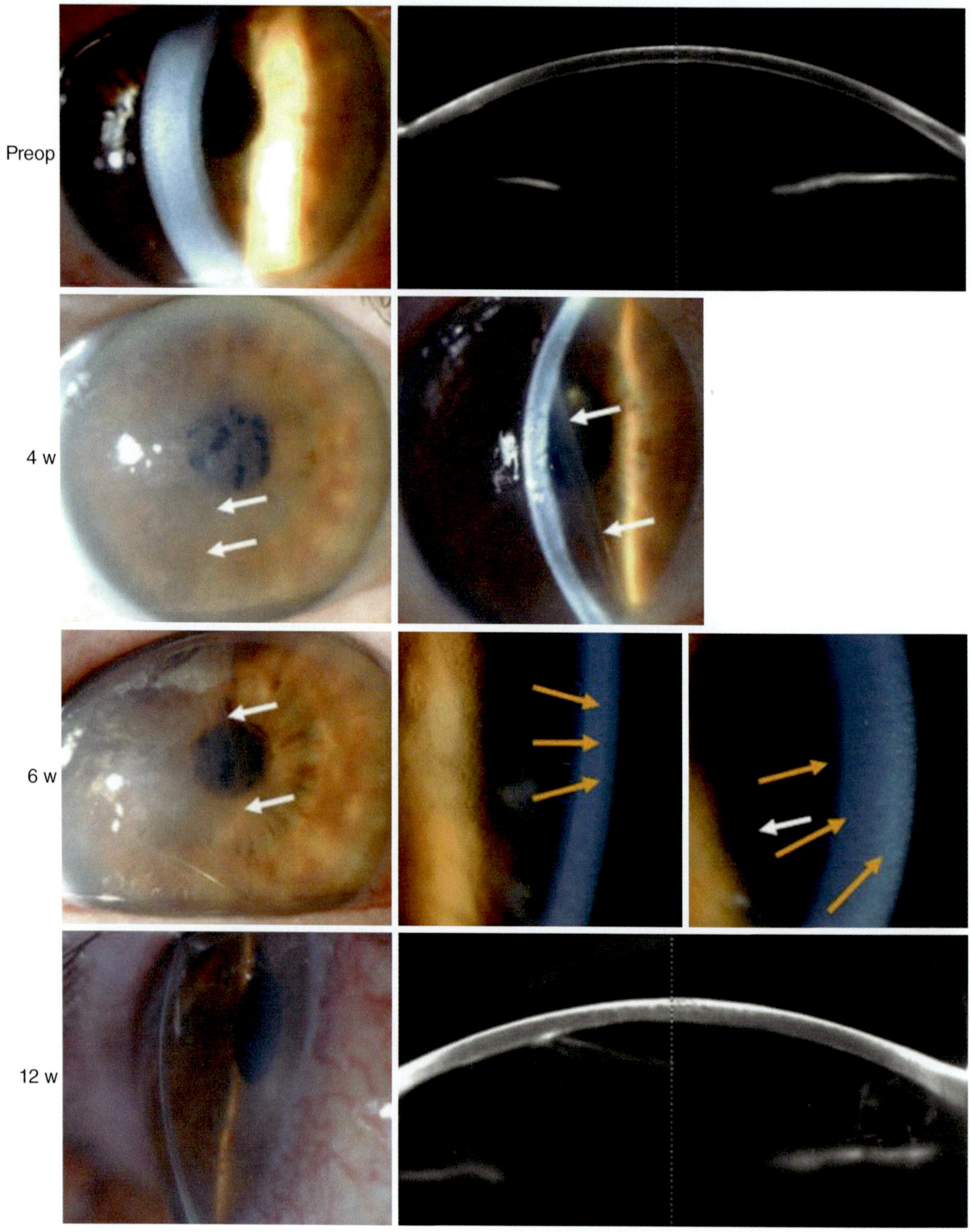


**Fig. 15.1** Collage displaying the change in corneal transparency after Descemet membrane endothelial keratoplasty (DMEK) complicated by postoperative partial graft detachment. (Top row, left and right) Before surgery, the cornea shows pathologic alterations consistent with Fuchs endothelial dystrophy. (Second row, left and right) 1 month after DMEK surgery, a Descemet roll is visible in the recipient anterior chamber [AC] (white arrows) and the transplanted cornea shows diffuse stromal edema in all quadrants. (Third row, left) At 6 weeks, the Descemet transplant shows a similar orientation and is still located on the temporal side of the AC. (Third row, middle and right) On the nasal side, a cellular wave front (orange arrows) is seen extending from the far nasal periphery toward the center. In the background, the edge of the Descemet roll is visible (white arrow). (Bottom left) At 12 weeks, the transplant is still in the same position, but the central cornea shows a marked improvement of its transparency and a near normal thickness. (Bottom right) Scheimpflug imaging (vertical beam orientation with the superior quadrant on the left) reveals a largely detached donor Descemet membrane with a touch at the 12-o'clock surgical position

upside-down (Fig. 15.2). The results suggested that a graft, if contacting the host cornea, could stimulate the transfer for endothelial cells from the donor to the recipient or possibly stimulate the migration and proliferation of recipient endothelial cells; thus, the concept of Descemet membrane endothelial transfer (DMET) was born [11].

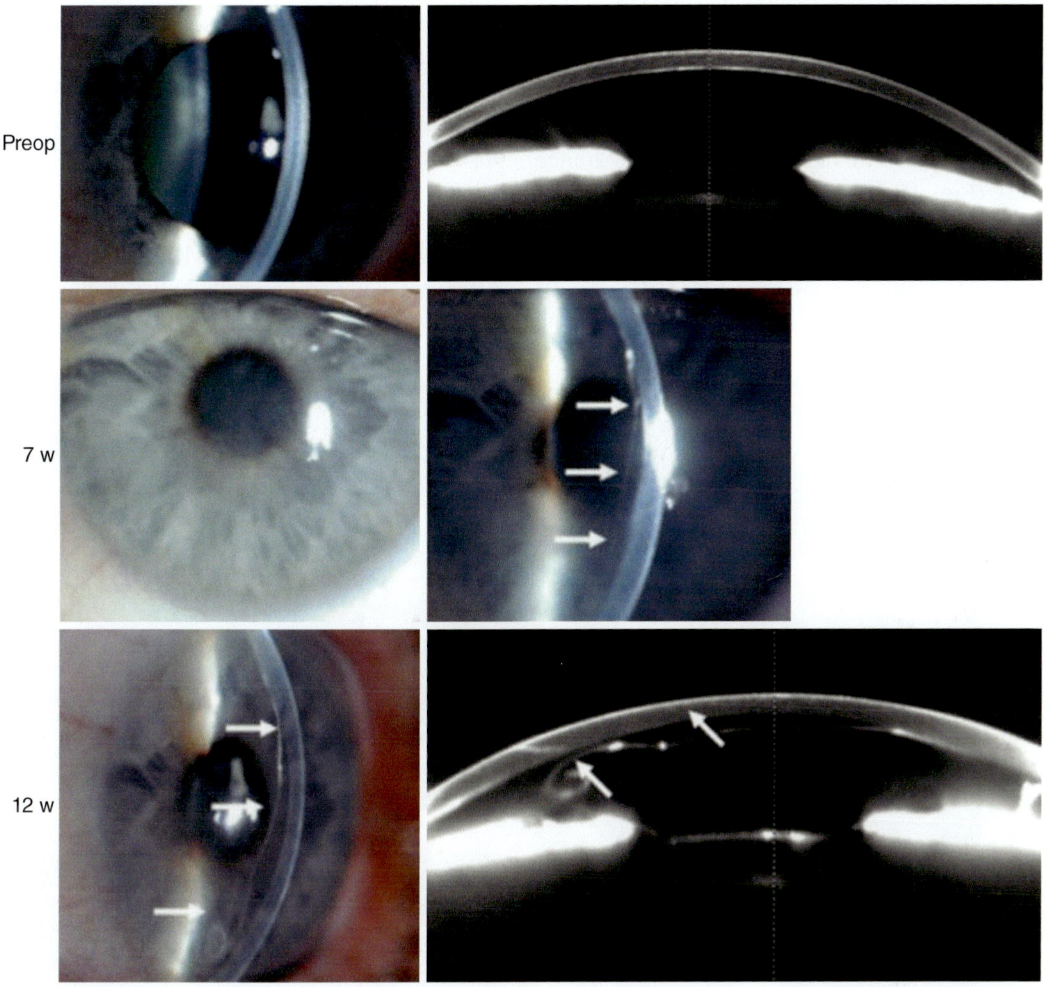


**Fig. 15.2** Collage displaying the change in corneal transparency after DMEK complicated by postoperative partial graft detachment. (Top left and right) Before surgery, the corneal condition was diagnosed as a Fuchs endothelial dystrophy. Seven weeks after DMEK surgery, the transplanted cornea shows (Middle left) diffuse stromal edema and (Middle right) a detached Descemet transplant (white arrows). (Bottom left) At 12 weeks, the transplant has the same orientation, but the central cornea has thinned to normal thickness with significant improvement of its transparency. (Bottom right) Scheimpflug imaging (oblique beam orientation with the inferotemporal quadrant on the left) reveals an upside-down detached donor Descemet membrane with a touch at the 12-o'clock surgical position

### 15.2.2 DMET Basics and Benefits

DMET was originally considered a simplified form of DMEK and aimed to provide similar visual outcomes and rates of corneal clearance. The surgery consisted of creating a large descemetorhexis and fixating a donor Descemet roll within a corneo-scleral wound to ensure contact between the graft and the host stroma, under the premise that contact was necessary to facilitate corneal clearance [12] (Fig. 15.3). By eliminating the need to unroll the graft, DMET was positioned as an alternative that would be less surgically demanding than conventional DMEK, as well as quicker and safer, since patients would no longer need a peripheral iridotomy and are no longer at risk for pupillary block glaucoma because an air bubble is not used to adhere the graft to the posterior cornea [11].

Dirisamer et al. [13] demonstrated in an early case series that DMET led to corneal clearance at 6 months postoperative in all patients with FED ($n = 10$) but in no patients with BK ($n = 6$). All documented cases of clearance began on the side opposite of the graft attachment [7, 14]. In patients with BK, postmortem histological evaluation of the cornea showed no evidence of endothelial cell migration after DMET [15]. With the difference in underlying pathology seeming to be

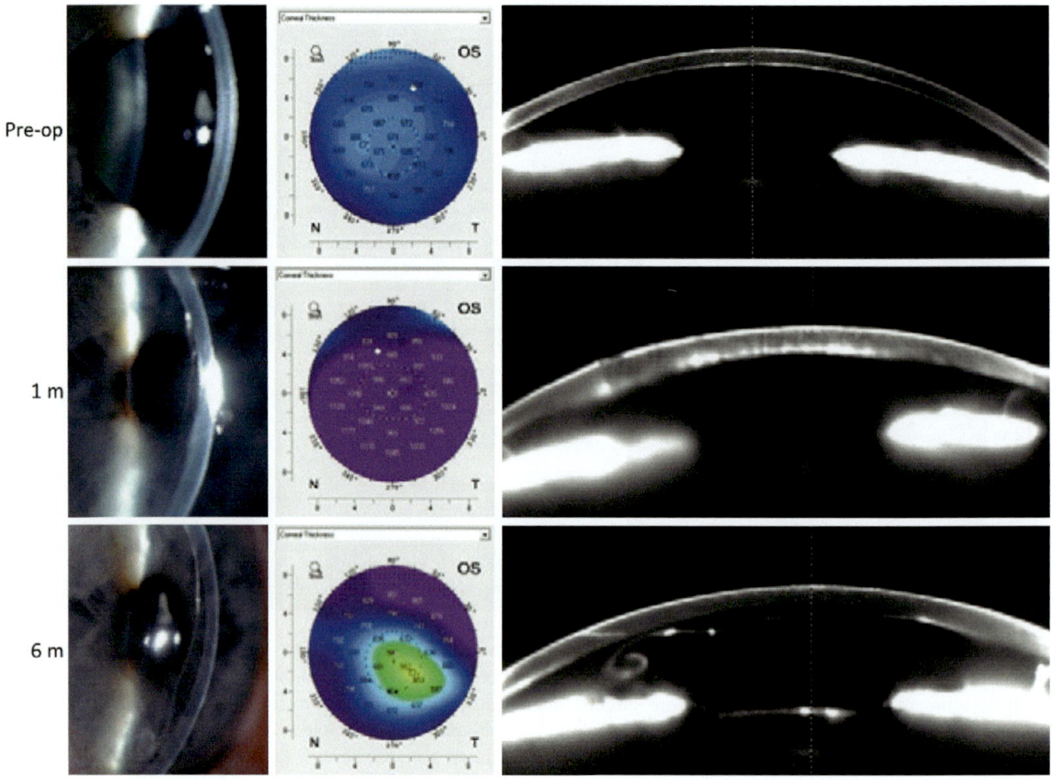


**Fig. 15.3** Collage of slit-lamp photographs, Pentacam pachymetry maps, and Scheimpflug images displaying the change in corneal transparency following Descemet membrane endothelial transfer (DMET) over time, operated on for Fuchs endothelial dystrophy. (Top row) Before surgery, the cornea shows pathologic alterations consistent with Fuchs endothelial dystrophy, and an increased corneal thickness. (Second row) At 1 month after surgery, the transplanted cornea shows diffuse stromal edema in all quadrants. (Third row) At 6 months, the Descemet graft is positioned upside-down with a small area of peripheral attachment, while the recipient cornea has a virtually normal clarity and pachymetry

a main contributor to the variation in primary surgical outcome, it insinuates that recipient endothelial cells, rather than donor endothelial cells, are mostly responsible for corneal deturgescence after DMET [11].

### 15.2.3 Endothelial Cell Function: Migration and Proliferation

The main question is the mechanism by which the recipient endothelial cells repopulate the posterior bare stroma: migration, proliferation, or both. Migration and enlargement of both donor and recipient endothelial cells is well documented and has been demonstrated on confocal microscopy [16, 17]. On the other hand, evidence of corneal endothelial cell proliferation has been slightly more elusive. It has been long believed that endothelial cells are stymied by a high concentration of transforming growth factor beta (TGF-β) in the anterior chamber and significant cell-cell contact inhibition, arresting them in G1 phase of the cell cycle and incapacitating them from proliferating [18, 19]. However, more recent studies have demonstrated potential stem-like corneal endothelial cells at the junctional region between the cornea and the trabecular meshwork [20].

### 15.2.4 Long-Term Results of DMET

Although DMET demonstrated initial promise, at least in cases of FED, Birbal et al. [21] reported the first long-term outcomes of DMET in 2018, which proved ultimately unsuccessful. While DMET indeed usually restored normal corneal clarity in patients with FED, the time needed to attain such an effect was significantly longer than with conventional DMEK. Most importantly, all initially successful DMET cases eventually experienced late corneal decompensation and failure, on average less than 1 year after surgery. As a result, the ultimate verdict for DMET is that the surgery is not likely a viable long-term solution to corneal endothelial dysfunction, either in patients with BK or FED (Fig. 15.4).

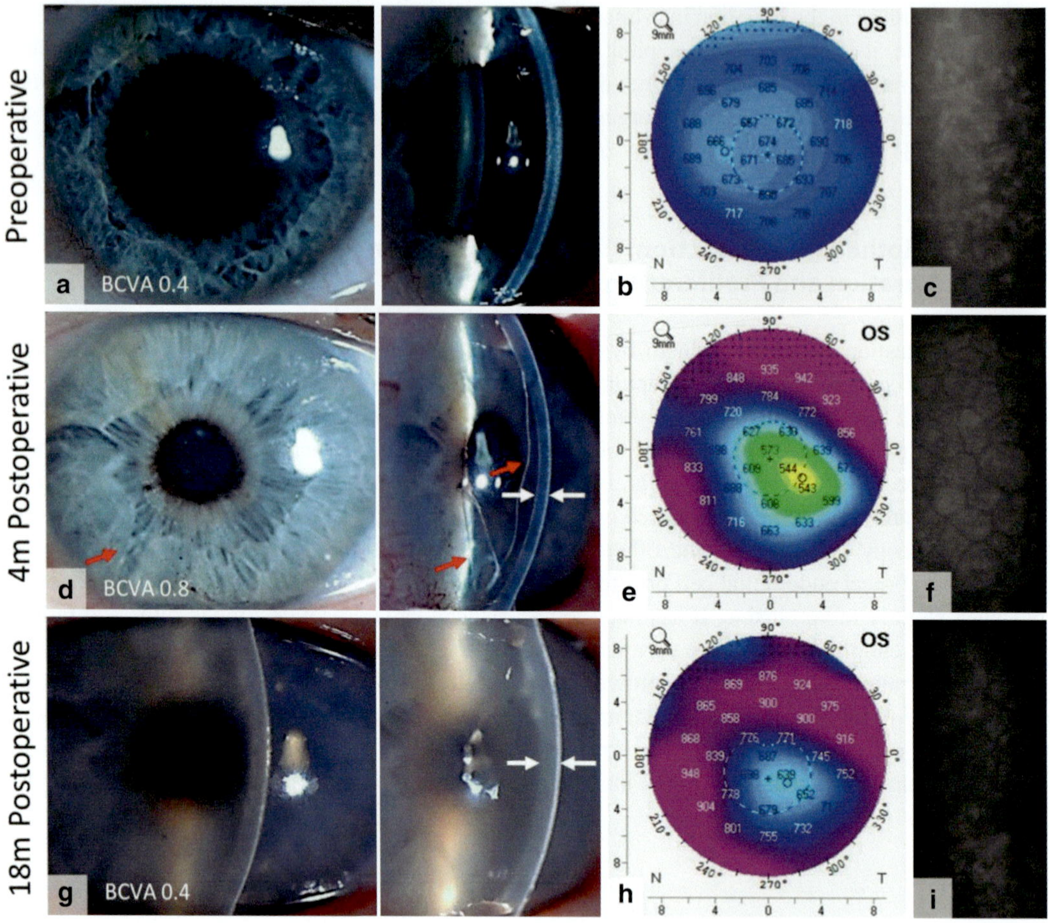


**Fig. 15.4** Slit-lamp images, pachymetry, and specular microscopy preoperatively (**a**, **b**, and **c**), at 4 months (**d**, **e**, and **f**) and at 18 months after DMET (**g**, **h**, and **i**). Note the initial corneal clearance at 4 months and the corneal decompensation at 18 months postoperatively (white arrows). The red arrows display the borders of the Descemet graft

## 15.3 Descemet Stripping Only

### 15.3.1 No Graft Needed?

Descemetorhexis without endothelial keratoplasty (DSO), or Descemet stripping only (DSO), is a procedure developed to further simplify surgical management for patients with endothelial dysfunction. As the name suggests, the operation consists of the removal of diseased endothelium and Descemet membrane without the insertion of a donor graft. Therefore, like DMET, it also aims to eliminate the two most problematic steps of conventional DMEK (graft unrolling and maintaining graft attachment postoperatively) [11]. Theoretically, by eliminating the need for transplantation entirely, the risk of allograft reaction and graft rejection would also be eliminated, as would the need for chronic anti-rejection medications and even chronic medical surveillance. By stripping the guttae-laden Descemet membrane and endothelium in patients with FED, the peripheral endothelium could repopulate the rest of the cornea because of decreased cell-cell contact inhibition. Additionally, an 8 mm descemetorhexis would leave almost half of the endothelial surface area intact, and because ECD is higher in the periphery, more than half of the native endothelial cells would remain after the operation [14, 22].

### 15.3.2 DSO Effectiveness

The premise of DSO was first demonstrated in early case reports of spontaneous corneal clearing following incidental intraoperative Descemet membrane detachment during cataract surgery [23, 24], but reports were scattered and conflicting, often showing failure of the cornea to clear [10]. Likewise, some of the first planned DSO operations showed mixed results [25–28]. And, similar to DMET, DSO is only positioned as an operation for patients with FED, not BK.

In early DSO, ophthalmologists experimented by making the descemetorhexis different sizes, with larger attempts being generally less successful than smaller ones. Results are mostly negative for a descemetorhexis greater than 8 mm [10] and are mixed at 6 mm [29]. However, in DSO cases with a 4 mm descemetorhexis, the published results have been mostly positive, with many cases showing initial corneal clearing [30]. This suggests that descemetorhexis size could be a critical variable in determining the success of the operation. Although, a small descemetorhexis would limit the number of patients that could potentially benefit from the surgery because it would be limited to those with FED with guttae isolated to the central cornea.

When compared in a retrospective cohort study [30] against 8 mm-diameter DMEK, 4 mm-diameter DSO had similar visual outcomes and rates of corneal clearance for those with FED. However, the time needed for visual rehabilitation (BCVA ≥20/40 [0.5]) is markedly longer in DSO (7.1 weeks) compared to DMEK (2.2 weeks). When rho-associated protein kinase (ROCK) inhibitors, such as ripasudil, are administered as standard postoperative course, DSO patients had a two-week faster visual recovery compared to those who did not receive ripasudil. Further, for DSO eyes receiving a ROCK inhibitor, peripheral ECD remained stable, while those receiving DSO alone saw a 10% drop in peripheral ECD [31]. ROCK inhibitors also improve corneal clarity in eyes that develop BK following DSO [30]. The mechanism of Descemet membrane stripping may influence postoperative endothelial cell migration; fewer corneas that underwent 360-degree scoring obtained corneal clearance (77%) than those that had 2 clock hours of scoring with removal of Descemet membrane using forceps (100%) [32]. This suggests that the act of scoring the stroma could impede endothelial cell migration, but larger studies are needed to validate these results.

## 15.4 Partial Transplantation

### 15.4.1 DMEK vs. DSO

Compared to DMEK, DSO presently possesses two shortcomings: it seems limited to patients with centrally located FED, and it entails a significantly longer recovery time. Moreover, no long-term results exist for the procedure, which calls into question whether the achieved corneal clarity will be transient (as with DMET) or durable. Perhaps a balance between DMEK and DSO exists that offers the quick corneal clearance of DMEK and the decreased immune response DSO, while also successfully treating many etiologies of endothelial decompensation and reducing the amount of donor tissue needed for the surgery [3–5]. Partial transplantations, such as hemi-DMEK and quarter-DMEK, were primarily created to increase the availability of donor endothelial tissue while providing the same visual outcomes of traditional DMEK.

### 15.4.2 Hemi-DMEK

Hemi-DMEK was introduced by Lam et al. [33] in 2014 with the goal of using one donor cornea for two endothelial keratoplasties. As opposed to traditional DMEK, which uses only the central portion of the Descemet-endothelial complex and leaves the peripheral rim (approximately half the tissue) to be discarded, hemi-DMEK uses a full-diameter graft that has been bisected (Fig. 15.5).

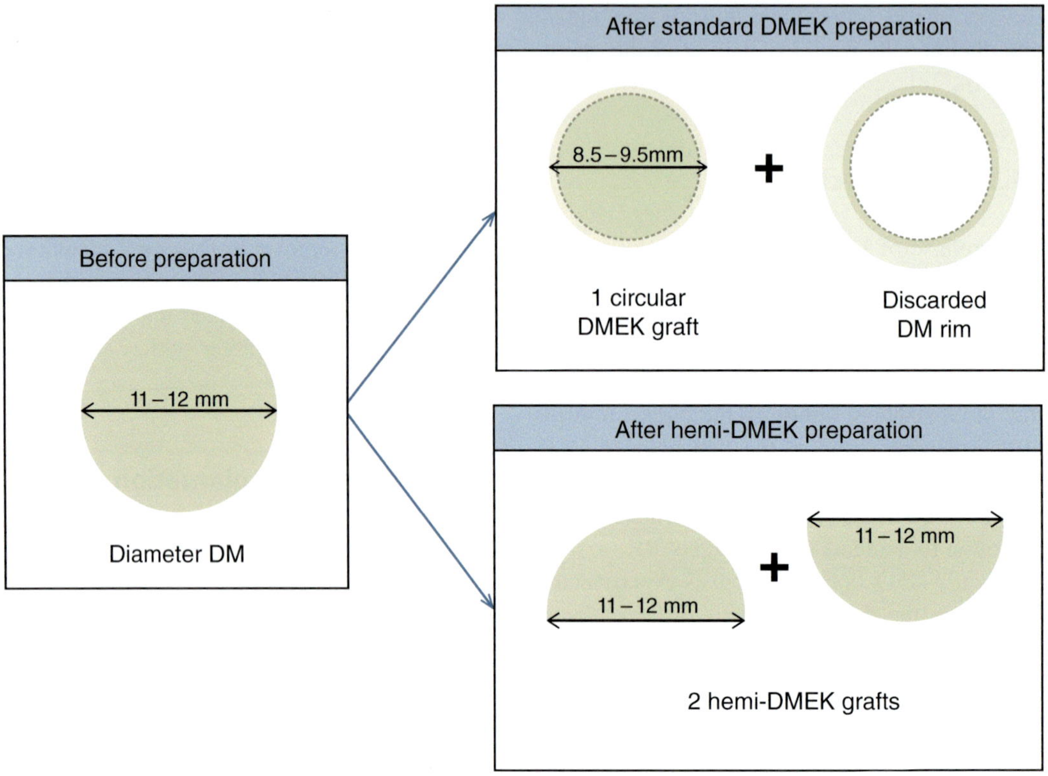


**Fig. 15.5** Schematic overview of cornea donor tissue before and after standard circular 8.5–9.5 mm Descemet membrane endothelial keratoplasty (DMEK) preparation and hemi-DMEK preparation

The half-moon grafts for hemi-DMEK are prepared by cutting a midline incision into a full-diameter cornea graft. After removing the trabecular meshwork from the periphery, each graft spontaneously coils with the endothelium on the outside of the roll, like in DMEK graft preparation [34].

The steps of hemi-DMEK surgery are similar to traditional DMEK, including creating an 8–9 mm circular descemetorhexis, unrolling the graft via a no-touch technique, and using an air bubble to hold the graft in place postoperatively [33, 35, 36]. During the unfolding of a hemi-DMEK graft, the widest aspect of the graft should be aligned with the longest horizontal meridian of the eye [33] (Fig. 15.6). Because of the incongruence between the shape of the graft and the descemetorhexis, a considerable portion of the stroma is left bare, which could be avoided by the creation of an elliptical descemetorhexis [35, 37].

### 15.4.3 Hemi-DMEK Effectiveness

Preliminary [35] and mid-term [37] studies show hemi-DMEK results parallel those achieved by conventional DMEK. Because a significant portion of the posterior stroma is left bare, corneal deturgescence occurs more slowly in these regions although the speed of visual recovery is not affected because the central cornea, which is covered with a hemi-DMEK graft, clears rapidly. Several studies have shown that ECD decreases by about 50% in the first month postoperatively. After 6 months, the rate of ECD decline seems to be comparable to DMEK: approximately 6–7% annually. The typically good visual outcomes normally seen after DMEK are expected after hemi-DMEK, with all eyes reaching a best corrected visual acuity (BCVA) ≥20/40 (0.5) at 3 months, and over half of operated eyes achieving a BCVA ≥20/20 (1.0) by 1 year.

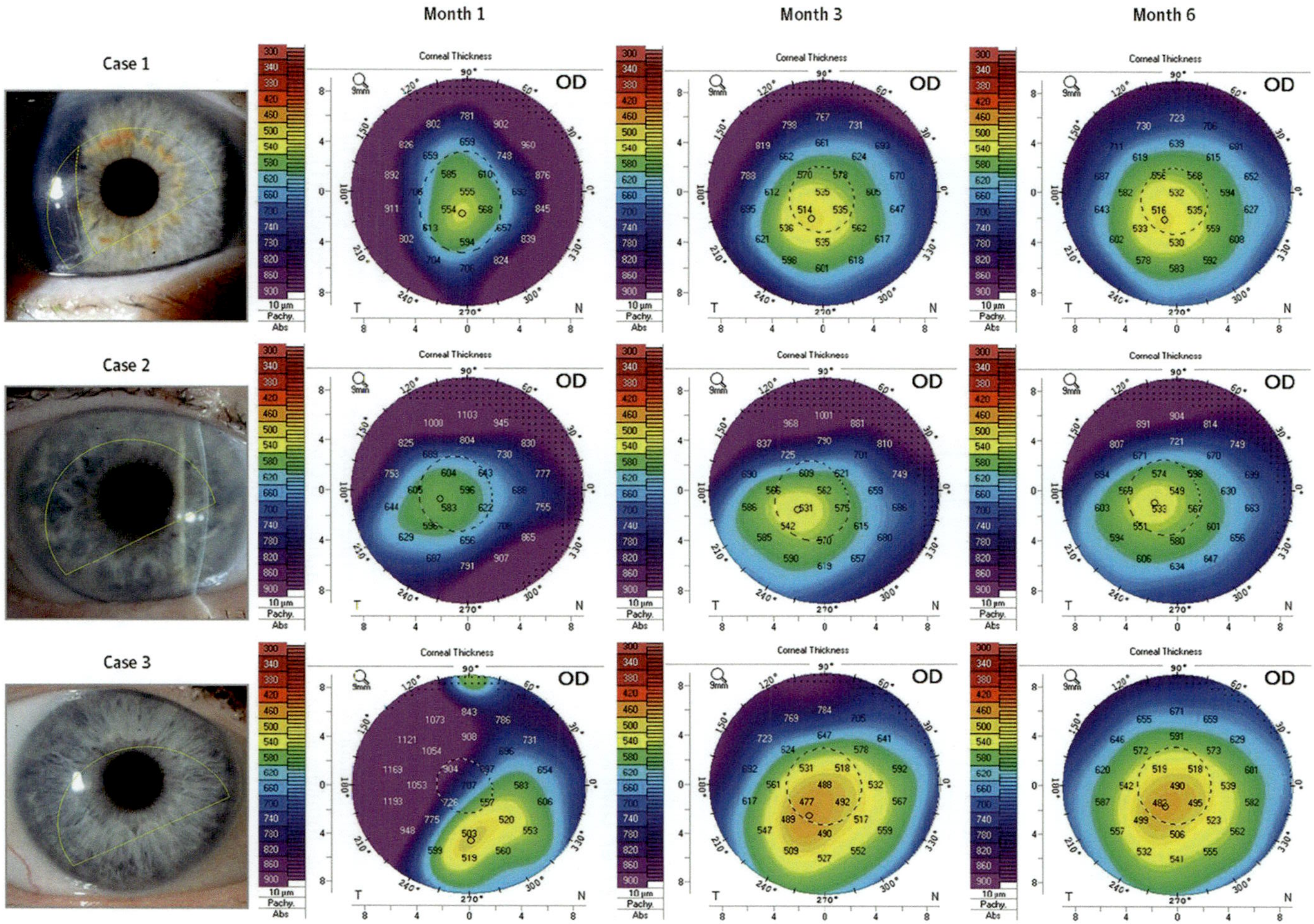


**Fig. 15.6** Corneal thickness (expressed in micrometers according to Pentacam software; Oculus) is indicated according to the color-coded information. The full yellow lines outline the approximate position of the hemi-DMEK graft, and the location of the peripheral graft detachment in case 1 is highlighted by a dotted yellow line. Note that corneal deturgescence starts in the graft's center and progresses outward from 1 month to 6 months

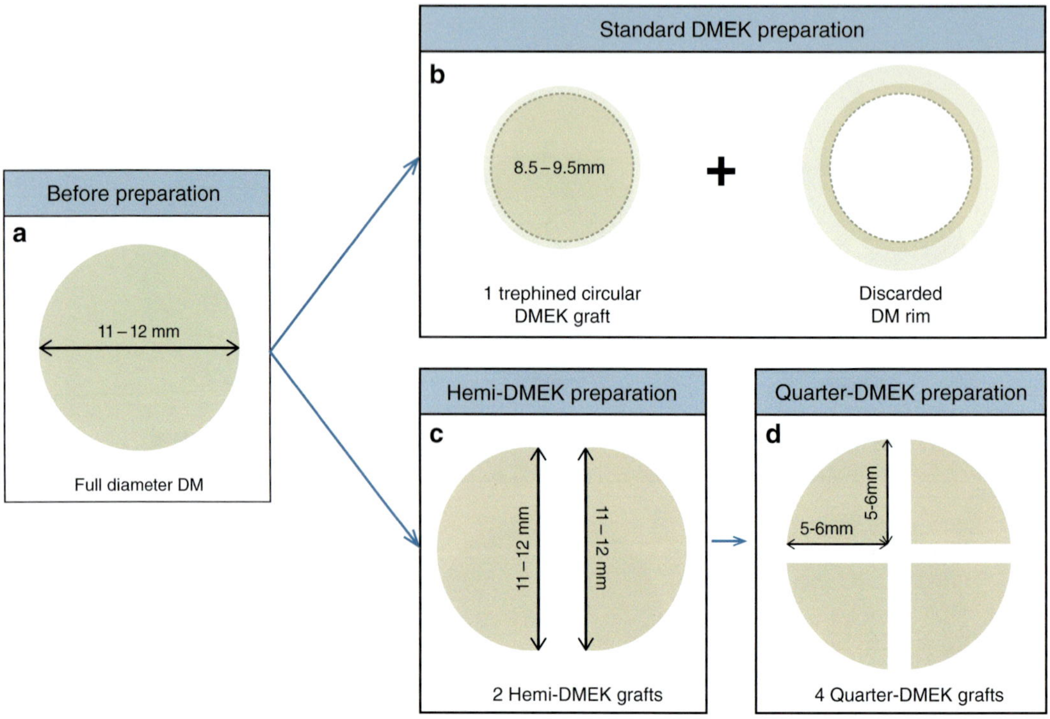


**Fig. 15.7** Diagram showing graft preparation from (**a**) a full-diameter corneo-scleral button to obtain (**b**) a single 8.5- to 9.5-mm standard DMEK graft or (**c**) two semicircular hemi-DMEK grafts and (**d**) four quarter-DMEK grafts

### 15.4.4 Quarter-DMEK

Considering the success of hemi-DMEK, which provides similar results as DMEK with half the donor tissue, questions arose about making endothelial transplantation grafting even more efficient. Quarter-DMEK grafts are prepared similarly to hemi-DMEK grafts, except an additional straight cut bisecting the graft is made perpendicular to the first straight cut, forming 4 "pie-shaped" transplantable pieces [38, 39] (Fig. 15.7).

### 15.4.5 Quarter-DMEK Effectiveness

Similar to hemi-DMEK, quarter-DMEK demonstrates potential as an alternative to conventional DMEK. Data from an early case report [40] and a larger case series [41] revealed 100% of operated patients obtained a BSCVA of ≥20/40 (0.5) by 3 months, and more than 90% were ≥20/25 (0.8) and 50% ≥20/20 (1.0) at 6 months (Fig. 15.8). As with hemi-DMEK, eyes undergoing quarter-DMEK demonstrate a 50% reduction in ECD in the first postoperative month, and thereafter rates of decline parallel conventional DMEK. Early reported complications include partial graft detachment requiring re-bubbling (33% of operated eyes in an early study), which may be attributable to the early learning curve of a new procedure, or to curvature incongruence, considering the central recipient cornea is aligned with the paracentral donor cornea [41].

When quarter-DMEK grafts are observed in vitro, cell migration is not uniform; it predominantly occurs along to radial cut edges of graft, with essentially no migration occurring in the far periphery, which could be attributed to the entanglement between collagen fibrils and endothelial cells in that region [39]. With initial corneal clearance and individual cell migration being more prevalent along the radial cut edges, it may be beneficial to shift those edges closer to the recipient central cornea than the edge of the far periphery in order to promote quicker central corneal deturgescence along the visual axis [39, 41].

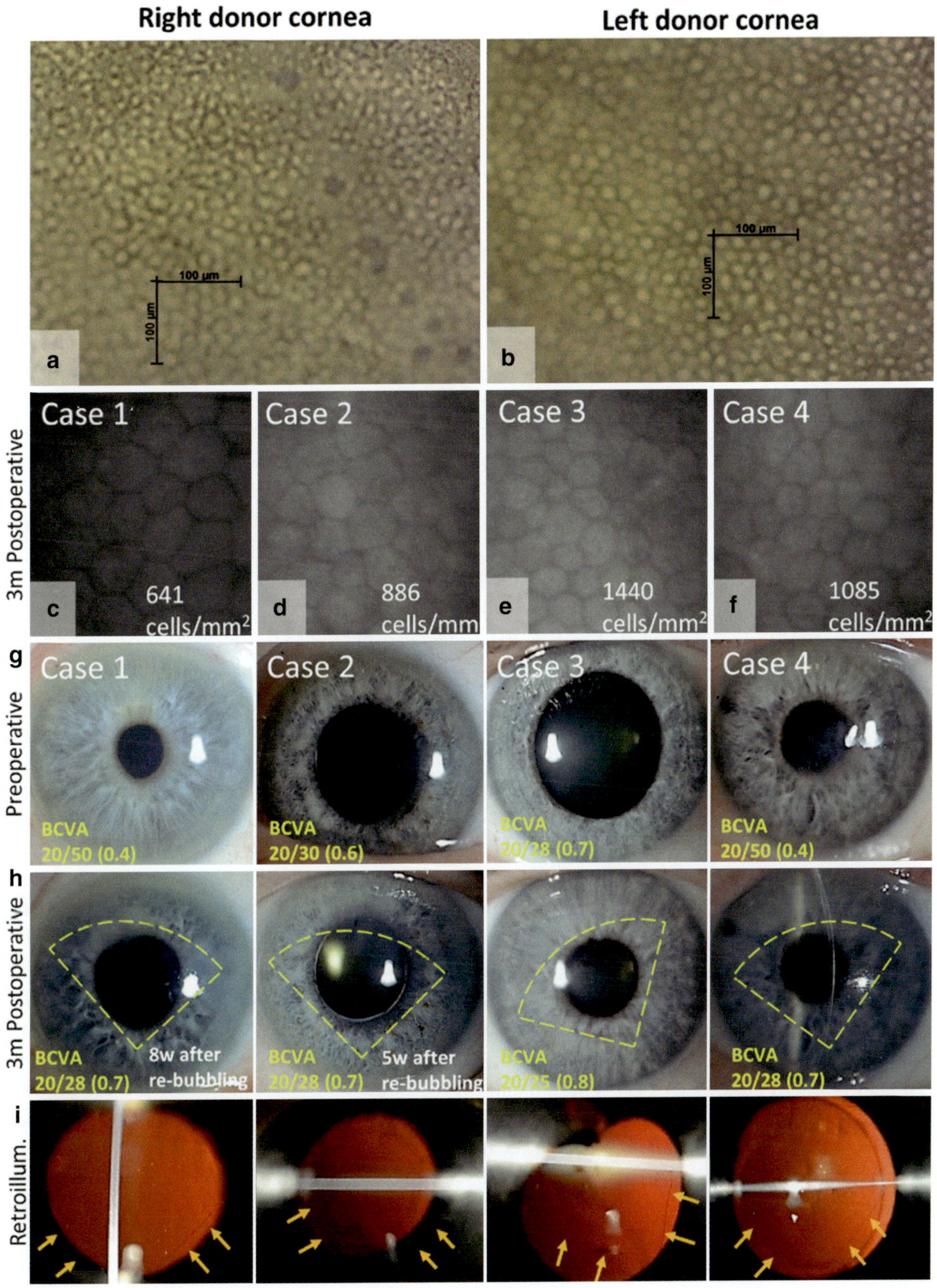


**Fig. 15.8** In vitro light microscopy images of the right (**a**) and left (**b**) donor cornea procured from the same 74-year-old male donor, and in vivo specular microscopy images (**c**–**f**) at 3 months postoperatively of the four recipient eyes that received Quarter-DMEK grafts from the right donor cornea (**c** and **d**) and the left donor cornea (**e** and **f**). Endothelial cell density (ECD) at this time-point was 641 cells/mm² (Case 1), 886 cells/mm² (Case 2), 1440 cells/mm² (Case 3), and 1085 cells/mm² (Case 4). Slit-lamp images of the four Quarter-DMEK eyes before (**g**), and 3 months (**h**) postoperatively. The orientation of the Quarter-DMEK grafts is outlined by orange arrows in the retro-illumination images (**i**) and the dashed lines in row (**h**). *BCVA* best corrected visual acuity at each time-point, *retroillum* retro-illumination

## 15.5 Cultured Corneal Endothelial Cells

### 15.5.1 Corneal Endothelial Cell Cultures

Although corneal endothelial cells may be resistant to proliferation in vivo due to the high concentration of TGF-β in the anterior chamber and their significant cell-cell contact inhibition [18, 19], they may proliferate in an in vitro environment [42, 43]. Zaniolo et al. [44] demonstrated that corneal endothelial cells could even be isolated and cultured from descemetorhexis tissue in FED patients. Culturing corneal endothelial cells could increase the tissue supply for the increasing global demand for endothelial keratoplasties. The proliferative capability varies substantially among endothelial cells, depending on age, disease state, and potentially location on the cornea [45]. Cultures with higher proliferative capacity are more susceptible to FGF-2-mediated endothelial-mesenchymal transformation [46]. While some strategies have been to administer therapies to reduce fibroblastic transformation, isolating higher quality endothelial cells through cell sorting by specific surface antibodies may be more promising [43, 47].

### 15.5.2 Endothelial Cell Transfer on Tissue Scaffolds

The first attempts to implant cultured corneal endothelial cells into eyes came in the form of tissue-engineered Descemet stripping endothelial keratoplasty (TE-DSEK) [47]. These manufactured scaffolds were created using a range of materials, including decellularized corneal stroma, collagen gel, Chitosan, and polylactides [48–50]. Thus far, all materials tried have elicited complications, such as inflammatory responses with scaffolds made from synthetic materials and rejection with scaffolds made from biologic materials [47]. Considering the insertion of endothelial cells on a tissue-engineered scaffold would entail an invasive surgery similar to DSAEK, this method may not represent improvement over DMEK (unless the transplanted cells could be cultured from the patient's own endothelium, in which case, there may be some benefit reflected in a reduced risk of allograft reaction) [47].

### 15.5.3 Injectable Endothelial Cell Therapy

To reduce the potential surgical morbidity from using a TE-DSEK graft, methods of injecting free-floating corneal endothelial cells into the anterior chamber have been proposed. Early animal experiments exhibit mixed results, with higher injected cell volumes demonstrating non-functioning endothelial multilayers with fibrotic transformation [51]. Multiple strategies, such as use of ROCK inhibitors and insertions of magnetic nanoparticles, have been developed to potentially reduce mesenchymal-endothelial transformation and increase endothelial monolayer formation [52].

Using in vitro models, Moysidis et al. [53] demonstrated that magnetic nanoparticles (MNP) endocytosed by corneal endothelial cells seem to improve monolayer formation and endothelial cell adherence to the posterior cornea, while not reducing cellular viability or function. While only 36% of control endothelial cells injected were attached to the cornea under the influence of gravity alone, 86% of MNP-loaded endothelial cells formed a monolayer, increasing ECD 2.4-fold. Additionally, manipulation of the magnetic field used to interact with the MNP-load endothelial cells allows for increased control of final endothelial cell location, making a uniform monolayer throughout the cornea more feasible. To date, no human trials have been performed.

In 2018, Kinoshita et al. [54] presented results of the first clinical trial testing the effects of injected allogenic cultured corneal endothelial cells in patients with corneal endothelial dystrophy ($n$ = 11). Corneal endothelial cell cultures were sorted using enzyme-linked immunosorbent assay or fluorescence-activated cell-sorting analysis to select cells with optimal proliferative capacity. All patients who were enrolled were diagnosed with BK and had no measurable ECD; they were treated with a descemetorhexis followed by the injection of approximately one million cultured corneal endothelial cells in a solution that contained the ROCK inhibitor Y-27632. For 3 h postoperatively, patients were positioned face down to assist in adhering the injected cells to the posterior cornea. At 24 weeks postoperatively, all patients achieved corneal clearance with an ECD greater than 500, with 82% improving to a BCVA ≥20/40 (0.5).

## 15.6 The Role of Rho Kinase Inhibitors

It remains uncertain whether ROCK inhibitors are useful adjuncts, or positively required components of therapy for eyes undergoing DSO or cultured endothelial injection, and—further—whether any ROCK inhibitor is satisfactory, or if only certain formulations will suffice. In two rabbit and primate models, eyes injected with endothelial cells but without the ROCK inhibitor demonstrated persistent corneal haze and a multilayer endothelium with fibroblastic changes [52, 55, 56]. Therefore, ROCK inhibitors may be required for treating corneal endothelial dysfunction with injected corneal endothelial cells.

ROCK inhibitors may also hasten corneal endothelial repopulation following DSO and decrease risk of developing BK following cataract surgery because of their suspected ability to promote corneal endothelial wound healing [31, 52, 57, 58]. When compared to a group of patients who received DSO alone, patients receiving ripasudil 0.4% drops four times per day for 2 months following DSO were more likely to achieve 20/40 (0.5) visual acuity (100 vs. 90%) and had faster corneal clearance (4.6 vs. 6.5 weeks), higher ECD (3 months: 859 vs. 552; 6 months: 934 vs. 672; 12 months: 1086 vs. 736), and better maintenance of peripheral ECD from baseline to 1 year postoperative (1239–1233 vs. 1257–1142) [31] (Fig. 15.9). By similar mechanism, use of ROCK inhibitors following cataract surgeries with incidental intraoperative Descemet stripping may hasten corneal clearance and limit the incidence of BK. In a recent case series, patients received 1 mM Y-27632 eye drops six times per day for 4 months then four times per day for 2 months; all ($n = 3$) achieved corneal clearance by 3 months [58].

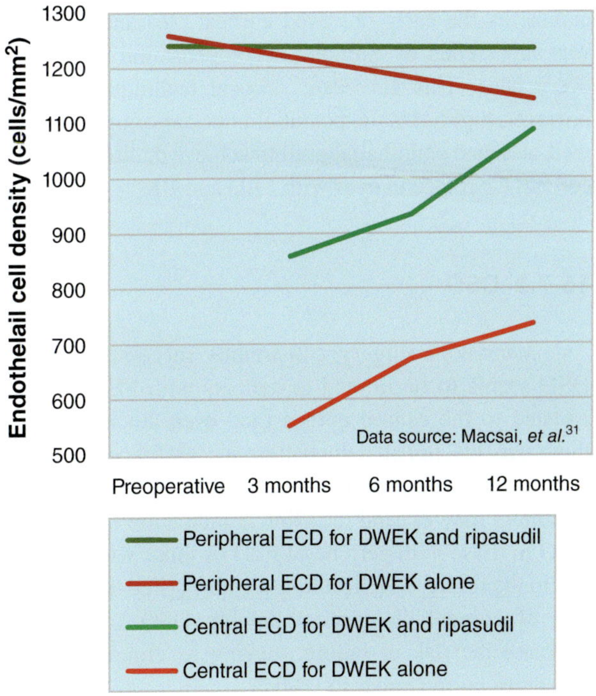


**Fig. 15.9** Trends of central and peripheral ECD over time following DWEK, or DSO, with and without the use of concurrent ripasudil use

Overall, ROCK inhibitors may promote endothelial cell proliferation and migration, monolayer formation, and maintenance of endothelial cell morphology. Little is known about the side effects of this medication, but transient guttae-like endothelial structures, abdominal pain, and constipation are among of the adverse effects described [52, 57, 58]. While Y-27632 is a ROCK inhibitor designed specifically for its use in the treatment of corneal endothelial dysfunction, ripasudil was approved in Japan in 2014 for the treatment of ocular hypertension and glaucoma (not for endothelial dysfunction, specifically) [53, 59]. Therefore, investigation of its use in endothelial disease could be worthwhile. Further randomized control trials to assess the effectiveness and dosage optimization of ROCK inhibitors is needed to determine their true role in endothelial regeneration.

## 15.7 Conclusions and Clinical Indications

### 15.7.1 DMET

As one of the first potential alternatives to DMEK, the inadvertently discovered DMET proved to have unsatisfactory long-term outcomes, as the early observed corneal clearance was superseded by eventual decompensation in every case. This candidate surgical technique, however, highlights the potential importance of a well-attached endothelial graft to achieve durable corneal clearance in eyes with FED and BK.

### 15.7.2 DSO

As a standalone surgery, consistently successful DSO seems to be limited to patients with FED isolated to the central cornea (and even among these patients, not all demonstrate successful corneal clearance). Postoperative use of ROCK inhibitors may expand the clinical indication for DSO to those with peripheral FED or those with BK in the future. ROCK inhibitors may speed the rate of corneal clearance following DSO and decrease the risk of failure, making its clinical outcomes more similar to DMEK.

Compared to conventional endothelial keratoplasty, DSO is a less technically challenging and reduces the need for donor cornea tissue. Because no graft is used, rejection is not a concern and long-term anti-rejection medications are not needed. Regions of the world with significant donor scarcity and limited access to care may benefit from this surgical option, along with patients predisposed to allograft reaction. Long-term outcomes for DSO, particularly DSO with postoperative ROCK inhibitor use, are still needed.

### 15.7.3 Hemi-DMEK and Quarter-DMEK

Hemi-DMEK and quarter-DMEK address the issue of global donor scarcity by doubling or quadrupling the pool of transplantable tissue. Their overall visual outcomes are similar to DMEK, with rapid central corneal clearance and restoration of visual function. Long-term studies are likewise needed for both Hemi- and Quarter-DMEK to assess the survival and viability of these grafts.

### 15.7.4 Cultured Corneal Endothelial Cells

To date, all human trials have used allogenic cells, but theoretically, autologous cells could be obtained and cultured to additionally reduce or eliminate allograft reaction. Injection of cultured corneal endothelial cells is a minimally invasive procedure but may lead to the creation of fibroblastic multilayers of endothelium when cells are injected in the absence of a ROCK inhibitor. The concomitant use of a ROCK inhibitor with injected corneal endothelial cells may be necessary for success of the procedure because of their assistance in monolayer formation, cell adhesions, and maintenance of cell morphology. While clinical outcomes seem promising, widespread use of cultured corneal endothelial cells could be limited by the strict regulation of advanced therapy medicinal products in many countries (Fig. 15.10).

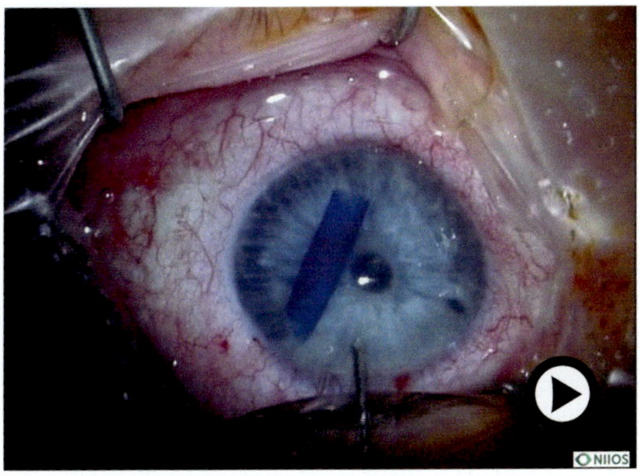


**Fig. 15.10** "Quarter-DMEK: quadrupling available tissue." Surgery Information: Quarter-DMEK performed by Lamis Baydoun, MD at the Netherlands Institute for Innovative Ocular Surgery in Rotterdam, The Netherlands. Producers: Philip Dockery, MD MPH; Jack Parker, MD PhD; Sorcha Ni Dhubhghaill, MD PhD; Lamis Baydoun, MD; Gerrit Melles, MD PhD. Narration and Animation: Philip Dockery, MD MPH. Music: "Divenire" by Ludovico Einaudi, performed by Jacob Ladegaard (https://doi.org/10.1007/000-dhw)

## References


1. Dapena I, Ham L, Melles GRJ. Endothelial keratoplasty: DSEK/DSAEK or DMEK—the thinner the better? Curr Opin Ophthalmol. 2009;20:299–307.
2. Terry MA. Endothelial keratoplasty: why aren't we doing Descemet membrane endothelial keratoplasty? Cornea. 2012;31:469–71.
3. Guam L, Reynolds I, Jones MN, et al. Tissue and corneal donation and transplantation in the UK. Br J Anaesth. 2012;108:43–7.
4. Vajpayee RB, Sharma N, Jhanji V, et al. One donor cornea for 3 recipients: a new concept for corneal transplantation surgery. Arch Ophthalmol. 2007;125:552–4.
5. Gain P, Jullienne R, He Z. Global survey of corneal transplantation and eye banking. JAMA Ophthalmol. 2016;134:167–73.
6. Romaniv N, Price PO, Price FW, et al. Donor Descemet membrane detachment after endothelial keratoplasty. Cornea. 2006;25:943–7.
7. Balachandran C, Ham L, Verschoor CA, et al. Spontaneous corneal clearance despite graft detachment in Descemet membrane endothelial keratoplasty. Am J Ophthalmol. 2009;148(2): 227–34.
8. Dirisamer M, Ham L, Dapena I, et al. Descemet membrane endothelial transfer: "free-floating" donor Descemet implantation as a potential alternative to "keratoplasty". Cornea. 2012;31(2):194–7.
9. Zafrakis P, Kymionis GD, Grentzelos MA, et al. Corneal graft detachment without corneal edema after Descemet stripping automated endothelial keratoplasty. Cornea. 2010;29:456–8.
10. Dirisamer M, Dapena I, Ham L, et al. Patterns of corneal clearance after Descemet membrane endothelial keratoplasty for Fuchs endothelial dystrophy. Am J Ophthalmol. 2011;152(4):543–55.
11. Lam FC, Bruinsma M, Melles GRJ. Descemet membrane endothelial transfer. Curr Opin Ophthalmol. 2014;25(4):353–7.
12. Dirisamer M, Dapena I, Ham L, et al. Patterns of corneal endothelialization and corneal clearance after Descemet membrane endothelial keratoplasty for Fuchs endothelial dystrophy. Am J Ophthalmol. 2011;152:543–55.
13. Dirisamer M, Ru-Yin Y, van Dijk K, et al. Recipient endothelium may relate to corneal clearance in Descemet membrane endothelial transfer. Am J Ophthalmol. 2012;154(2):290–6.
14. Van den Bogerd B, Dhubhghaill SN, Koppen C, et al. A review of the evidence for in vivo corneal endothelial regeneration. Surv Ophthalmol. 2018;63(2):149–65.
15. Parker JS, Verdijk RM, Muller RM, et al. Histopathology of failed Descemet membrane endothelial transfer. Eye Contact Lens. 2017;44(1):361–4.
16. Jacobi C, Zhivov A, Korbmacher J, et al. Evidence of endothelial cell migration after Descemet membrane endothelial keratoplasty. Am J Ophthalmol. 2011;152:537–42.
17. Lagali H, Stenevi U, Claesson M, et al. Donor and recipient endothelial cell population of the transplanted human cornea: a two-dimensional imaging study. Invest Ophthalmol Vis Sci. 2010;51:1898–904.
18. Joyce NC, Meklir B, Joyce SJ, et al. Cell cycle protein expression and proliferative status in human corneal cells. Invest Ophthalmol Vis Sci. 1996;37:645–55.
19. Joyce N. Proliferative capacity of corneal endothelial cells. Exp Eye Res. 2012;95(1):16–23.
20. Whikehart DR, Parikh CH, Vaughn AV, et al. Evidence suggesting the existence of stem cells for the human corneal endothelium. Mol Vis. 2005;11:816–24.
21. Birbal RS, Parker JS, Dirisamer M, et al. Descemet membrane endothelial transfer: ultimate outcome. Cornea. 2018;37(2):141–4.
22. Amann J, Holley GP, Lee SB, et al. Increased endothelial cell density in paracentral and peripheral regions of the human cornea. Am J Ophthalmol. 2003;135(5):584–90.
23. Choo SY, Zahidin AZ, Then KY. Spontaneous corneal clearance despite graft detachment in Descemet membrane endothelial keratoplasty. Am J Ophthalmol. 2010;149(3):531.
24. Watson SL, Abiad G, Coroneo MT. Spontaneous resolution of corneal oedema following Descemet's detachment. Clin Ex Ophthalmol. 2006;34:797–9.
25. Moloney G, Chan UT, Hamilton A, et al. Descemetorhexis for Fuchs' dystrophy. Can J Ophthalmol. 2015;50(1):68–72.
26. Moloney G, Petsoglou C, Ball M, et al. Descemetorhexis without grafting for fuchs endothelial dystrophy—supplementation with topical ripasudil. Cornea. 2017;36:642–8.

27. Shah RD, Randleman JB, Grossniklaus HE. Spontaneous corneal clearing after Descemet's stripping without endothelial replacement. Ophthalmology. 2012;119:256–60.
28. Bleyen I, Saelens IA, van Dooren BT, et al. Spontaneous clearing after Descemet's stripping. Ophthalmology. 2013;120:215.
29. Koenig SB. Planned descemetorhexis without endothelial keratoplasty in eyes with Fuchs corneal endothelial dystrophy. Cornea. 2015;34(9):1149–51.
30. Huang MJ, Kaine S, Dhaliwal DK. Descemetorhexis without endothelial keratoplasty verses DMEK for treatment for Fuchs endothelial corneal dystrophy. Cornea. 2018;37(12):1479–983.
31. Macsai MS, Shiloach M. Use of topical rho kinase inhibitors in the treatment of Fuchs dystrophy after Descemet stripping only. Cornea. 2019;38(5):529–34.
32. Davies E, Jurkunas U, Pineda R. Predictive factors for corneal clearance after descemetorhexis without endothelial keratoplasty. Cornea. 2018;37(2):137–40.
33. Lam FC, Baydoun L, Dirisamer M, et al. Hemi-Descemet membrane endothelial keratoplasty transplantation: a potential method for increasing the pool of endothelial graft tissue. JAMA Ophthalmol. 2014;132(12):1469–73.
34. Lie JT, Lam FC, Groeneveld-van Beek EA, et al. Graft preparation for hemi-Descemet membrane endothelial keratoplasty (hemi-DMEK). Br J Ophthalmol. 2016;100:4204.
35. Gerber-Hollbach N, Parker JS, Baydoun L, et al. Preliminary outcome of hemi-Descemet membrane endothelial keratoplasty for Fuchs endothelial dystrophy. Br J Ophthalmol. 2016;100(11):1564–8.
36. Dapena I, Moutsouris K, Droutsas K, et al. Standardized 'no touch' technique of Descemet membrane endothelial keratoplasty. Arch Ophthalmol. 2011;129:29–35.
37. Birbal RS, Hsien S, Zygoura V, et al. Outcomes of hemi-Descemet membrane endothelial keratoplasty for Fuchs endothelial corneal dystrophy. Cornea. 2018;37(7):854–8.
38. Baydoun L, Zygoura H, Birbal RS, et al. Clinical feasibility of using multiple grafts from a single donor for quarter-DMEK. Acta Ophthalmol. 2018;37(5):667–71.
39. Miron A, Spinozzi D, Bruinsma M, et al. Asymmetrical endothelial cell migration from in vitro quarter-Descemet membrane endothelial keratoplasty grafts. Acta Ophthalmolog. 2018;96(8):828–33.
40. Muller TM, Lavy I, Baydoun L, et al. Case report of quarter-Descemet membrane endothelial keratoplasty for Fuchs endothelial dystrophy. Cornea. 2017;36(1):104–7.
41. Zygoura V, Baydoun L, Ham L, et al. Quarter-Descemet membrane endothelial keratoplasty (quarter-DMEK) for Fuchs endothelial dystrophy: 6 months clinical outcome. Br J Ophthalmol. 2018;102(10):1425–30.
42. Baum JL, Niedra R, Davis C, et al. Mass culture of human corneal endothelial cell. Arch Ophthalmol. 1979;97:1136–40.
43. Soh YQ, Peh GS, Mehta JS. Translational tissues for human corneal endothelial tissue engineering. J Tissue Eng Regen Med. 2017;11(9):2425–42.
44. Zaniolo K, Bostan C, Rochette Drouin O, et al. Culture of human corneal endothelial cells isolated from corneas with Fuchs endothelial corneal dystrophy. Exp Eye Res. 2012;94:22–31.
45. Zhu C, Joyce NC. Proliferative response of corneal endothelial cells from young and older donors. Invest Ophthalomol Vis Sci. 2004;45:1743–51.
46. Lee JG, Kay EP. FGF-2-mediated signal transduction during endothelial mesenchymal transformation in corneal endothelial cells. Exp Eye Res. 2006;83(6):1309–16.
47. Fuest M, Hin-Fai Yam G, Swee-Lim Peh G, et al. Corneal cell therapy—an overview. Der Ophthalmol. 2017;114(8):705–15.
48. Koizumi N, Sadamoto Y, Okumura N, et al. Cultivated corneal endothelial transplantation in a primate: possible future clinical applications in corneal endothelial regenerative medicine. Cornea. 2008;27(1):48–55.
49. Fan T, Ma X, Zhao J, et al. Transplantation of tissue-engineered human corneal endothelium in cat models. Mol Vis. 2013;19:400–7.
50. Young TH, Wang IJ, Hu FR, et al. Fabrication of a bioengineered corneal endothelial cell sheet using chitosan/polycaprolactone blend membranes. Colloids Surf B Biointerfaces. 2014;116:403–10.
51. Bostan C, Theriault M, Forget KJ, et al. In vitro functionality of a corneal endothelium transplanted by cell-injection therapy in a feline model. Invest Ophthalmol Vis Sci. 2016;57:1620–34.
52. Okumura N, Kinoshita S, Koizumi N. The role of rho kinase inhibitors in corneal endothelial dysfunction. Curr Pharm Des. 2017;23(4):660–6.
53. Moysidis SN, Alvarex-Delfin K, Peschansky VJ, et al. Magnetic field-guided cell delivery with nanoparticle-loaded human corneal endothelial cells. Nanomedicine. 2015;11(3):499–509.
54. Kinoshita S, Koizumi N, Ueno M, et al. Injection of cultured cells with a ROCK inhibitor for bullous keratopathy. N Engl J Med. 2018;378(11):995–1003.
55. Okumura N, Koizumi N, Ueno M, et al. ROCK inhibitor converts corneal endothelial cells into a phenotype capable of regenerating in vivo tissue. Am J Pathol. 2012;181:268–77.
56. Okumura N, Sakamoto Y, Fujii K, et al. Rho kinase inhibitors enables cell-based therapy for corneal endothelial dysfunction. Sci Rep. 2016;6:26113.
57. Okumura N, Koizumi N, Kay EP, et al. The ROCK inhibitor eye drop accelerates corneal endothelium wound healing. Invest Ophthalmol Vis Sci. 2013;54(4):2493–502.
58. Okumura N, Inoue R, Okazaki Y, et al. Effects of rho kinase inhibitor eye drop Y-27632 on corneal endothelial wound healing. Invest Ophthalmol Vis Sci. 2015;56:6067–74.
59. Garnock-Jones KP. Ripasudil: first global approval. Drugs. 2014;74(18):2211–5.

# OCT in PDEK and DMEK

# 16

Dhivya Ashok Kumar, Amar Agarwal,
and Soosan Jacob

## 16.1 Introduction

Graft adherence is considered as the single important factor for better functional outcome after successful endothelial keratoplasty [1, 2]. Graft detachment has been described as a common complication after endothelial keratoplasty techniques like DMEK and DSAEK [1–3]. Though thinner grafts are more susceptible to incomplete graft adhesion after primary positioning; early and possibly better visual recovery may be possible only with thin grafts [4]. Clinical slit lamp examination has always been the gold standard method of evaluation of graft position postoperatively. However, in eyes with corneal edema or corneal haze, the position of graft and delineation of graft is difficult. Optical coherence tomography technique aids in easy visualization and proper documentation of posterior corneal layers [5–7]. Spectral domain optical coherence tomography (OCT) has been used in corneal evaluation for Descemet's membrane evaluation and has been used widely for follow-up and prognosis assessment [7].

Endothelial keratoplasty has evolved over the last decade, especially the newer techniques like Descemet's membrane endothelial keratoplasty (DMEK), and the Pre-Descemet's endothelial keratoplasty (PDEK) has the advantage of thinner grafts. OCT is based on the principle of "Michelson's interferometry" which can be either time domain or spectral domain. Recently swept source and enhanced depth OCT is also introduced for evaluation in ophthalmology. In our clinical practice, we have used both time domain and spectral domain OCT for corneal evaluation. Spectral domain has the advantage of higher resolution and many instruments have both anterior and posterior segment modules in combined setup. We would be sharing our experiences on the use of OCT in endothelial keratoplasty in this section.

## 16.2 Optical Coherence Tomography

A Cirrus HD Fourier domain OCT prototype system with an anterior segment module (Fig. 16.1) (model 4000, Carl Zeiss Meditec AG) was used in one of our study. The system has been described and used for posterior segment examination can also be used for corneal examination using the anterior segment module [8–11]. It consists of an in-built anterior segment focus adjustment lens and has an 840 nm wavelength superluminescent laser diode as the optical source. The axial resolution is 5 mm and the transverse resolution is 25 mm in tissue. It has a scanning speed of up to 27,000 A-scans/s. The

D. A. Kumar · A. Agarwal (✉) · S. Jacob
Dr. Agarwal's Eye Hospital and Eye Research Centre, Chennai, India



S. Jacob (ed.), *Mastering DMEK and PDEK*, https://doi.org/10.1007/978-981-97-3469-6_16

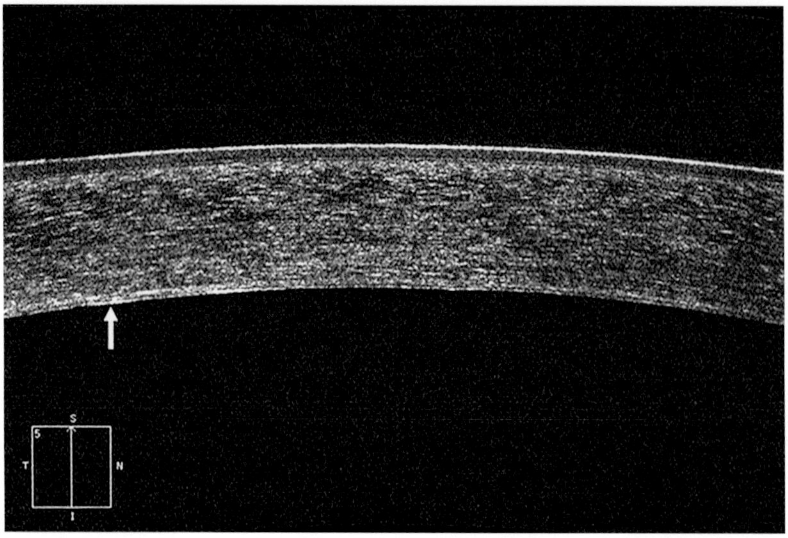


**Fig. 16.1** Spectral or Fourier domain optical coherence tomography showing cornea post-endothelial keratoplasty (arrow)

scanning depth in tissue is 2.0 mm and the optical power at the cornea, less than 725 mW. The forehead and the chin of the patient were positioned in the dual headrest and chinrest with automated right–left sensors. The patient was asked to focus on the target through the eye being examined. Before the scan acquisition, the patient confirmed that he or she saw a green star-shaped target against a black background through the imaging aperture. After the 3-D motorized patient alignment unit and table heights were adjusted, the cornea was brought into focus. An anterior segment 5-line raster pattern (Fig. 16.2) had 5 lines (length 3.0 mm), with a distance of 250 mm between the lines. The noninvasive nature and higher resolution as compared to other imaging techniques like ultrasound, magnetic resonance imaging and computerized tomography, made OCT as one of the standard diagnostic tests in many ocular disorders.

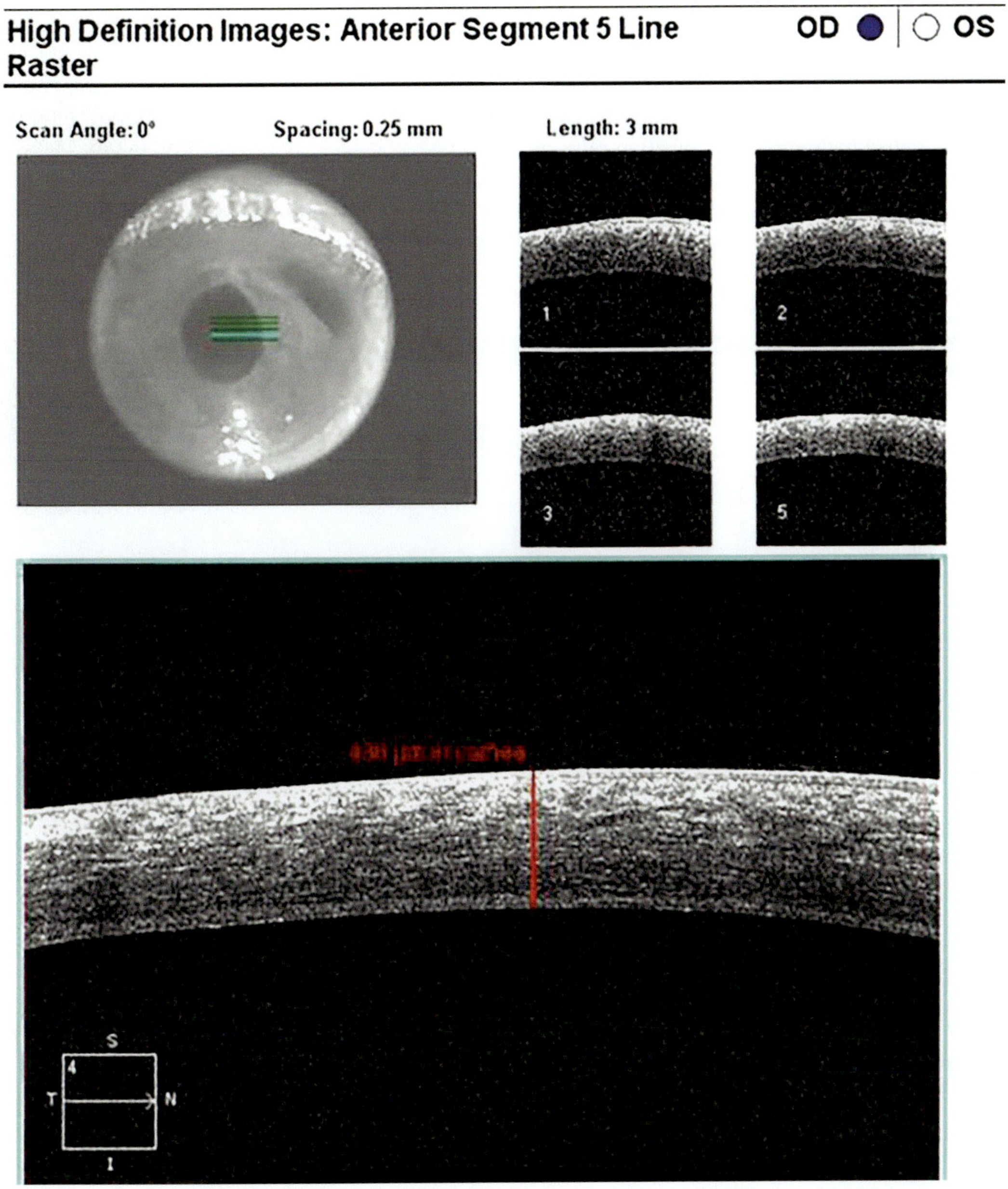


**Fig. 16.2** Fourier domain optical coherence tomography showing the scan being taken in the anterior segment raster pattern

## 16.3 Preoperative Assessment

Anterior OCT has equal role in pre-assessment of eyes undergoing endothelial keratoplasty. Due to its noncontact nature, short acquisition time, and user friendly system, it has been used widely. Preoperative evaluation will be required for serial analysis of worsening of endothelial decompensation such as increasing corneal thickness, progressing subepithelial haze, advancing hypertrophic epithelium, and persistent bullae (Fig. 16.3). It also helps in assessing the anterior chamber details like chamber depth, angles, pupil, and iris lens diaphragm status for proper preoperative anatomical evaluation in corneal haze.

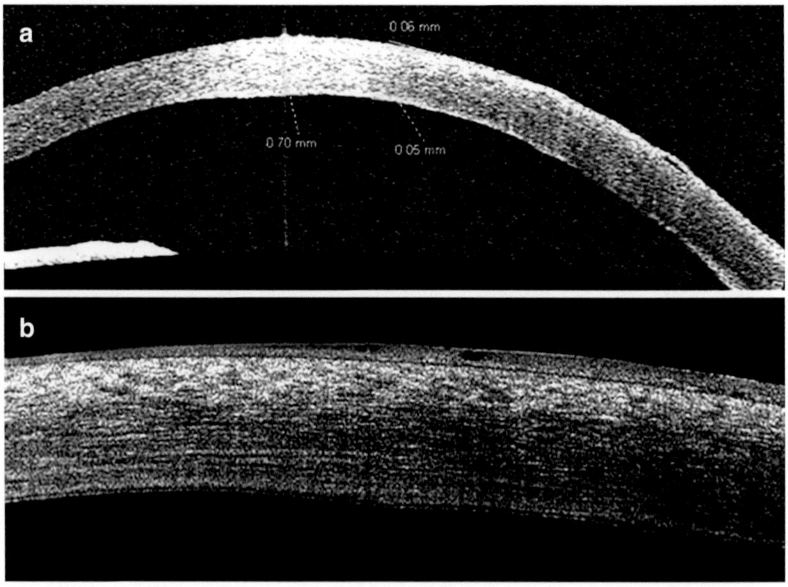


**Fig. 16.3** Time domain (**a**) and spectral domain OCT (**b**) showing the preoperative assessment in eyes with endothelial decompensation showing corneal edema, hypertrophic epithelium, subepithelial haze, and microbullae

## 16.4 OCT in PDEK

Twelve eyes of 12 patients who had PDEK for pseudophakic bullous keratopathy were studied [12]. The mean age was 63 years ±7.2. The donor age ranged from 1 to 65 years. The graft size ranged from 7.5 to 8.0 mm. The mean graft thickness at 1 day was 37.3 ± 3.5 μm (range 32 to 44 μm) (Fig. 16.4). The mean graft thickness at 7 days, 30 days, and 90 days was 35.5 ± 3.4 μm (range 32 to 40 μm), 33 ± 1.8 μm (range 32 to 36 μm), and 30.3 ± 2.6 μm (range 28 to 36 μm), respectively. There was a statistically significant difference in the graft thickness over the time period ($p = 0.000$, Friedman test). The graft was attached in 8 of 12 eyes at 1 day. Out of 4 eyes with graft detachment (Fig. 16.5), the detachment was grade I in 2 eyes, grade II in 1 eye, and grade III in 1 eye respectively. The mean detachment depth was 26 ± 10.3 μm. No eye had complete

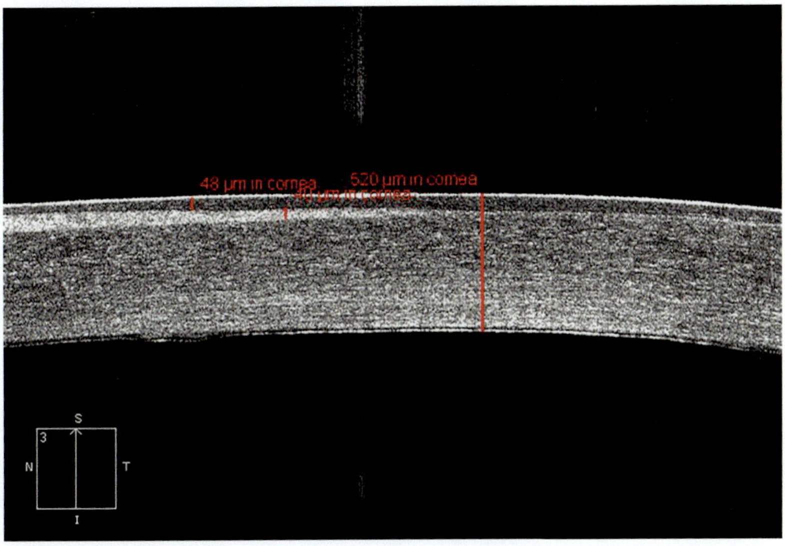


**Fig. 16.4** Fourier domain OCT image of postoperative pre-Descemet's endothelial keratoplasty showing the graft in situ

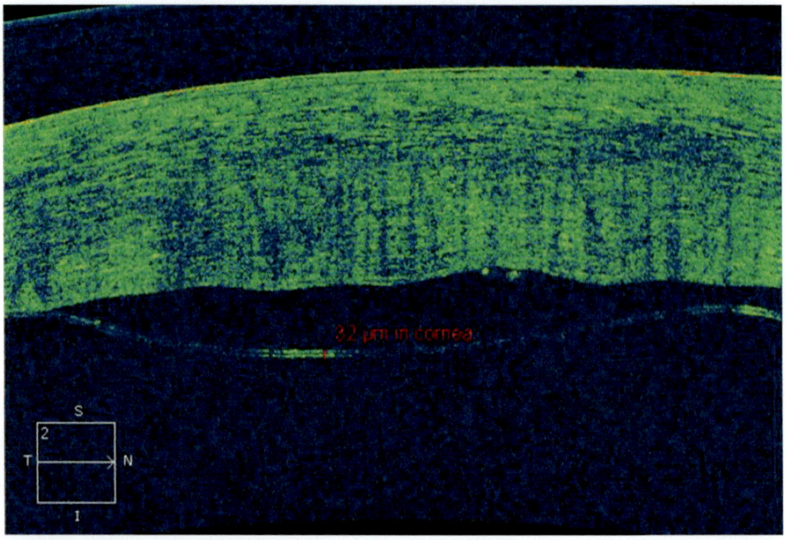


**Fig. 16.5** Color-coded Fourier domain OCT showing the graft detachment

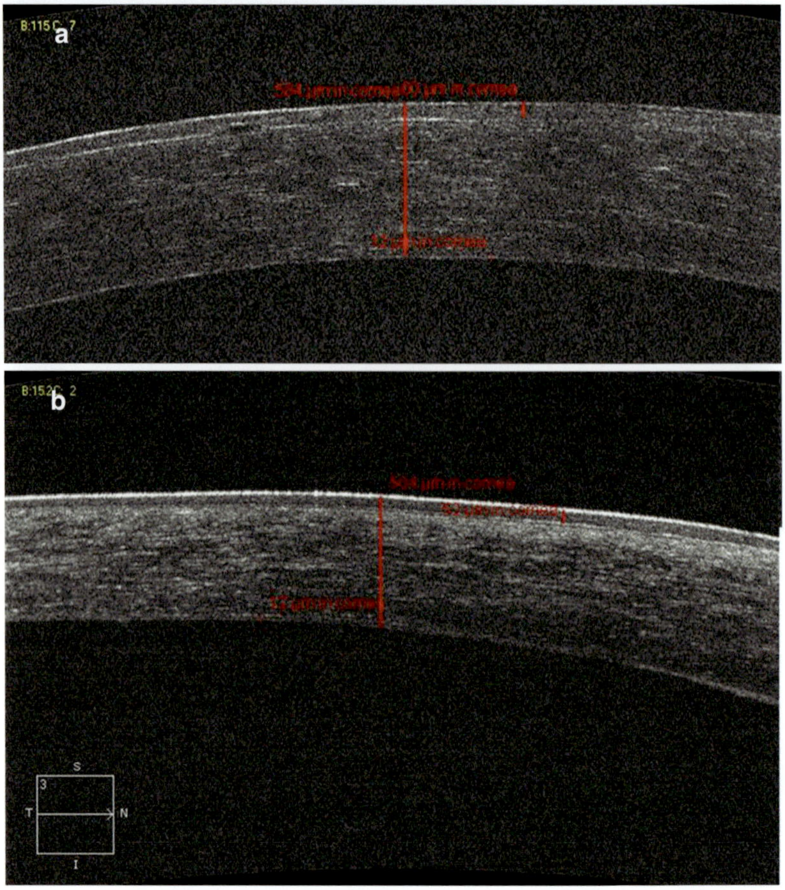


**Fig. 16.6** Epithelial thickness as seen by optical coherence tomography after PDEK showing change from preoperative (**a**) to postoperative status (**b**)

graft detachment or lenticule drop. One eye had minimal interface haze by 1 month postoperatively. The mean epithelial thickness of 44.4 ± 9.8 μm at 7 days decreased to 37.5 ± 6.2 μm by 90 days (Fig. 16.6). The 1-day postoperative corneal edema (mean 621 ± 46.4 μm) showed

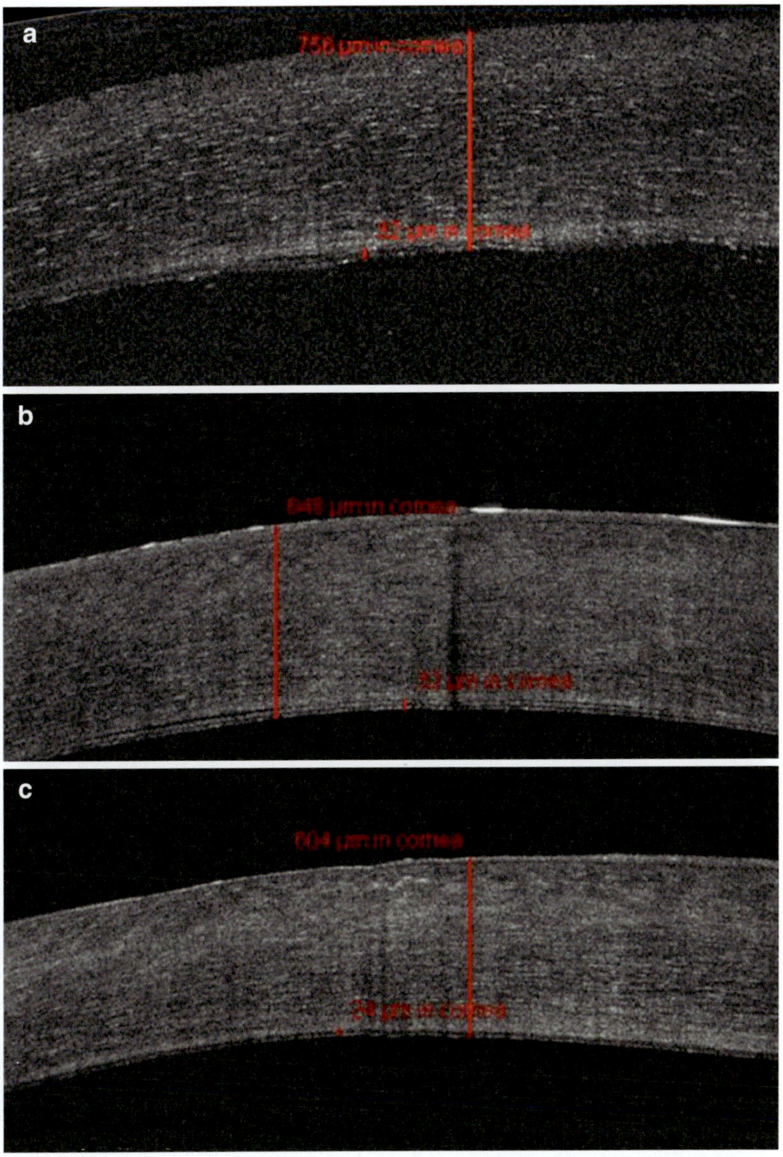


**Fig. 16.7** Optical coherence tomography showing the reduction in corneal edema from **a** (1 week postoperative PDEK) to **b, c** (1 month and 2 months postoperative period)

significant resolution by 7 days ($p = 0.000$) (Fig. 16.7). There was a statistically significant improvement in visual acuity from preoperatively to postoperatively ($p = 0.002$). The final corrected distance visual acuity (CDVA) was 0.61 ± 0.2. There was no significant correlation between the graft thickness and the CDVA at 1 day ($p = 0.402$) or 90 days ($p = 0.649$).

## 16.5 OCT in DMEK

Anterior segment time domain OCT has been widely used to see graft position after DMEK (Fig. 16.8) [13, 14]. Because of the stromal haze at times on the immediate postoperative period after DMEK, it will be challenging for the surgeon to differentiate between detached graft and

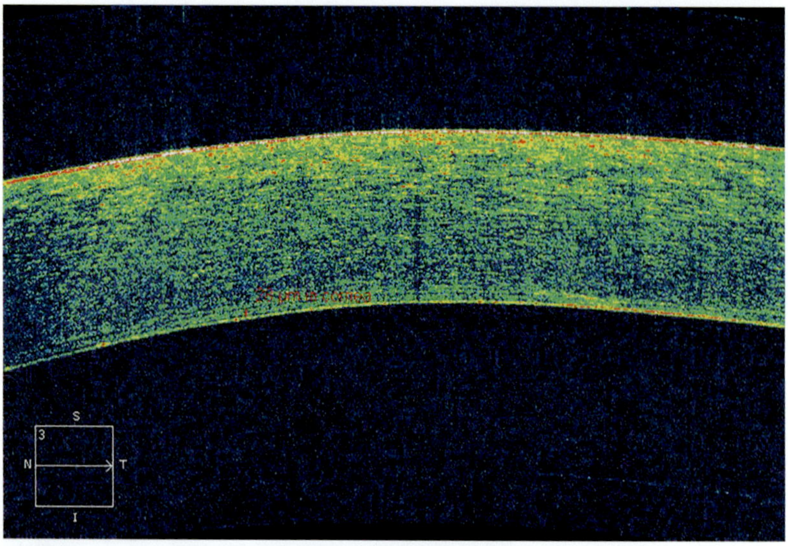


**Fig. 16.8** Fourier domain OCT image of the post-Descemet's membrane endothelial keratoplasty showing the graft in situ

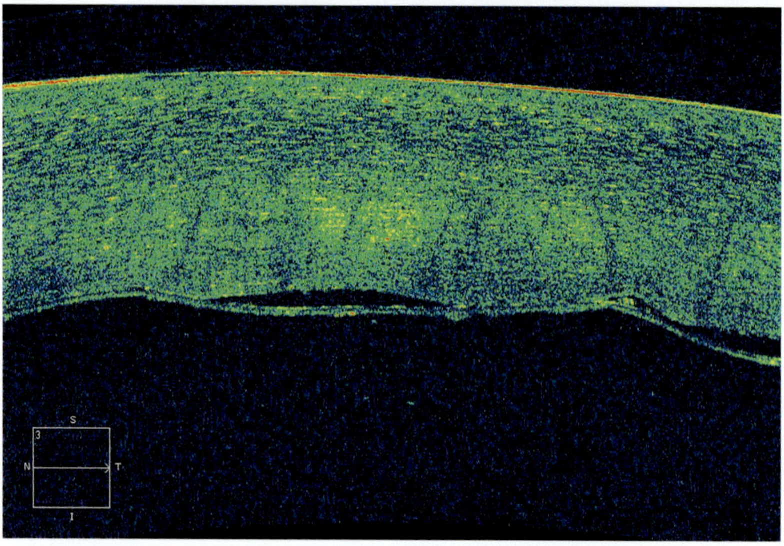


**Fig. 16.9** Fourier domain OCT image of post-Descemet's membrane endothelial keratoplasty graft detachment

delayed clearance. Postoperative graft status was evaluated from obtained OCT images and classified as group I: completely attached grafts or with a minimal edge detachment (Fig. 16.9); group II: graft detachments over one third of the graft surface area, not affecting the visual axis; group III: graft detachments over one third of the graft surface area; and group IV: completely detached grafts, commonly seen as a "free-floating" Descemet-roll in the anterior chamber [14]. This technique has superseded perforating keratoplasty, in many cases sparing unaffected stromal tissue. Advantages of this tissue-selective approach include better visual outcome owing to maintenance of the corneal structural configuration, faster visual recovery after initial surgery, and fewer intraoperative complications, in particular, expulsive hemorrhage. Yeh et al. in their study reported that 1-hour anterior segment OCT scans were more accurate at predicting the final 6-months graft adherence status than those at 1 week or 1 month [14]. The combined information of the 1-hour and 1-week OCT scans may facilitate decision making about surgical reintervention after DMEK. One can use postoperative OCT for serial evaluation of graft position and resolution of corneal edema by documentation of central corneal thickness.

## 16.6 Intraoperative OCT and DMEK

Intraoperative OCT has the additional advantage of direct visualization of graft position in real time during the surgery [15]. Such OCT can be either hand-held device or integrated with operating microscope. Operating microscope-integrated OCT has several advantages, such as online visualization of all surgical steps without the necessity of interrupting the procedure for focus and alignment for OCT and realignment under the microscope [16]. Intraoperative OCT study in DMEK as reported by Cost et al. showed that correct graft orientation was confirmed by intraoperative OCT prior to unscrolling in 100% of cases [15]. Intraoperative OCT may facilitate the transition for beginner surgeons by increasing surgeon confidence and reducing the risk of iatrogenic graft failure. Serial evaluation starting from intraoperative period to postoperative follow-up can help in evaluation of stromal irregularities and lines.

## 16.7 Mouse Sign in OCT

We present a unique sign of graft inversion seen in endothelial keratoplasty eyes [17]. One end of the graft formed a thick convex scroll detaching outward, downward, and upward, and the other end was attached to the edematous cornea forming the "mouse" configuration (Fig. 16.10). Graft reversal is identified when the endothelial side of the donor graft faces the recipient cornea while the Descemet's membrane (DM) faces the iris lens diaphragm. In a series, we reported three cases of similar configuration of graft after pre-Descemet's endothelial keratoplasty which did not respond for air injection [17]. The rebubbling attempts failed in all cases because the graft regained the same configuration each time after manipulation (Fig. 16.11). The probable reasons that have been reported for the rolling of the grafts are (1) the uncorrected rolled or curled edges at the end of surgery, (2) insufficient air support inside the chamber, (3) inverse graft positioning, (4) stromal irregularities or incomplete recipient DM removal. Graft edema, tendency to form tight scroll, and premature loss of air support are the probable reasons for this configuration. There are many techniques suggested to identify and avoid graft reversal intraoperatively. Bimanual infusion technique, endoilluminator-assisted endothelial keratoplasty, F mark, S mark,

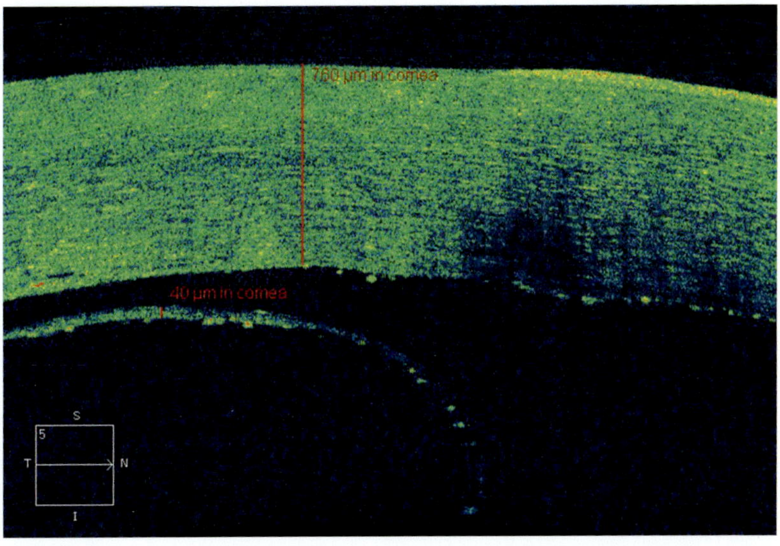


**Fig. 16.10** "Mouse sign" seen by Fourier domain OCT following the pre-Descemet's endothelial keratoplasty

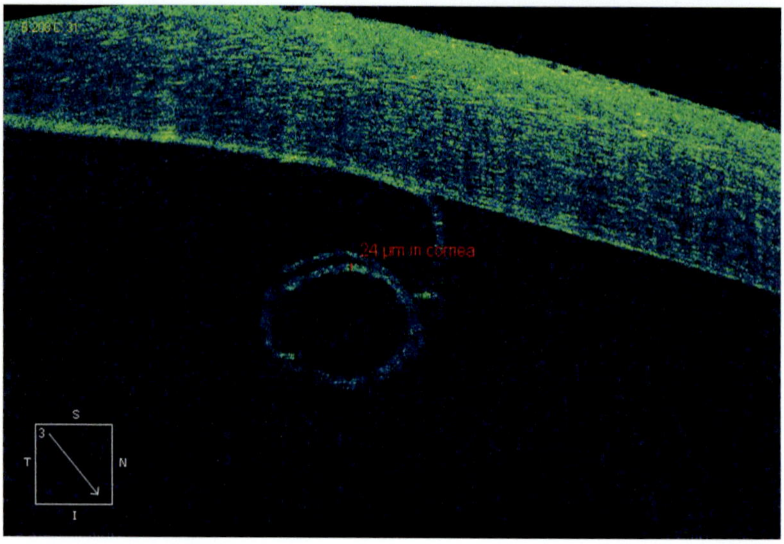


**Fig. 16.11** "Mouse sign" seen by Fourier domain OCT following the pre-Descemet's endothelial keratoplasty after air injection showing inverted graft

intraoperative OCT, triangular mark, Taco configuration, Venn diagram, and Mourtiser's sign are the clinical methods used to identify the orientation of the endothelial graft intraoperatively. Dirisamer et al. studied a series of graft displacements and grouped them into various presentations; they noted that the upside down graft showed reverse corneal clearance and interface spikes [18]. They also observed that 11% of the graft detachments were due to invert grafting. This new sign of inverted graft can give hint to the surgeon that repeat air injection may not help such cases.

## 16.8 Conclusion

Optical coherence tomography can be widely used for any indication starting from corneal thickness assessment, Descemet's membrane detachment identification, graft position assessment, graft thickness determination, and graft detachments grading. Being a noncontact method, OCT has a vital role from preoperative assessment like corneal thickness, scar assessment, and epithelial thickness to postoperative follow-up after endothelial keratoplasty. Be it PDEK or DMEK, all endothelial keratoplasties final outcome depends on the graft attachment to the donor site which is very crucial especially in the immediate postoperative time. Intraoperative and immediate postoperative OCT can thus be used genuinely to evaluate these grafts.

## References

1. Dirisamer M, van Dijk K, Dapena I, et al. Prevention and management of graft detachment in Descemet membrane endothelial keratoplasty. Arch Ophthalmol. 2012;130(3):280–91.
2. Guerra FP, Anshu A, Price MO, et al. Descemet's membrane endothelial keratoplasty: prospective study of 1-year visual outcomes, graft survival, and endothelial cell loss. Ophthalmology. 2011;118(12):2368–73.
3. Shih CY, Ritterband DC, Rubino S, Palmiero PM, Jangi A, Liebmann J, et al. Visually significant and nonsignificant complications arising from Descemet stripping automated endothelial keratoplasty. Am J Ophthalmol. 2009;148(6):837–43.
4. Kaiserman I, Bahar I, Rootman DS. Optical coherence tomography of Descemet membrane separation by the big bubble technique. Cornea. 2007;26(9):1115–7.
5. Hayashi T, Yamaguchi T, Yuda K, Kato N, Satake Y, Shimazaki J. Topographic characteristics after Descemet's membrane endothelial keratoplasty and Descemet's stripping automated endothelial keratoplasty. PLoS One. 2017;12(11):e0188832.
6. Lim LS, Aung HT, Aung T, Tan DT. Corneal imaging with anterior segment optical coherence tomography for lamellar keratoplasty procedures. Am J Ophthalmol. 2008;145(1):81–90.
7. Siebelmann S, Gehlsen U, Le Blanc C, Stanzel TP, Cursiefen C, Steven P. Detection of graft detachments immediately following Descemet membrane endothelial keratoplasty (DMEK) comparing time domain

and spectral domain OCT. Graefes Arch Clin Exp Ophthalmol. 2016;254(12):2431–7.
8. Suh LH, Yoo SH, Deobhakta A, Donaldson KE, Alfonso EC, Culbertson WW, et al. Complications of Descemet's stripping with automated endothelial keratoplasty: survey of 118 eyes at one institute. Ophthalmology. 2008;115(9):1517–24.
9. Dapena I, Ham L, Melles GR. Endothelial keratoplasty: DSEK/DSAEK or DMEK—the thinner the better? Curr Opin Ophthalmol. 2009;20(4):299–307.
10. Moreno-Montanes J, Olmo N, Alvarez A, Garcıa N, Zarranz-Ventura J. Cirrus high-definition optical coherence tomography compared with stratus optical coherence tomography in glaucoma diagnosis. Invest Ophthalmol Vis Sci. 2010;51:335–43.
11. Gupta V, Gupta P, Singh R, Dogra MR, Gupta A. Spectral domain cirrus high-definition optical coherence tomography is better than time-domain stratus optical coherence tomography for evaluation of macular pathologic features in uveitis. Am J Ophthalmol. 2008;145:1018–22.
12. Kumar DA, Dua HS, Agarwal A, Jacob S. Postoperative spectral-domain optical coherence tomography evaluation of pre-Descemet endothelial keratoplasty grafts. J Cataract Refract Surg. 2015;41(7): 1535–6.
13. Moutsouris K, Dapena I, Ham L, et al. Optical coherence tomography, Scheimpflug imaging and slit-lamp biomicroscopy in the early detection of graft detachment after Descemet membrane endothelial keratoplasty. Cornea. 2011;30:1369–75.
14. Yeh RY, Quilendrino R, Musa FU, Liarakos VS, Dapena I, Melles GR. Predictive value of optical coherence tomography in graft attachment after Descemet's membrane endothelial keratoplasty. Ophthalmology. 2013 Feb;120(2):240–5.
15. Cost B, Goshe JM, Srivastava S, Ehlers JP. Intraoperative optical coherence tomography-assisted descemet membrane endothelial keratoplasty in the DISCOVER study. Am J Ophthalmol. 2015;160(3):430–7.
16. Saad A, Guilbert E, Grise-Dulac A, Sabatier P, Gatinel D. Intraoperative OCT-assisted DMEK: 14 consecutive cases. Cornea. 2015;34(7):802–7.
17. Kumar DA, Sood S, Agarwal A. Mouse sign on optical coherence tomography of detached endothelial graft indicates graft inversion. J Ophthalmic Vis Res. 2018;13(3):344–7.
18. Dirisamer M, van Dijk K, Dapena I, Ham L, Oganes O, Frank LE, et al. Prevention and management of graft detachment in Descemet membrane endothelial keratoplasty. Arch Ophthalmol. 2012;130:280–91.

# 17 Comparison of Clinical Outcomes of All Endothelial Keratoplasty: A Systematic Review of Literature

Dhivya Ashok Kumar

## 17.1 Introduction

Endothelial keratoplasty (EK) techniques have nearly replaced the penetrating keratoplasty in the last two decades [1–5]. Graft rejection is one of the key causes for secondary failure whose prevalence is high following full-thickness keratoplasty [6, 7]. On the other hand, the lamellar keratoplasties, where the diseased cornea alone is transplanted, have fewer incidences of rejection [8]. Endothelial grafts have the advantage of harbouring less or no stromal tissue adherent to the endothelium; hence, the incidence of failure due to immune rejection has been reported to be less [1–5]. Other superior benefits of endothelial grafts are the ease of surgery, early visual rehabilitation, and less suture-related astigmatism. With the introduction of pneumatic dissection, the donor tissue harvesting has been made simpler for the surgeons without advanced instrumentation [6–8]. Restoring the function in a decompensated cornea by means of Descemet's membrane endothelial keratoplasty (DMEK), Descemet's stripping automated endothelial keratoplasty (DSAEK), ultrathin DSAEK and recently Pre-Descemet's endothelial keratoplasty (PDEK) are in vogue [7–14]. In this chapter, we do a literature search and limited meta-analysis of surgical outcomes of the recent EK techniques, namely the Descemet's membrane endothelial keratoplasty (DMEK), Descemet's stripping automated endothelial keratoplasty (DSAEK), ultrathin DSAEK and Pre-Descemet's endothelial keratoplasty (PDEK).

## 17.2 Meta-Analysis and Systematic Review

Meta-analysis is a quantitative, epidemiological study design used to systematically assess the previous research on EK studies to derive conclusions on the clinical outcomes. Studies related to EK with keyword Descemet's membrane endothelial keratoplasty (DMEK), Descemet's stripping automated endothelial keratoplasty (DSAEK), ultrathin DSAEK and recently Pre-Descemet's endothelial keratoplasty (PDEK) were searched. Pubmed, Google scholars, and Cochrane database studies and the data were analysed. Only articles published in English were considered. Systematic reviews, meta-analyses, randomized controlled trials, case series, and audits comparing DMEK, DSAEK/DSEK, and PDEK irrespective of location were included. There were no restrictions on preexisting conditions of patients or indications for surgery.

D. A. Kumar (✉)
Dr. Agarwal's Eye Hospital and Eye Research Centre, Chennai, India



S. Jacob (ed.), *Mastering DMEK and PDEK*, https://doi.org/10.1007/978-981-97-3469-6_17

## 17.3 Literature Review in Clinical Outcomes of EK

In a meta-analysis by Pavlovic et al., 11 clinical studies in DMEK were analysed [15]. A total of 11 studies with a total of 723 eyes (350 DMEK and 373 DSAEK) were included. No significant difference was found regarding the total detachment rate, graft failure, and rejection. One out of 340 eyes of DMEK showed total detachment and 5 out of 363 eyes of DSAEK showed total detachment ($p = 0.28$). Six out of 280 eyes of DMEK showed graft failure; 1 out of 313 eyes of DSAEK developed graft failure ($p = 0.18$). No rejection was observed in 158 eyes undergoing DMEK; four cases of rejection occurred in 196 eyes undergoing DSAEK ($p = 0.37$). No significant difference was found regarding endothelial cell loss ($p = 0.48$). There was a significantly higher partial detachment rate with DMEK: 88 out of 340 eyes undergoing DMEK showed partial detachment; 16 out of 363 eyes undergoing DSAEK showed partial detachment ($p = 0.00001$). DMEK was superior in best corrected visual acuity after 6 months ($p = 0.001$), subjective evaluation of visual acuity ($P = 0.001$), patient satisfaction ($p = 0.001$), and was the method preferred by patients ($p = 0.001$).

Another meta-analysis by Saquin Li et al., 19 studies were eligible, and 1124 eyes and 1254 eyes were included in the DMEK and Descemet's stripping endothelial keratoplasty (DSEK) groups, respectively [16]. The overall pooled estimates showed a significantly better postoperative BCVA, a comparable endothelial cell density (ECD), and an increased graft detachment rate in the DMEK group compared with the DSEK group (BCVA: mean difference (MD) = −0.15, 95% CI = −0.19 to −0.11, $p < 0.001$; ECD: MD = 14.88, 95% CI = −181.50 to 211.27, $P = 0.882$; graft detachment rate: OR = 4.56, 95% CI = 2.43 to 8.58, $p < 0.001$) [16]. Except for the postoperative ECD, which was changed to be higher in the DSEK group than the DMEK group, the learning curve did not have a marked effect on the comparison outcome of the BCVA and graft detachment rate based on the estimates pooled from studies that collected data during the DMEK learning phase (ECD (learning curve): MD = −361.24, 95% CI = −649.42 to −73.07, $p = 0.014$) [16].

In a study by Marques et al., a total of 10 retrospective studies of moderate methodological quality were included [17]. There were total 947 eyes. They compared the outcomes of DMEK with DSAEK in Fuchs' endothelial dystrophy. The BCVA was better with DMEK at all evaluated time points (0.16 logMAR at 12 months) compared to DSAEK (0.30 logMAR, $p < 0.001$). DMEK had a 60% lower rate of rejection (risk ratio (RR) 0.4, 95% CI (0.24, 0.67), $p = 0.0005$), but required more rebubbling (RR = 2.48, 95% CI (1.32, 4.64), $p = 0.005$). DMEK had more primary graft failures and less endothelial cell density loss, but statistical difference was not reached. More patients were satisfied after DMEK (odds ratio = 10.29, 95% CI (3.55, 29.80), $p < 0.0001$) [17].

In a systematic review of endothelial keratoplasty by Singh et al., DMEK is superior to DSAEK for the following outcomes: visual acuity, central corneal thickness, and patient satisfaction [18]. There was a statistically significant difference in the mean spectacle-corrected visual acuity at 6 months for DMEK (mean = 0.161, SD = 0.129) and DSAEK eye (mean = 0.293, SD = 0.153) conditions; t (297) = 8.042, $P < 0.0001$. The pooled mean difference was −0.13 (95% confidence interval, −0.16 to −0.09) and $I$ = 44%, indicating better visual acuity for DMEK [18]. Mean postoperative ECD showed statistically no significant difference in the mean values for DMEK (mean = 1855, SD = 442) and DSAEK eye (mean = 1872, SD = 429) conditions; t (336) = 0.375, $P = 0.708$. A higher proportion of patients prefer DMEK to DSAEK. However, DSAEK was superior to DMEK with respect to the need for rebubbling as the rebubbling rate was higher in the DMEK group. They concluded that although DMEK was associated with a higher rate of rebubbling, better visual outcomes were seen in DMEK.

In a comparative trial of DMEK with DSAEK by Hamzglou et al., they compared the results of the first 100 eyes of DSAEK and DMEK that were performed at a single institution [19]. They concluded that the DMEK provided better visual recovery and comparable 6 months endothelial cell loss. The DMEK group had a higher although not statistically significant, percentage of rebubbling procedures.

A systematic review by Stuart et al., analysis was performed for primary and secondary outcomes after endothelial keratoplasty [20]. The primary outcome was best corrected visual acuity (BCVA) measured in logarithm of the Minimum Angle of Resolution (logMAR). Secondary outcomes were endothelial cell count, graft rejection, primary graft failure, and graft dislocation. The study analysed four non-randomized studies which consisted 72 adult patients with Fuchs' endothelial dystrophy with decompensated cornea who had received DSAEK in the first eye followed by DMEK in the fellow eye. They noted at 1 year, using DMEK in cases of endothelial failure may result in better BCVA compared with DSAEK (mean difference (MD) −0.14, 95% confidence interval (CI) −0.18 to −0.10 logMAR, 4 studies, 140 eyes, low-certainty evidence). None of the participants had severe visual loss (BCVA of 1.0 logMAR or more; very low-certainty evidence). No primary graft failure and only one graft rejection was recorded. The most common complications reported were graft dislocations, which were recorded in one or two out of 100 participants with DSAEK but were more common using DMEK although that difference could not be precisely estimated (risk ratio (RR) 5.40, 95% CI 1.51–19.3; 4 studies, 144 eyes, very low-certainty evidence) [20].

Droutas et al. compared the DMEK and DSAEK in specific matched pairs and noted that DMEK patients showed faster rehabilitation and higher BSCVA at all postoperative visits [21]. On clinical outcome, central corneal thickness decreased from 718 μm (range, 566–1041 μm) to 533 μm (range, 460–605 μm) after DMEK and from 650 μm (range, 527–749 μm) to 605 μm (range, 486–650 μm) after DSAEK. Endothelial cell density decreased from 2448 cells/mm (range, 2106–3000 cells/mm) to 1263 cells/mm (range, 589–2282 cells/mm) after DMEK and from 2348 cells/mm (range, 2156–2781 cells/mm) to 1327 cells/mm (range, 664–1972 cells/mm) after DSAEK.

While comparing the ultrathin DSAEK with DMEK, both had not differed significantly in mean BSCVA, but the percentage of eyes achieving 20/25 Snellen vision was significantly higher with DMEK [22]. Endothelial cell loss did not differ significantly between the treatment groups, and both techniques induced a minimal hyperopic shift. Another study by Dickman et al., comparing DASEK with UT-DSAEK showed that compared with DSAEK, UT-DSAEK results in faster and better recovery of BSCVA with similar refractive outcomes, endothelial cell loss, and incidence of complications [23]. Thickness does have improved functional outcome as reported in thinner grafts. A review study by Busin et al. concluded that UT-DSAEK is a procedure that shared the improved visual outcome and lower immunologic rejection rate of DMEK over DSAEK, while minimizing all types of postoperative complications [24].

There are no recent studies comparing PDEK with DMEK or DSEAK. In the case series on PDEK by Kumar et al., there was no significant difference between PDEK and control eyes in the total corneal densitometry in the entire depth of the cornea ($p$ = 0.662) [25]. Agarwal et al. reported PDEK using infant donors and noted that there was improvement in the visual acuity in all the patients [26]. The mean donor endothelial cell density was 3073 ± 68 cells per square millimetre, and the mean postoperative specular count at 6 months was 2230 ± 43 cells per square millimetre. The mean percentage loss of endothelial cells at 6 months was 27 ± 2%. In another series of 10 eyes by Jacob et al., good clinical visual outcome and endothelial cell loss was 38.6% was reported in air pump-assisted PDEK [27]. Kumar et al. observed PDEK grafts by optical coherence tomography and noted that there was no significant correlation between the graft thickness and the BCVA at 1 day ($p$ = 0.402) or 90 days ($p$ = 0.649) [28]. There was a statistically significant improvement in visual acuity from preoperatively to postoperatively ($p$ = 0 0.002). The final BCVA was 0.61 ± 0.2 [28].

In a comparative study between in DSAEK and DMEK, Droutas et al. noted that DMEK showed lower corneal densitometry and better BCVA compared with DSAEK in the first 6 postoperative months [29]. A study comparing the effect of DASEK on DMEK graft versus primary DSAEK noted that the there was an increase in central corneal light scattering after secondary DSAEK performed after a failed DMEK as compared to primary DSAEK [30].

With respect to high-order aberrations changes, DMEK results in less posterior corneal HOA compared with ultrathin DSAEK. It has been shown that DMEK decreases and ultrathin DSAEK increases posterior corneal HOA compared with presurgical values [31]. At 3, 6, and 12 months after surgery, the posterior corneal surface had significantly less coma ($P \leq 0.003$) and total HOA ($P \leq 0.001$) in DMEK compared with ultrathin DSAEK (4.0- and 6.0-mm OZ).

## 17.4 Conclusion

Melles et al. introduced the Descemet membrane endothelial keratoplasty in 2006. The advantage of the DMEK is that it eliminated the stromal interface, allowing perfect anatomical replacement of the diseased endothelium by a healthy donor. Agarwal et al. introduced the PDEK procedure, which had the advantage of procurement of graft from young donors. Ultrathin DSAEK improved visual outcome and lower immunologic rejection over DSAEK. Every other endothelial keratoplasty in the last two decades have their inherent advantages. However, the limitations are minimal. Graft procurement, less tissue wastage, storage facility, and skill transfer are the other parameters that will also affect the availability of these techniques widely to patients. Nevertheless, the popular EK techniques in the recent past have shown promising functional and anatomical outcomes. Long-term results are yet to be observed in the future years in newer modifications.

## References


1. Melles GR, Eggink FA, Lander F, et al. A surgical technique for posterior lamellar keratoplasty. Cornea. 1998;17:618–26.
2. Terry MA, Ousley PJ. Deep lamellar endothelial keratoplasty in the first United States patients: early clinical results. Cornea. 2001;20:239–43.
3. Terry MA, Ousley PJ. Small-incision deep lamellar endothelial keratoplasty (DLEK). Cornea. 2005;24:7.
4. Gorovoy MS. Descemet-stripping automated endothelial keratoplasty. Cornea. 2006;25:886–9.
5. Bahar I, Kaiserman I, McAllum P, Slomovic A, Rootman D. Comparison of posterior lamellar keratoplasty techniques to penetrating keratoplasty. Ophthalmology. 2008;115:1525–33.
6. Price MO, Gorovoy M, Price FW Jr, Benetz BA, Menegay HJ, Lass JH. Descemet's stripping automated endothelial keratoplasty: three-year graft and endothelial cell survival compared with penetrating keratoplasty. Ophthalmology. 2013;120(2):246–51.
7. Zhang YM, Wu SQ, Yao YF. Long-term comparison of full-bed deep anterior lamellar keratoplasty and penetrating keratoplasty in treating keratoconus. J Zhejiang Univ Sci B. 2013;14(5):438–50.
8. Kymionis GD, Mikropoulos DG, Portaliou DM, Boboridis KG, Voudouragkaki IC, Dragoumis ND, Konstas AG. New perspectives on lamellar keratoplasty. Adv Ther. 2014;31(5):494–511.
9. Rodríguez-Calvo-de-Mora M, Quilendrino R, Ham L, et al. Clinical outcome of 500 consecutive cases undergoing Descemet's membrane endothelial keratoplasty. Ophthalmology. 2015;122:464–70. https://doi.org/10.1016/j.ophtha.2014.09.004.
10. Heinzelmann S, Böhringer D, Eberwein P, Reinhard T, Maier P. Outcomes of Descemet membrane endothelial keratoplasty, Descemet stripping automated endothelial keratoplasty and penetrating keratoplasty from a single centre study. Graefes Arch Clin Exp Ophthalmol. 2016;254:515–22. https://doi.org/10.1007/s00417-015-3248-z.
11. Agarwal A, Dua HS, Narang P, Kumar DA, Agarwal A, Jacob S, Agarwal A, Gupta A. Pre-Descemet's endothelial keratoplasty (PDEK). Br J Ophthalmol. 2014;98:1181. https://doi.org/10.1136/bjophthalmol-2013-304639.
12. Busin M, Madi S, Santorum P, Scorcia V, Beltz J. Ultrathin Descemet's stripping automated endothelial keratoplasty with the microkeratome double-pass technique: two-year outcomes. Ophthalmology. 2013;120(6):1186–94.
13. Lekhanont K, Pisitpayat P, Cheewaruangroj N, Jongkhajornpong P, Nonpassopon M, Anothaisintawee T. Outcomes of Descemet membrane endothelial keratoplasty in Bangkok, Thailand. Clin Ophthalmol. 2021;15:2239–51.
14. Hayashi T, Kobayashi A, Takahashi H, Oyakawa I, Kato N, Yamaguchi T. Optical characteristics after

Descemet membrane endothelial keratoplasty: 1-year result. PLoS One. 2020;15(10):e0240458.
15. Pavlovic I, Shajari M, Herrmann E, Schmack I, Lencova A, Kohnen T. Meta-analysis of postoperative outcome parameters comparing Descemet membrane endothelial keratoplasty versus Descemet stripping automated endothelial keratoplasty. Cornea. 2017;36(12):1445–51.
16. Li S, Liu L, Wang W, Huang T, Zhong X, Yuan J, Liang L. Efficacy and safety of Descemet's membrane endothelial keratoplasty versus Descemet's stripping endothelial keratoplasty: a systematic review and meta-analysis. PLoS One. 2017;12(12):e0182275.
17. Marques RE, Guerra PS, Sousa DC, Gonçalves AI, Quintas AM, Rodrigues W. DMEK versus DSAEK for Fuchs' endothelial dystrophy: a meta-analysis. Eur J Ophthalmol. 2019;29(1):15–22.
18. Singh A, Zarei-Ghanavati M, Avadhanam V, Liu C, Singh A, et al. Systematic review and meta-analysis of clinical outcomes of Descemet membrane endothelial keratoplasty versus Descemet stripping endothelial keratoplasty/Descemet stripping automated endothelial keratoplasty. Cornea. 2017;36(11):1437–43.
19. Hamzaoglu EC, Straiko MD, Mayko ZM, Sáles CS, Terry MA, Hamzaoglu EC, et al. The first 100 eyes of standardized Descemet stripping automated endothelial keratoplasty versus standardized Descemet membrane endothelial keratoplasty. Ophthalmology. 2015;122(11):2193–9.
20. Stuart AJ, Romano V, Virgili G, Shortt AJ, Stuart AJ, et al. Descemet's membrane endothelial keratoplasty (DMEK) versus Descemet's stripping automated endothelial keratoplasty (DSAEK) for corneal endothelial failure. Cochrane Database Syst Rev. 2018;6(6):CD012097.
21. Droutsas K, Lazaridis A, Papaconstantinou D, Brouzas D, Moschos MM, Schulze S, Sekundo W, Droutsas K, et al. Visual outcomes after Descemet membrane endothelial keratoplasty versus Descemet stripping automated endothelial keratoplasty-comparison of specific matched pairs. Cornea. 2016;35(6):765–71.
22. Dunker SL, Dickman MM, Wisse RPL, Nobacht S, Wijdh RHJ, Bartels MC, Tang ML, van den Biggelaar FJHM, Kruit PJ, Nuijts RMMA, Dunker SL, et al. Descemet membrane endothelial keratoplasty versus ultrathin Descemet stripping automated endothelial keratoplasty: a multicenter randomized controlled clinical trial. Ophthalmology. 2020;127(9):1152–9.
23. Dickman MM, Kruit PJ, Remeijer L, van Rooij J, Van der Lelij A, Wijdh RH, van den Biggelaar FJ, Berendschot TT, Nuijts RM, Dickman MM, et al. A randomized multicenter clinical trial of ultrathin Descemet stripping automated endothelial keratoplasty (DSAEK) versus DSAEK. Ophthalmology. 2016;123(11):2276–84.
24. Busin M, Albé E, Busin M, et al. Does thickness matter: ultrathin Descemet stripping automated endothelial keratoplasty. Curr Opin Ophthalmol. 2014;25(4):312–8.
25. Kumar DA, Agarwal A, Jaganathasai N. Densitometry analysis of corneal backscatter after pre-Descemet endothelial keratoplasty for pseudophakic bullous keratopathy. Cornea. 2020;39(1):30–8.
26. Agarwal A, Agarwal A, Narang P, Kumar DA, Jacob S. Pre-Descemet endothelial keratoplasty with infant donor corneas: a prospective analysis. Cornea. 2015;34(8):859–65.
27. Jacob S, Narasimhan S, Agarwal S, Agarwal A, Saijimol AI. Air pump-assisted graft centration, graft edge unfolding, and graft uncreasing in young donor graft pre-Descemet endothelial keratoplasty. Cornea. 2017;36(8):1009–13.
28. Kumar DA, Dua HS, Agarwal A, Jacob S. Postoperative spectral-domain optical coherence tomography evaluation of pre-Descemet endothelial keratoplasty grafts. J Cataract Refract Surg. 2015;41(7):1535–6.
29. Droutsas K, Lazaridis A, Giallouros E, Kymionis G, Chatzistefanou K, Sekundo W. Scheimpflug densitometry after DMEK versus DSAEK-two-year outcomes. Cornea. 2018;37(4):455–61.
30. Arnalich-Montiel F, Hernández-Verdejo JL, Oblanca N, Muñoz-Negrete FJ, De Miguel MP, Arnalich-Montiel F, et al. Comparison of corneal haze and visual outcome in primary DSAEK versus DSAEK following failed DMEK. Graefes Arch Clin Exp Ophthalmol. 2013;251(11):2575–84.
31. Duggan MJ, Rose-Nussbaumer J, Lin CC, Austin A, Labadzinzki PC, Chamberlain WD, Duggan MJ, et al. Corneal higher-order aberrations in Descemet membrane endothelial keratoplasty versus ultrathin DSAEK in the Descemet endothelial thickness comparison trial: a randomized clinical trial. Ophthalmology. 2019;126(7):946–57.

# 18 Rock Inhibitors

Amardeep Singh

## 18.1 Introduction

In ophthalmology, a growing interest in Rho-kinases (ROCKs) and their inhibitors over the last decade has generated a multitude of scientific studies. Collectively, these studies have demonstrated the implication of the ROCK signalling pathway in the pathogenesis of some ocular diseases, especially those affecting the cornea, optic nerve, and retina. Pharmacological ROCK inhibition is already an established and approved modality of treatment in patients with primary open-angle glaucoma (POAG) or ocular hypertension (OHT). In the cornea, ROCK inhibition appears to contribute to maintenance of epithelial integrity and limbal stem cell health, prevention of corneal vascularization, and promotion of endothelial cell survival. Diseases affecting the various layers of the cornea may be amenable to medical therapies alone, but invasive therapies are not infrequently required. A familiar clinical problem is corneal endothelial decompensation where topical eye drops consisting of hypertonic sodium chloride may initially be effective in dehydrating the stroma. However, as the condition progresses some form of corneal transplantation procedure will be required to improve visual acuity. Corneal transplantation is often successful in restoring corneal transparency, but tags along with it a long list of potential complications, such as glaucoma and immunological rejection. Moreover, there is a global shortage of donor tissue which limits the number of procedures that can be performed. Thus, there is a constant need for innovative thinking and discovery of new ways to address this problem. ROCK inhibition may help bridge the gap between medical and surgical therapy of several commonly encountered eye diseases, such as Fuchs endothelial dystrophy and pseudophakic bullous keratopathy. In this bargain, dependence on cornea grafts will lessen and ultimately allow for the treatment of a wider spectrum of patients, including those where transplantation is (relatively) contraindicated, for example, concurrent glaucoma.

Corneal disease and glaucoma are related in such a way that one often affects the other. For instance, ocular hypertension may occur in up to 50% of patients after penetrating keratoplasty [1]. In turn, ocular hypertension is negatively correlated with corneal endothelial cell survival and higher risk of graft failure [2, 3]. Thus, for a corneal surgeon, knowledge of mechanisms responsible for elevated IOP in cornea patients is critical. ROCK inhibition may have dual functions in the same patient (e.g. promoting corneal

A. Singh (✉)
Department of Ophthalmology, Skåne University Hospital, Lund University, Lund, Sweden

Department of Ophthalmology, Rigshospitalet-Glostrup, Glostrup, Denmark

Department of Clinical Medicine, Faculty of Health and Medical Sciences, University of Copenhagen, Copenhagen, Denmark



S. Jacob (ed.), *Mastering DMEK and PDEK*, https://doi.org/10.1007/978-981-97-3469-6_18

endothelial cells survival and simultaneously reducing IOP). The purpose of this chapter is to describe the ROCK signalling pathways and their implications in ocular diseases. Findings from preclinical and clinical studies on the ROCK pathway and its inhibition will be discussed in the context of ocular disease with special weight on corneal disease and glaucoma. Finally, selected ophthalmic formulations containing ROCK inhibitors will be discussed.

## 18.2 Protein Kinases and Rock Signalling Pathways

About 30 years ago, the Rho-associated protein kinase or Rho-associated coiled-coin-containing protein kinase (ROCK) was identified as an effector of the small GTPase Rho [4–7]. The Ras homologous (Rho) proteins are members of the GTPase family of small, monomeric molecules that control several complex cellular processes. When Rho is activated by guanine triphosphate (GTP), it interacts with one of its many effector molecules, for example, Rho-associated protein kinase or Rho-associated coiled-coin-containing protein kinase (ROCK). A kinase is an enzymatic protein structure that adds phosphate groups ($PO_4^{3-}$) to other molecules, for example, amino acids, lipids, and nucleotides subsequently affecting downstream cell signalling mechanisms. The Rho-associated protein kinase or Rho-associated coiled-coin-containing protein kinase (ROCK) is specifically directed towards phosphorylation of the amino acids serine and threonine. Since ROCK is a downstream effector of the Rho GTPases (molecular switches controlling the transduction of external signals to cytoplasmic and nuclear effectors), it regulates multiple physiological functions, including cell contraction, migration, proliferation, angiogenesis, chemotaxis, neural protection, regulation of cell polarity, gene transcription, enzymatic activities, modulation of actomyosin cytoskeletal rearrangements, and vasodilation [8–11].

ROCK exists in two isoforms, ROCK-I (ROCK-β) and ROCK-II (ROCK-α) [7, 10]. ROCK-I genes are located on chromosome 18 (18q11.1) and ROCK-II genes are located on chromosome 2 (2p24) [12]. Both isoforms are highly homologous, with an overall amino acid sequence identity of 65% and small molecular weight (160 kDa) [9, 13, 14]. Both contain an N-terminal kinase domain and an identical ATP-binding pocket. ROCK-I is ubiquitously expressed with a preferential expression of ROCK-I in circulating inflammatory cells and ROCK-II in vascular cells, brain and skeletal muscle [15]. In human eyes, both isoforms have been detected in the cornea, trabecular meshwork, ciliary muscle, and optic nerve head [16, 17]. As a consequence, ROCK signalling is believed to be involved in numerous physiological functions of the eye.

Modulation of the ROCK signalling pathway may be achieved by two means: (1) pharmacological, which is discussed in detail later, and (2) non-pharmacological, for example, ageing, which is associated with increase in ROCK activity, and exercise and smoking, which have inhibitory and promoting effects on the ROCK pathway, respectively [18–21].

## 18.3 Rock Signalling in Corneal Health and Disease

Structural integrity and optical transparency of the cornea are essential prerequisites for transmission and accurate refraction of light. Disruption of the corneal layers as observed in epithelial defects will usually affect visual quality in a significant manner. An epithelial defect is readily replaced by new cells originating from the stem cells at the corneoscleral limbus [22]. These stem cells also act as a barrier to translimbal migration of blood vessels and cells with conjunctival phenotype onto the corneal surface. Thus, depletion of limbal epithelial stem cells results in an unhealthy epithelial layer and corneal neovascularization [22–24]. Other than stem cell failure, an imbalance between pro-angiogenic and anti-angiogenic factors in favour of the former (e.g. due to inflammation) can cause proliferation and migration of vascular endothelial cells onto the corneal stroma [25]. The ROCK signalling pathway is involved in the process of angiogenesis, primarily through suppression of the inflammatory response, but also by reducing oxidative damage and inhibiting vascular growth endothelial factor (VEGF) [26–29]. Decompensation of the corneal endothelium layer leads to loss of corneal transparency and visual impairment. A state of relative stromal dehydration is a prerequisite for corneal transparency and is dependent on functional epithelial and endothelial layers. Together these two layers serve as a mechanical barrier to fluid diffusion and actively pump water molecules away from the stroma. Below follows a discussion on current knowledge on ROCK inhibition in the behaviour of corneal epithelial, limbal stem cell, and endothelial cells since these are the areas most extensively investigated.

## 18.4 Epithelium and Limbal Stem Cells

More than 25 years ago, SundarRaj and co-authors discovered that ROCK-I is distributed in limbal and corneal epithelium in rabbits [30]. Ten years later, the same group found that inhibiting the ROCK pathway prevented cell replication (G1/S transition) in rabbit corneal epithelial cells [31], suggesting a supportive role of the ROCK pathway in cell cycle progression. On the contrary, Yin and co-authors reported enhanced cell proliferation and epithelial differentiation in immortalized human corneal epithelial cells upon exposure to Y-27632, an inhibitor of ROCK [16]. However, cell migration and adhesion, and tight-junction barrier formation were negatively modulated indicating an equivocal role of the ROCK pathway in epithelial function. In mice with alkali-induced corneal burns, topical ROCK inhibitor application led to faster resolution of epithelial defects [28]. This may, in part, be explained by the role of the ROCK pathway in limbal stem cell function. In rabbit limbal epithelial cells, Y-27632 increases their cloning efficiency by improving adherence to other cells and decreasing accumulation of reactive oxygen species, thereby preventing the detrimental effects of reactive oxygen species on stem cell function [32, 33]. In limbal explants from human donor eyes, Y-27632 promoted proliferation of limbal epithelial cell proliferation [34]. Thus, inhibition of the ROCK pathway may promote regeneration of the corneal epithelium and limbal stem cell function.

## 18.5 Neovascularization

Corneal neovascularization is usually a non-specific response to chronic inflammation or hypoxia. Although an adaptive response in nature, the growth of new vessels originating from existing vessels of the pericorneal plexus are often associated with unfavourable consequences, such as visual impairment, perpetuation of inflammation with scarring, oedema and leakage of lipids or exudate, and worsening the prognosis of graft survival following transplantation [24]. Vascularization of the cornea occurs when there is an imbalance between pro-angiogenic factors, such as vascular endothelial growth factor (VEGF), and anti-angiogenic factors, such as soluble VEGF Receptor-2 [35]. Fasudil (also known as HA-1077), a selective ROCK inhibitor approved in China and Japan for management of cerebral vasospasm, is an inhibitor of corneal neovascularization. When applied topically to mice with alkali-induced corneal burns, Fasudil significantly reduces the degree of neovascularization compared to placebo, possibly by virtue of its anti-inflammatory effect which protects endothelial cells from inflammatory damage, and reduced reactive oxygen species production [28]. AMA0526, another inhibitor of ROCK significantly reduces corneal neovascularization in an alkali-burn mice model in a similar fashion as dexamethasone with additional antifibrotic effect [36]. Thus, there is evidence from preclinical studies to imply that ROCK inhibition may be as effective or more effective in the treatment of corneal neovascularization as currently employed topical drugs, such as dexamethasone. The notion that ROCK inhibition can do this without the side-effects of topical steroids, such as elevated IOP and cataract formation is especially appealing.

## 18.6 Endothelium

The corneal endothelium consists of a monolayer of hexagonal cells which undergo continuous reduction of cell density at the rate of approximately 0.6% per annum due to age-related apoptosis. To compensate for this loss, adjacent living cells migrate and enlarge to cover the area of lost cells. However, when cell density falls below a threshold value, endothelial decompensation will lead to corneal oedema [37]. Cataract extraction using phacoemulsification stresses the endothelium and may tip the balance towards endothelial decompensation leading to pseudophakic bullous keratopathy. Traditionally, corneal endothelial cells have been considered to have limited regenerative potential, but recent evidence challenges this line of thought [38, 39]. Stem cell markers have been located in the periphery of the endothelium and in the transition zone between the trabecular meshwork and outer edge of the corneal endothelium [40–43]. The presence of stem cells in close proximity to the corneal endothelium is highly suggestive of its regenerative potential [44]. Since ROCK signalling pathways have an established role in cellular proliferation, adhesive capabilities and inhibition of apoptosis (but not necrosis), it is hardly surprising that their role in endothelial proliferation has received their fair share of attention [45, 46]. Not all studies, however; are able to replicate the positive effects of ROCK inhibitors on cell proliferation [47]. A possible explanation for this discrepancy could be the variation in the concentration of ROCK inhibitors used in different studies [47, 48]. The current knowledge on the importance of ROCK inhibition on the regenerative potential of corneal endothelial cells has generated two different directions of research; one focusing on tissue engineering therapy (i.e. transplanting cultivated corneal endothelial cells either as suspension or sheet to recipient corneas), and another on pharmaceutical treatment (i.e. topical or intraocular administration of ROCK inhibitors). Cultured corneal endothelial cells on a substrate have been transplanted into animal models resulting in regeneration of the endothelial cell layer and corneal transparency [49–51]. Transplantation of a cell sheet, which acts like a lamellar graft has obvious advantages over transplantation of cell suspensions without a guiding substrate; however, when a ROCK inhibitor is added to the cell suspension, the cells attain a sense of direction, are less likely to undergo apoptosis, and more likely to adhere onto a substrate [52]. Thus, in rabbits and cynomolgus monkeys with experimental corneal endothelial dysfunction, injection of cell suspensions consisting of cultured corneal endothelial cells successfully regenerated the endothelium and promoted corneal clarity when ROCK inhibitors were added to the cell suspension [53, 54]. In terms of pharmaceutical treatment, topical application of Y-27632 has been shown to be efficacious in facilitating healing of iatrogenic corneal endothelial defects in monkeys, rabbits, and dogs [55, 56]. At least in rabbits, regeneration of the endothelium with Y-27632 is associated with expression of functionality markers, such as ZO-1 or tight-junction protein-1 and $Na^+/K^+$ -ATPase, suggestive of a healthy cell phenotype [53]. Conversely, absence of ROCK inhibition leads to endothelial reconstruction with a stratified fibroblastic phenotype without expression of functionality markers. The anti-apoptotic ability of ROCK inhibitors has potential clinical value, especially in procedures where cell death is anticipated, such as routine phacoemulsification of the lens which stresses the endothelium. When human corneal endothelial cells from donor corneoscleral tissue were subjected to phacoemulsification energy, the rate of endothelial cell apoptosis was significantly reduced in tissue that had been stored in the presence of a ROCK inhibitor [57]. Assuming that the same applies in patients undergoing cataract surgery, the concept of using intraoperative or perioperative administration of topical or intracameral ROCK inhibitors is particularly attractive considering that it is potentially a cost-effective and simple way to prevent endothelial cell decompensation in susceptible patients. The first published case of Y-27632 application on a living human cornea was presented by Koizumi and co-authors in 2013. Here, a 52-year-old Japanese man with Fuchs endothelial dystrophy was managed with pre-pupillary endothelial denudation by transcorneal freezing using a steel rod on the corneal surface for 15 s and 50 µm Y-27632 (10 mM) eye drops six times daily for 1 week [58]. On this treatment, the cornea cleared, central corneal thickness decreased, the endothelial cell density increased from 757 to 1549 cells/$mm^2$, and the best corrected visual acuity in the worse eye went from 20/63 to 20/20 and 20/16 after 2 weeks and 6 months, respectively. In a clinical study by the same group, 8 patients with either central or diffuse corneal oedema were given Y-27632 eye drops (10 mM) six times daily for 7 days after denudation of the central endothelium with a cryoprobe. A clear, but non-significant trend was seen for a reduction in central corneal thickness in patients with central, but not diffuse, oedema [59]. When interpreting these results, however, it is useful to know that denudation of the endothelium alone may promote spontaneous remodelling, as exemplified by reports of successful repopulation of the endothelium by descemetorhexis without graft transplantation [60–65]. In a recent study, 18 patients with Fuchs endothelial dystrophy and BCVA of 0.4 or less underwent Descemet stripping with or without topical ripasudil 0.4% QID postoperatively for 2 months [66]. All patients had >1000 cells/$mm^2$ outside the central area preoperatively and received sodium chloride ointment at bedtime for 2 months. All patients achieved a BCVA of 0.5 or more by 6 months although the ripasudil group demonstrated significantly quicker recovery of vision (4.6 vs. 6.5 weeks) and significantly higher average endothelial cell count for at least 1 year (1086 vs 736 cells/$mm^2$). The central cornea thickness did not differ in the two groups at 12 months. One patient experienced severe abdominal pain and constipation within 3 days of starting topical ripasudil and subsequently discontinued treatment. Another patient in the ripasudil group initially did well at the 3- and 6-month postoperative visits with BCVA 0.5; however, at the 1-year visit, her vision decreased to 0.1 due to endothelial decompensation and DMEK was performed resulting in vision improvement to 0.8 at 3 months after surgery. This study suggests that Descemet stripping alone with or without postoperative topical ROCK inhibition is a possible alternative to graft transplantation in patients with endothelial decompensation and peripheral endothelial cell count >1000 µm. In another study, ROCK inhibitors have been used with some success as a form of salvage therapy in eyes unresponsive to Descemet stripping alone [65]. There is currently no study comparing Descemet stripping alone with or without ROCK inhibition with Descemet striping followed by graft transplantation. Currently, the use of ROCK inhibitors for corneal endothelial diseases is off label.

Building on their preclinical research on tissue engineering in rabbits and monkeys where corneal endothelial cells supplemented with Y-27632 underwent repopulation and self-organization into healthy endothelium when injected into the anterior chamber, Kinoshita and co-authors published a landmark proof-of-concept uncontrolled single-group clinical study in 2018. In this study, 11 human subjects with pseudophakic bullous keratopathy, BCVA <0.5, and no detectable corneal endothelial cells on specular microscopy were managed with intracameral injection of cultured human donor CECs supplemented with Y-27632 followed by prone position for 3 h. Prior to injection, a central 8-mm-diameter descemetorhexis was performed using a silicone needle. After 24 weeks, the mean cell density increased to 1924 cells per $mm^2$, corneal thickness was reduced, and corneal transparency was restored. This treatment was reported to be safe without any postoperative intraocular inflammation or immunogenic reaction. One of 11 patients, experienced elevated intraocular pressure to 27 mmHg 8 months after treatment and was managed with trabeculotomy. This technique holds the potential to bring about a paradigm shift in the way we manage corneal endothelial decompensation as it appears to be safe, effective, minimally invasive, and surgically easier to execute when compared to corneal transplantation. However, the study generates some important questions which probably need to be addressed before the novel technique can be adopted by clinicians [67]: (1) What is the precise contribution of ROCK inhibition in corneal endothelial cell regeneration? This question was not answered by the original study as there was no control group where corneal endothelial cells without prior ROCK inhibitor exposure were injected. However, as discussed above, there is some evidence that ROCK inhibition in itself guides injected cells to repopulate the endothelium. (2) What is the origin of the repopulated endothelial cells? This question is interesting from an academic point of view. In an open letter by Dana, several possible origins have been proposed: donor-cell integration, migration of peripheral cells, paracrine effects, ROCK inhibition, or a combination of these factors. [67] (3) Are there risks associated with injected cells that do not adhere to the posterior corneal surface, such as ocular hypertension due to trabecular meshwork clogging, or ectopic tumour formation? Studies on a larger scale and longer follow-up are called for in order to uncover this important concern.

## 18.7 Rock Signalling in Intraocular Pressure Regulation and Glaucoma

Glaucoma is a potentially devastating complication of penetrating, lamellar and endothelial keratoplasty. The most recognized modifiable risk factor for glaucoma development and progression is increased intraocular pressure. The significance of detecting and managing glaucoma in patients where keratoplasty has been performed or is planned cannot be overemphasized. Ocular hypertension is not a rare entity in the post-keratoplasty period and may commonly be secondary to pupil block due to air bubble in the anterior chamber, retained viscoelastic, steroid response, peripheral anterior synechiae, or trabecular meshwork collapse in aphakic patients. While other known complications of keratoplasty, such as induced astigmatism, rejection and macular oedema may be responsive to treatment, uncontrolled ocular hypertension is a gateway to disastrous and irreversible visual impairment. In turn, ocular hypertension significantly increases the risk of graft failure, probably because of its detrimental effects on the endothelium [68]. Studies have also found that benzalkonium chloride (BAK), found in some antihypertensive eye drops, as well as filtrating surgery have a negative impact on endothelial survival [69]. The risk of glaucoma in keratoplasty is probably similar for all types of keratoplasties [70]. It is important to realize while measuring IOP on a transplanted cornea that the reading will usually be imprecise due to altered biomechanics (Fig. 18.1).

Intraocular pressure regulation is a complex homeostatic process balanced by rate of aqueous humour production in the ciliary body and rate of efflux through the trabecular meshwork (TM) or the uveoscleral route. Anatomically, the TM consists of a spongy connective tissue containing collagen and elastin fibres surrounded by endothelial-like trabecular cells (trabeculocytes) which rest on a basement membrane. Its juxtacanalicular tissue (JCT) portion is the site of greatest resistance to aqueous humour outflow. Physiologically, the trabeculocytes display smooth muscle-like properties, due to expression of actin and myosin. Relaxation of the TM results in increased aqueous humour outflow [71–73]. This dynamic regulation of aqueous humour outflow is partly regulated by ROCK I and II isotypes which are expressed in the TM. The beneficial role of ROCK inhibition in glaucoma may be related to decreased IOP through TM cytoskeleton leading to TM contraction [10, 74–77]. In cultured human TM cells, exposure to Y-27632 is reported to be non-toxic [78]. Many ROCK inhibitors, including Y-27632, fasudil, AR-12286, netarsudil, H-1152, Y-39983, and AMA-0076 significantly decrease outflow resistance in porcine and rabbit eyes, and IOP in rabbits and monkeys [79–84].

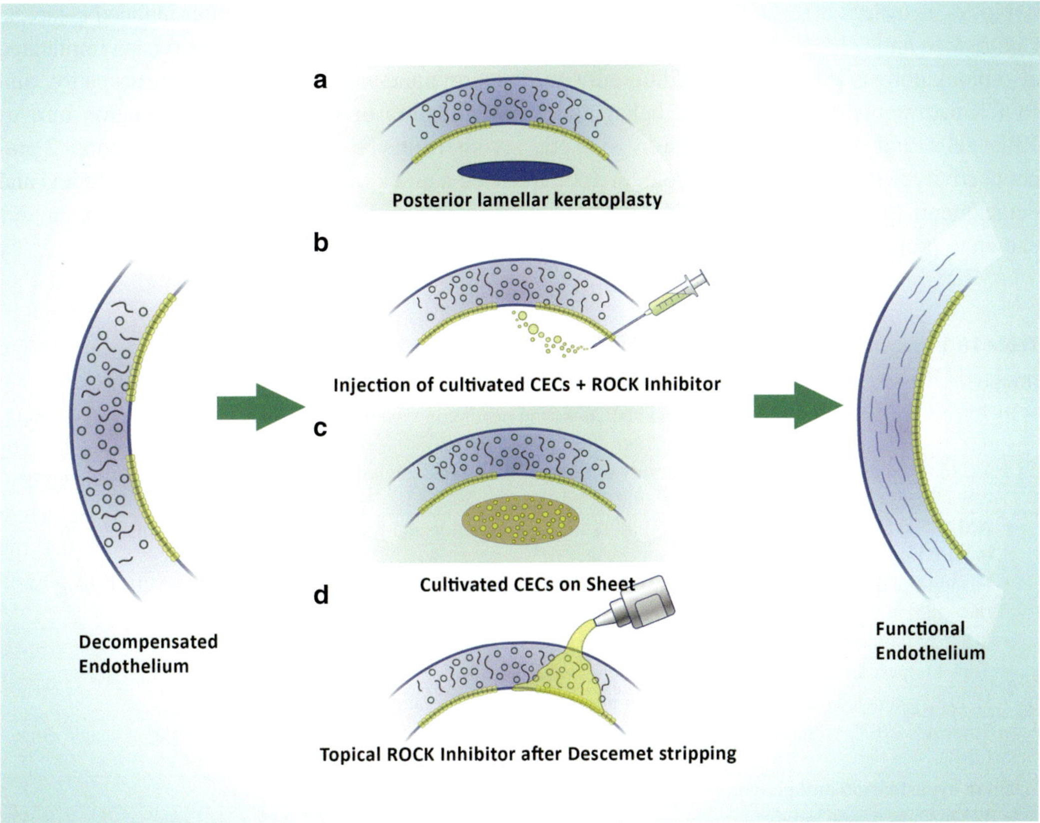


**Fig. 18.1** Surgical options in the management of corneal endothelial decompensation: (**a**) Posterior lamellar keratoplasty, for example, DSAEK, DMEK, or PDEK is currently the gold standard. (**b**) Corneal endothelial cells (CECs) are cultivated from donor cornea and ROCK inhibitor is added. The cell suspension is then injected into the anterior chamber. (**c**) Cultivated CECs are spread on a sheet made of collagen or amnion and inserted into the anterior chamber. (**d**) Topical ROCK inhibitor is applied onto the cornea for several weeks. In all cases, denudation of the endothelium is performed prior to the procedure. Descemet stripping alone (not illustrated in this figure) is also an option of management

## 18.8 Rock Signalling in Other Eye Conditions

It is hardly surprising that ROCK signalling plays a part in other eye conditions considering the ubiquity of ROCK signalling proteins in the eye. ROCK signalling plays a vital role in microvasculopathy of the diabetic retina by modulating endothelial cell migration, survival, and cell permeability. ROCK inhibition promotes vascular endothelial cell survival by protecting them from inflammatory damage, reducing retinal hypoxia, retinal pigment epithelium breakdown, and lessening reactive oxygen species production [85–90]. In a randomized clinical trial, intravitreal co-administration of fasudil and bevacizumab for diabetic maculopathy was more effective in oedema resorption compared to administration of bevacizumab alone [91]. In a retrospective analysis, topically administered ripasudil for POAG significantly reduced foveal thickness in patients with diabetic macular oedema compared to patients without treatment. However, visual acuity did not differ amongst the groups [92]. Animal studies have confirmed favourable effects of ROCK inhibition in experimental retinal vein occlusion [93] and experimental age-related macular degeneration, where it blocks neovascularization and inflammation. Contrary to anti-VEGF agents, ROCK inhibitors also block fibrosis [88, 94, 95]. Additionally, the ROCK pathway is implicated in the behaviour of RPE cells and photoreceptor-neuron synaptic connectivity which may play a role in retinal detachment [96–98]. Recently, Y-27632 was shown to prevent anterior subcapsular cataract in mice with ultraviolet radiation-induced cataracts [99]. ROCK inhibitors have also been implicated in myopia, non-arteritic optic neuropathy, and modulation of intraocular inflammation in eyes with uveitis [100–105]. Tables 18.1 and 18.2 provide a quick overview of selected preclinical and clinical studies with ROCK inhibitors in eye disease.

**Table 18.1** Summary of selected preclinical studies involving rock inhibitors

| |
|---|
| Cornea |
| • Topical Y-27632 promoted corneal endothelial wound healing in vivo (rabbits) and in vitro (monkeys) [41, 45, 47] |
| • Y-27632 did not affect proliferative ability of human corneal endothelial cells, but altered cell shape, increased cell adhesion and enhanced wound healing ex vivo and in vitro [43] |
| • AMA0526 inhibited endothelial cell proliferation and migration and prevented corneal neovascularization in vitro [32] |
| • Fasudil eye drops inhibited alkali burn-induced corneal neovascularization and promoted epithelial healing in mice [25] |
| • Y-27632 promoted ex vivo and in vitro proliferation of human limbal epithelial cells [30] |
| • Topical ripasudil promoted corneal endothelial wound healing in cultured cells [92, 93] |
| • H-1152 promoted corneal endothelial cell migration and proliferation in adult porcines [130] |
| • Topical Y-27632 promoted corneal endothelial cell regeneration following transcorneal freezing in beagle dogs [46] |
| **Ocular hypertension and glaucoma** |
| • Y-27632 decreased intraocular pressure by increasing aqueous outflow [79–84, 123, 131–134] |
| • Ripasudil increased retinal ganglion cell survival after damage to optic nerve in mice [135] |
| • Ripasudil promoted retinal ganglion cell regeneration in cats [136] |
| **Retina** |
| • Fasudil protects rat retina from ischemia-reperfusion injury by inhibiting apoptosis and inducible nitric oxide synthase expression [137] |
| • Selective ROCK-II inhibition decreases M2-like macrophages and choroidal neovascularization [94] |
| • Y-27632 protects against retinitis pigmentosa in rats [138] |
| • Ripasudil, but not fasudil inhibits retinal angiogenesis in vitro (human retinal microvascular endothelial cells) and in vivo (mice) [95] |
| • Promotes human retinal pigment epithelium survival in vitro [139] |
| • Stabilizes rod-photoreceptor synapses after experimental retinal detachment in pigs [97] |
| • Protects against diabetic retinopathy by reducing leakage and neovascularization in rodents [88] |
| • Promotes retinal ganglion cell survival and axon regeneration after optic nerve injury in rodents [140] |
| • Intraocular injection reduces retinal hypoxia and retinal pigment epithelial barrier breakdown in rats [89] |
| • Prevents retinal oedema, reduces size of non-perfusion area, and improves retinal blood blow in murine retinal vein occlusion model [93] |
| • Protects Müller cells against cellular injury caused by oxidative stress and hypoxia [138] |
| **Cataract** |
| • Prevents anterior subcapsular cataracts in mice [99] |
| • Reduces endothelial cell loss during phacoemulsification in ex vivo human donor tissue [57] |
| **Uveitis** |
| • Anti-inflammatory effect against ocular inflammatory disease, including acute uveitis and possibly uveitis glaucoma [102] |
| • Favourable effects in anterior uveitis, possibly due to reorganized blood–aqueous barrier [103] |

(continued)

**Table 18.1** (continued)

| |
|---|
| **Optic nerve** |
| • Topical application of ripasudil increased blood flow to optic nerve in normal rats [105] |
| • Rabbits given fasudil for non-arteritic anterior ischemic optic neuropathy exhibited neuronal repair, alleviation of retinal ganglion cell loss after traumatic optic nerve injury [100] |
| • Intravitreal ripasudil protects against tumour necrosis factor-alpha-induced axon loss in rats [141] |

**Table 18.2** Summary of selected clinical studies involving ROCK inhibitors

| |
|---|
| **Cornea** |
| • Topical Y-27632 after transcorneal freezing for Fuchs endothelial dystrophy successfully reversed stromal oedema, increased endothelial cell density, and improved visual acuity in a 52-year-old male with Fuchs endothelial dystrophy [58] |
| • Intracameral injection of human corneal endothelial cells supplemented with Y-27632 increased corneal endothelial cell density after 24 months in 11 subjects with bullous keratopathy [142] |
| • Topical Y-27632 given six times daily for 7 days following debridement of central 2 mm of endothelium with cryoprobe resulted in a clear, but non-significant trend for reduction in central corneal thickness in patients with central, but not diffuse, stromal oedema [59] |
| • Topical ripasudil four times daily for 2 months after Descemet stripping only with ripasudil (i.e. without graft) resulted in faster recovery of visual acuity and higher endothelial cell count compared to Descemet stripping without ripasudil [66] |
| **Glaucoma** |
| • Ripasudil lowered intraocular pressure (IOP) when added to timolol to a similar level as the additive IOP lowering observed with brimonidine or dorzalamide, albeit with a higher incidence of conjunctival hyperaemia [118, 143–145] |
| • AR-12286 decreased IOP by up to −7.0 mmHg in normal subjects in phase 1 trial [146] and −4.5 mmHg in subjects with ocular hypertension (OHT)/primary open-angle glaucoma (POAG) in phase 2 trial [119] |
| • SNJ-1656 significantly reduced IOP up to $-3.0 \pm 1.2$ mmHg in healthy adults in phase 1 study [118] and −3.0 to −3.5 mmHg in patients with OHT or POAG in phase 2 study [120] |
| • In patients with baseline IOP < 26 mmHg, netarsudil was more effective and lowering IOP than latanoprost [114] |
| • Netarsudil lowers IOP by about 2 mmHg when added to latanoprost [147] |
| • A combination of latanoprost and netarsudil (Rocklatan) demonstrated superior IOP reduction over latanoprost and netarsudil. Rocklatan decreased IOP by 30% or more in >60% of patients. Compared to latanoprost, nearly three times as many patients reached 14 mmHg [117] |
| • Fasudil decreased IOP by about 16% in patients with unilateral end-stage POAG with peak effect 2–4 h after application [148] |
| • Ripasudil effective as an adjunctive therapy for lowering IOP in POAG [125] |
| **Retina** |
| • Topically administered ripasudil significantly reduced foveal thickness in eyes with diabetic macular oedema that received ripasudil for the treatment of primary open-angle glaucoma compared to controls that received no treatment. No change in visual acuity was observed between the groups [92] |
| • In patients with centre-involving diabetic macular edema, intravitreal fasudil and bevacizumab resulted in a greater proportion gaining at least 15 ETRDS letters at month 6 compared to intravitreal bevacizumab alone (54.5 vs. 10%, $p = 0.026$) [91] |
| **Optic nerve** |
| • Intravitreal injection of fasudil improved vision, decreased peripapillary retinal fibre layer thickness, and reduced mean index of visual field in patients with nonarteritic anterior ischemic optic neuropathy [100] |

## 18.9 Rock Inhibitors

Drug delivery to the eye is achievable through topical, intraocular, or systemic means. As there are concerns regarding safety of ROCK inhibitors when given systemically [106], such as vasodilation and hypotension, topical and intraocular means are generally preferred. In freshly excised porcine eyes, topical administration of the ROCK inhibitor Y-27632 penetrates the stroma to reach the endothelium. Topical delivery can be facilitated by using a mucoadhesive film, which results in a three-fold greater penetration of Y-27632 into the corneas of freshly excised porcine eyes [107]. Not surprisingly, intraocular administration (intracameral or intravitreal) is the most effective route of ROCK delivery to the eye [95, 108, 109].

Although most preclinical studies have employed Y-27632 to inhibit the ROCK signalling pathway, this ROCK inhibitor is currently not approved for clinical use. Two different clinical studies have demonstrated efficacy of intracameral or topical Y-27632 in patients with Fuchs endothelial dystrophy (discussed earlier). In ophthalmology, two different ROCK inhibitors have gained approval by governmental authorities for use in ocular hypertension and/or glaucoma: Netarsudil and Ripasudil. Although not approved for use in ophthalmology, Fasudil (HA-1077) was the first ROCK inhibitor to be approved in Japan and China for use in cerebral vasospasm. Table 18.3 presents an overview of three formulations of ROCK inhibitors currently approved for use in ophthalmology.

- **Netarsudil 0.02%** (Rhopressa, Aerie pharmaceuticals, NC, USA) was FDA approved in 2017 to treat ocular hypertension (OHT) and primary open-angle glaucoma (POAG) and is awaiting approval in the EU under the trade name Rhokiinsa. In addition to being a potent ROCK inhibitor, Netarsudil also inhibits the norepinephrine transporter. This unique feature of netarsudil probably contributes to IOP lowering by decreasing aqueous humour production and episcleral venous pressure [84, 110–112]. Netarsudil reduces IOP within 2 h of instillation and maintains IOP reduction for 24 h allowing for once-daily application [113]. In a phase 3 trial, netarsudil was not as effective as latanoprost in reducing IOP, except for patients with lower baseline IOP (26 mmHg or less). Adverse effects, such as conjunctival hyperaemia were significantly more commonly encountered with netarsudil than latanoprost [114]. The phase 3 ROCKET 1 and 2 trials did not find netarsudil to be non-inferior to timolol, except when baseline IOP was <25 mmHg [115]. The main problem with netarsudil is relatively higher incidence of adverse effects, such as conjunctival hyperaemia, perilimbal microhaemorrhages, cornea verticillata, and eye pruritus. In March 2019, a fixed combination of netarsudil and latanoprost (Rocklatan, Aerie Pharmaceuticals, NC, USA) was FDA approved for use in OHT and POAG. In the phase 3 multicentre trials, MERCURY 1 and MERCURY 2, Rocklatan demonstrated superior IOP reducing action compared to latanoprost and netarsudil alone. Compared to patients on latanoprost monother-

**Table 18.3** ROCK inhibitors

| | Ripasudil 0.4% | Netarsudil 0.02% | Netarsudil 0.02% + latanoprost 0.005% |
|---|---|---|---|
| Alternative names | K-115 | AR-13503, AR-13324 | – |
| Trade names | Glanatec | Rhopressa (USA), Rhokiinsa (EU) | Rocklatan |
| Chemical structure | $C_{15}H_{18}FN_3O_2S$ | $C_{28}H_{27}N_3O_3$ | $C_{26}H_{40}O_5 + C_{28}H_{27}N_3O_3$ |
| Approval status | Granted by PMDA (Japan) for OHT/POAG | Granted by FDA (USA) for OHT/POAG | Granted by FDA (USA) for OHT/POAG |

Abbreviations: *OHT* ocular hypertension, *POAG* primary open-angle glaucoma apy, nearly three times as many patients on Rocklatan reached an IOP of 14 mmHg. However, a significant proportion of patients receiving Rocklatan or netarsudil monotherapy discontinued treatment due to adverse effects [116, 117].

- **Ripasudil 0.4%** (Glanatec, Kowa Co. Ltd., Aichi, Japan) is approved for the treatment of OHT and POAG in Japan. In a phase 3 trial, ripasudil 0.4% lowered IOP on average by 2.6 mmHg at trough and 3.7 mmHg at peak in patients with OHT or POAG compared to placebo after 52 weeks [118]. This reduction was even more obvious on patients with baseline IOP > or = 21 mmHg. In patients already taking timolol, ripasudil has an additive effects on IOP reduction [118].

Other ROCK inhibitors, such as SNJ-1656 and AR-12286 have shown to be efficacious as IOP lowering agents in clinical trials [119, 120]. A critical issue with most topical ROCK inhibitors is the relatively high incidence of adverse effects. Conjunctival hyperaemia and allergic conjunctivitis are also very common in patients taking for IOP lowering purposes [118]. Approximately one-third of patients taking ripasudil 0.4% for glaucoma stop taking the drug within 2 years due to blepharitis [121]. The rates of adverse events appear similar across the array of different ROCK inhibitors and tend to disappear following cessation of therapy [117, 122]. Recently, a highly selective ROCK inhibitor ITRI-E-212 was introduced as being efficacious in lowering IOP in rabbits while having a good ocular tolerability profile with lower incidence of local adverse effects [123]. Generally, ocular ROCK inhibitors are considered systemically safe though some patients have encountered systemic side-effects after commencing topical therapy, such as abdominal pain and skin rash [124, 125].

## 18.10 Conclusion

The last few decades have witnessed a growing interest in the ROCK signalling pathways. Eye drops that inhibit ROCK proteins have been approved for use in ocular hypertension and glaucoma. ROCK inhibitors are not approved for use in corneal disease as of yet, but this is expected to change in the future with accumulation of more studies on the topic. In 2017, the Cornea Research Foundation of America announced a new investigational study to assess the role of netarsudil 0.02% in reducing corneal transplant complications, especially elevated intraocular pressure. A search for ongoing and completed clinical trials on *clinicaltrials.gov* returns a number of active and inactive registered trials looking ROCK inhibitors in eye disease; the primary focus is on corneal endothelial dysfunction and OHT/POAG. Cellular processes governed by ROCK signalling pathways (e.g. adhesion, apoptosis) are known to underlie the pathogenesis of several eye conditions; this combined with the ubiquity of ROCK proteins in the eye (and rest of the body) is therefore suggestive of countless clinical applications. The future perspectives for ROCK inhibition are manifold. Two examples are stem cell therapy and allograft rejection, both of which are affected partly by the ROCK signalling pathway. ROCK inhibition enhances recovery and growth of human embryonic stem cells which possess the ability to grow and differentiate into corneal endothelial-like cells in vitro [126, 127]. From animal models of rejection following renal and cardiac transplantation, studies suggest that ROCK inhibitors can inhibit rejection [128, 129]. An expansion of our understanding of the ROCK signalling pathways in the eye combined with development of highly specific ROCK inhibitors with lower incidence of adverse side-effects will surely lead to a better integration of ROCK inhibitors in clinical ophthalmology.

## References

1. Orucoglu F, Blumenthal EZ, Frucht-Pery J, Solomon A. Risk factors and incidence of ocular hypertension after penetrating keratoplasty. J Glaucoma. 2014;23(9):599–605.
2. Aldave AJ, Rudd JC, Cohen EJ, Rapuano CJ, Laibson PR. The role of glaucoma therapy in the need for repeat penetrating keratoplasty. Cornea. 2000;19(6):772–6.
3. Banitt M, Lee RK. Management of patients with combined glaucoma and corneal transplant surgery. Eye (Lond). 2009;23(10):1972–9.

4. Manser E, Leung T, Salihuddin H, Zhao ZS, Lim L. A brain serine/threonine protein kinase activated by Cdc42 and Rac1. Nature. 1994;367(6458):40–6.
5. Leung T, Manser E, Tan L, Lim L. A novel serine/threonine kinase binding the Ras-related RhoA GTPase which translocates the kinase to peripheral membranes. J Biol Chem. 1995;270(49):29051–4.
6. Matsui T, Amano M, Yamamoto T, et al. Rho-associated kinase, a novel serine/threonine kinase, as a putative target for small GTP binding protein Rho. EMBO J. 1996;15(9):2208–16.
7. Ishizaki T, Naito M, Fujisawa K, et al. p160ROCK, a Rho-associated coiled-coil forming protein kinase, works downstream of Rho and induces focal adhesions. FEBS Lett. 1997;404(2–3):118–24.
8. Kaibuchi K. Regulation of cytoskeleton and cell adhesion by Rho targets. Prog Mol Subcell Biol. 1999;22:23–38.
9. Etienne-Manneville S, Hall A. Rho GTPases in cell biology. Nature. 2002;420(6916):629–35.
10. Riento K, Guasch RM, Garg R, Jin B, Ridley AJ. RhoE binds to ROCK I and inhibits downstream signaling. Mol Cell Biol. 2003;23(12):4219–29.
11. Jaffe AB, Hall A. Rho GTPases: biochemistry and biology. Annu Rev Cell Dev Biol. 2005;21:247–69.
12. Loirand G. Rho kinases in health and disease: from basic science to translational research. Pharmacol Rev. 2015;67(4):1074–95.
13. Nakagawa O, Fujisawa K, Ishizaki T, Saito Y, Nakao K, Narumiya S. ROCK-I and ROCK-II, two isoforms of Rho-associated coiled-coil forming protein serine/threonine kinase in mice. FEBS Lett. 1996;392(2):189–93.
14. Feng Y, LoGrasso PV, Defert O, Li R. Rho kinase (ROCK) inhibitors and their therapeutic potential. J Med Chem. 2016;59(6):2269–300.
15. Fukata M, Kuroda S, Nakagawa M, et al. Cdc42 and Rac1 regulate the interaction of IQGAP1 with beta-catenin. J Biol Chem. 1999;274(37):26044–50.
16. Yin J, Yu FS. Rho kinases regulate corneal epithelial wound healing. Am J Physiol Cell Physiol. 2008;295(2):C378–87.
17. Goldhagen B, Proia AD, Epstein DL, Rao PV. Elevated levels of RhoA in the optic nerve head of human eyes with glaucoma. J Glaucoma. 2012;21(8):530–8.
18. Matsumoto A, Manthey HD, Marsh SA, et al. Effects of exercise training and RhoA/ROCK inhibition on plaque in ApoE−/− mice. Int J Cardiol. 2013;167(4):1282–8.
19. Munoz A, Correa CL, Villar-Cheda B, Costa-Besada MA, Labandeira-Garcia JL. Aging-related increase in Rho kinase activity in the Nigral region is counteracted by physical exercise. J Gerontol A Biol Sci Med Sci. 2016;71(10):1254–7.
20. Munoz VR, Gaspar RC, Kuga GK, et al. The effects of aging on Rho kinase and insulin signalling in skeletal muscle and white adipose tissue of rats. J Gerontol A Biol Sci Med Sci. 2020;75(3):432–6.
21. Munoz VR, Gaspar RC, Kuga GK, da Rocha AL. Exercise increases Rho-kinase activity and insulin signaling in skeletal muscle. J Cell Physiol. 2018;233(6):4791–800.
22. Dua HS, Azuara-Blanco A. Limbal stem cells of the corneal epithelium. Surv Ophthalmol. 2000;44(5):415–25.
23. Folkman J. Angiogenesis in cancer, vascular, rheumatoid and other disease. Nat Med. 1995;1(1):27–31.
24. Chang JH, Gabison EE, Kato T, Azar DT. Corneal neovascularization. Curr Opin Ophthalmol. 2001;12(4):242–9.
25. Stromblad S, Cheresh DA. Cell adhesion and angiogenesis. Trends Cell Biol. 1996;6(12):462–8.
26. Hoang MV, Whelan MC, Senger DR. Rho activity critically and selectively regulates endothelial cell organization during angiogenesis. Proc Natl Acad Sci USA. 2004;101(7):1874–9.
27. Hyvelin JM, Howell K, Nichol A, Costello CM, Preston RJ, McLoughlin P. Inhibition of Rho-kinase attenuates hypoxia-induced angiogenesis in the pulmonary circulation. Circ Res. 2005;97(2):185–91.
28. Zeng P, Pi RB, Li P, et al. Fasudil hydrochloride, a potent ROCK inhibitor, inhibits corneal neovascularization after alkali burns in mice. Mol Vis. 2015;21:688–98.
29. Qiu MK, Wang SQ, Pan C, et al. ROCK inhibition as a potential therapeutic target involved in apoptosis in hemangioma. Oncol Rep. 2017;37(5):2987–93.
30. SundarRaj N, Kinchington PR, Wessel H, et al. A Rho-associated protein kinase: differentially distributed in limbal and corneal epithelia. Invest Ophthalmol Vis Sci. 1998;39(7):1266–72.
31. Chen J, Guerriero E, Lathrop K, SundarRaj N. Rho/ROCK signaling in regulation of corneal epithelial cell cycle progression. Invest Ophthalmol Vis Sci. 2008;49(1):175–83.
32. Valko M, Leibfritz D, Moncol J, Cronin MT, Mazur M, Telser J. Free radicals and antioxidants in normal physiological functions and human disease. Int J Biochem Cell Biol. 2007;39(1):44–84.
33. Zhou Q, Duan H, Wang Y, Qu M, Yang L, Xie L. ROCK inhibitor Y-27632 increases the cloning efficiency of limbal stem/progenitor cells by improving their adherence and ROS-scavenging capacity. Tissue Eng Part C Methods. 2013;19(7):531–7.
34. Sun CC, Chiu HT, Lin YF, Lee KY, Pang JH. Y-27632, a ROCK inhibitor, promoted Limbal epithelial cell proliferation and corneal wound healing. PLoS One. 2015;10(12):e0144571.
35. Ambati BK, Nozaki M, Singh N, et al. Corneal avascularity is due to soluble VEGF receptor-1. Nature. 2006;443(7114):993–7.
36. Sijnave D, Van Bergen T, Castermans K, et al. Inhibition of Rho-associated kinase prevents pathological wound healing and neovascularization after corneal trauma. Cornea. 2015;34(9):1120–9.
37. Van den Bogerd B, Dhubhghaill SN, Koppen C, Tassignon MJ, Zakaria N. A review of the evidence

for in vivo corneal endothelial regeneration. Surv Ophthalmol. 2018;63(2):149–65.
38. Wollensak G, Green WR. Analysis of sex-mismatched human corneal transplants by fluorescence in situ hybridization of the sex-chromosomes. Exp Eye Res. 1999;68(3):341–6.
39. Lagali N, Stenevi U, Claesson M, et al. Donor and recipient endothelial cell population of the transplanted human cornea: a two-dimensional imaging study. Invest Ophthalmol Vis Sci. 2010;51(4):1898–904.
40. Whikehart DR, Parikh CH, Vaughn AV, Mishler K, Edelhauser HF. Evidence suggesting the existence of stem cells for the human corneal endothelium. Mol Vis. 2005;11:816–24.
41. McGowan SL, Edelhauser HF, Pfister RR, Whikehart DR. Stem cell markers in the human posterior limbus and corneal endothelium of unwounded and wounded corneas. Mol Vis. 2007;13:1984–2000.
42. He Z, Campolmi N, Gain P, et al. Revisited microanatomy of the corneal endothelial periphery: new evidence for continuous centripetal migration of endothelial cells in humans. Stem Cells. 2012;30(11):2523–34.
43. Hirata-Tominaga K, Nakamura T, Okumura N, et al. Corneal endothelial cell fate is maintained by LGR5 through the regulation of hedgehog and Wnt pathway. Stem Cells. 2013;31(7):1396–407.
44. Galvis V, Tello A, Gutierrez AJ. Human corneal endothelium regeneration: effect of ROCK inhibitor. Invest Ophthalmol Vis Sci. 2013;54(7):4971–3.
45. Peh GS, Adnan K, George BL, et al. The effects of Rho-associated kinase inhibitor Y-27632 on primary human corneal endothelial cells propagated using a dual media approach. Sci Rep. 2015;5:9167.
46. Goldstein AS, Aldrich BT, Skeie JM, et al. Assessing the effects of ripasudil, a novel Rho kinase inhibitor, on human corneal endothelial cell health. J Ocul Pharmacol Ther. 2018;34:692–9.
47. Pipparelli A, Arsenijevic Y, Thuret G, Gain P, Nicolas M, Majo F. ROCK inhibitor enhances adhesion and wound healing of human corneal endothelial cells. PLoS One. 2013;8(4):e62095.
48. Diao YM, Hong J. Rho-associated protein kinase inhibitor, Y-27632, significantly enhances cell adhesion and induces a delay in G1 to S phase transition in rabbit corneal endothelial cells. Mol Med Rep. 2015;12(2):1951–6.
49. Ishino Y, Sano Y, Nakamura T, et al. Amniotic membrane as a carrier for cultivated human corneal endothelial cell transplantation. Invest Ophthalmol Vis Sci. 2004;45(3):800–6.
50. Mimura T, Yamagami S, Yokoo S, et al. Cultured human corneal endothelial cell transplantation with a collagen sheet in a rabbit model. Invest Ophthalmol Vis Sci. 2004;45(9):2992–7.
51. Koizumi N, Sakamoto Y, Okumura N, et al. Cultivated corneal endothelial cell sheet transplantation in a primate model. Invest Ophthalmol Vis Sci. 2007;48(10):4519–26.
52. Okumura N, Ueno M, Koizumi N, et al. Enhancement on primate corneal endothelial cell survival in vitro by a ROCK inhibitor. Invest Ophthalmol Vis Sci. 2009;50(8):3680–7.
53. Okumura N, Koizumi N, Ueno M, et al. ROCK inhibitor converts corneal endothelial cells into a phenotype capable of regenerating in vivo endothelial tissue. Am J Pathol. 2012;181(1):268–77.
54. Okumura N, Sakamoto Y, Fujii K, et al. Rho kinase inhibitor enables cell-based therapy for corneal endothelial dysfunction. Sci Rep. 2016;6:26113.
55. Okumura N, Koizumi N, Ueno M, et al. Enhancement of corneal endothelium wound healing by Rho-associated kinase (ROCK) inhibitor eye drops. Br J Ophthalmol. 2011;95(7):1006–9.
56. Miyagi H, Kim S, Li J, Murphy CJ, Thomasy SM. Topical Rho-associated kinase inhibitor, Y27632, accelerates corneal endothelial regeneration in a canine cryoinjury model. Cornea. 2019;38(3):352–9.
57. Achiron A, Feldman A, Karmona L, et al. Prophylactic exposure of human corneal endothelial cells to Rho-associated kinase inhibitor reduced apoptosis rate after phacoemulsification: ex vivo study. J Cataract Refract Surg. 2018;44(10):1261–6.
58. Koizumi N, Okumura N, Ueno M, Nakagawa H, Hamuro J, Kinoshita S. Rho-associated kinase inhibitor eye drop treatment as a possible medical treatment for Fuchs corneal dystrophy. Cornea. 2013;32(8):1167–70.
59. Okumura N, Kinoshita S, Koizumi N. Application of Rho kinase inhibitors for the treatment of corneal endothelial diseases. J Ophthalmol. 2017;2017:2646904.
60. Shah VC. Reorientation of inverted endothelial graft during Descemet stripping automated endothelial keratoplasty. Cornea. 2012;31(9):1075–7.
61. Moloney G, Chan UT, Hamilton A, Zahidin AM, Grigg JR, Devasahayam RN. Descemetorhexis for Fuchs' dystrophy. Can J Ophthalmol. 2015;50(1):68–72.
62. Borkar DS, Veldman P, Colby KA. Treatment of Fuchs endothelial dystrophy by Descemet stripping without endothelial keratoplasty. Cornea. 2016;35(10):1267–73.
63. Iovieno A, Neri A, Soldani AM, Adani C, Fontana L. Descemetorhexis without graft placement for the treatment of Fuchs endothelial dystrophy: preliminary results and review of the literature. Cornea. 2017;36(6):637–41.
64. Malyugin BE, Izmaylova SB, Malyutina EA, Antonova OP, Gelyastanov AM. Clinical and functional results of one-step phaco surgery and central descemetorhexis for cataract and Fuchs primary endothelial corneal dystrophy. Vestn oftalmol. 2017;133(6):16–22.
65. Moloney G, Petsoglou C, Ball M, et al. Descemetorhexis without grafting for Fuchs endothelial dystrophy-supplementation with topical ripasudil. Cornea. 2017;36(6):642–8.

66. Macsai MS, Shiloach M. Use of topical Rho kinase inhibitors in the treatment of Fuchs dystrophy after Descemet stripping only. Cornea. 2019;38(5):529–34.
67. Dana R. A new frontier in curing corneal blindness. N Engl J Med. 2018;378(11):1057–8.
68. Sugar A, Tanner JP, Dontchev M, et al. Recipient risk factors for graft failure in the cornea donor study. Ophthalmology. 2009;116(6):1023–8.
69. Price FW Jr, Wellemeyer M. Long-term results of Molteno implants. Ophthalmic Surg. 1995;26(2):130–5.
70. Naveiras M, Dirisamer M, Parker J, et al. Causes of glaucoma after descemet membrane endothelial keratoplasty. Am J Ophthalmol. 2012;153(5):958–966.e951.
71. Thieme H, Nuskovski M, Nass JU, Pleyer U, Strauss O, Wiederholt M. Mediation of calcium-independent contraction in trabecular meshwork through protein kinase C and Rho-A. Invest Ophthalmol Vis Sci. 2000;41(13):4240–6.
72. Nakamura Y, Hirano S, Suzuki K, Seki K, Sagara T, Nishida T. Signaling mechanism of TGF-beta1-induced collagen contraction mediated by bovine trabecular meshwork cells. Invest Ophthalmol Vis Sci. 2002;43(11):3465–72.
73. Nakamura Y, Sagara T, Seki K, Hirano S, Nishida T. Permissive effect of fibronectin on collagen gel contraction mediated by bovine trabecular meshwork cells. Invest Ophthalmol Vis Sci. 2003;44(10):4331–6.
74. Feng J, Ito M, Kureishi Y, et al. Rho-associated kinase of chicken gizzard smooth muscle. J Biol Chem. 1999;274(6):3744–52.
75. Fukiage C, Mizutani K, Kawamoto Y, Azuma M, Shearer TR. Involvement of phosphorylation of myosin phosphatase by ROCK in trabecular meshwork and ciliary muscle contraction. Biochem Biophys Res Commun. 2001;288(2):296–300.
76. Waki M, Yoshida Y, Oka T, Azuma M. Reduction of intraocular pressure by topical administration of an inhibitor of the Rho-associated protein kinase. Curr Eye Res. 2001;22(6):470–4.
77. Rao VP, Epstein DL. Rho GTPase/Rho kinase inhibition as a novel target for the treatment of glaucoma. BioDrugs. 2007;21(3):167–77.
78. Koga T, Koga T, Awai M, Tsutsui J, Yue BY, Tanihara H. Rho-associated protein kinase inhibitor, Y-27632, induces alterations in adhesion, contraction and motility in cultured human trabecular meshwork cells. Exp Eye Res. 2006;82(3):362–70.
79. Honjo M, Tanihara H, Inatani M, et al. Effects of Rho-associated protein kinase inhibitor Y-27632 on intraocular pressure and outflow facility. Invest Ophthalmol Vis Sci. 2001;42(1):137–44.
80. Rao PV, Deng PF, Kumar J, Epstein DL. Modulation of aqueous humor outflow facility by the Rho kinase-specific inhibitor Y-27632. Invest Ophthalmol Vis Sci. 2001;42(5):1029–37.
81. Rao PV, Deng P, Sasaki Y, Epstein DL. Regulation of myosin light chain phosphorylation in the trabecular meshwork: role in aqueous humour outflow facility. Exp Eye Res. 2005;80(2):197–206.
82. Nishio M, Fukunaga T, Sugimoto M, et al. The effect of the H-1152P, a potent Rho-associated coiled coil-formed protein kinase inhibitor, in rabbit normal and ocular hypertensive eyes. Curr Eye Res. 2009;34(4):282–6.
83. Van de Velde S, Van Bergen T, Sijnave D, et al. AMA0076, a novel, locally acting Rho kinase inhibitor, potently lowers intraocular pressure in New Zealand white rabbits with minimal hyperemia. Invest Ophthalmol Vis Sci. 2014;55(2):1006–16.
84. Wang RF, Williamson JE, Kopczynski C, Serle JB. Effect of 0.04% AR-13324, a ROCK, and norepinephrine transporter inhibitor, on aqueous humor dynamics in normotensive monkey eyes. J Glaucoma. 2015;24(1):51–4.
85. Arita R, Hata Y, Nakao S, et al. Rho kinase inhibition by fasudil ameliorates diabetes-induced microvascular damage. Diabetes. 2009;58(1):215–26.
86. Bryan BA, Dennstedt E, Mitchell DC, et al. RhoA/ROCK signaling is essential for multiple aspects of VEGF-mediated angiogenesis. FASEB J. 2010;24(9):3186–95.
87. Lahne M, Li J, Marton RM, Hyde DR. Actin-cytoskeleton- and rock-mediated INM are required for photoreceptor regeneration in the adult zebrafish retina. J Neurosci. 2015;35(47):15612–34.
88. Hollanders K, Hove IV, Sergeys J, et al. AMA0428, a potent rock inhibitor, attenuates early and late experimental diabetic retinopathy. Curr Eye Res. 2017;42(2):260–72.
89. Rothschild PR, Salah S, Berdugo M, et al. ROCK-1 mediates diabetes-induced retinal pigment epithelial and endothelial cell blebbing: contribution to diabetic retinopathy. Sci Rep. 2017;7(1):8834.
90. Mohammad G, AlSharif HM, Siddiquei MM, Ahmad A, Alam K, Abu El-Asrar AM. Rho-associated protein kinase-1 mediates the regulation of inflammatory markers in diabetic retina and in retinal Muller cells. Ann Clin Lab Sci. 2018;48(2):137–45.
91. Ahmadieh H, Nourinia R, Hafezi-Moghadam A, et al. Intravitreal injection of a Rho-kinase inhibitor (fasudil) combined with bevacizumab versus bevacizumab monotherapy for diabetic macular oedema: a pilot randomised clinical trial. Br J Ophthalmol. 2018;103:922–7.
92. Minami Y, Song YS, Ishibazawa A, et al. Effect of ripasudil on diabetic macular edema. Sci Rep. 2019;9(1):3703.
93. Hida Y, Nakamura S, Nishinaka A, Inoue Y, Shimazawa M, Hara H. Effects of ripasudil, a ROCK inhibitor, on retinal edema and nonperfusion area in a retinal vein occlusion murine model. J Pharmacol Sci. 2018;137(2):129–36.
94. Zandi S, Nakao S, Chun KH, et al. ROCK-isoform-specific polarization of macrophages associated

with age-related macular degeneration. Cell Rep. 2015;10(7):1173–86.
95. Yamaguchi M, Nakao S, Arita R, et al. Vascular normalization by ROCK inhibitor: therapeutic potential of ripasudil (K-115) eye drop in retinal angiogenesis and hypoxia. Invest Ophthalmol Vis Sci. 2016;57(4):2264–76.
96. Croze RH, Thi WJ, Clegg DO. ROCK inhibition promotes attachment, proliferation, and wound closure in human embryonic stem cell-derived retinal pigmented epithelium. Transl Vis Sci Technol. 2016;5(6):7.
97. Townes-Anderson E, Wang J, Halasz E, et al. Fasudil, a clinically used ROCK inhibitor, stabilizes rod photoreceptor synapses after retinal detachment. Transl Vis Sci Technol. 2017;6(3):22.
98. Tsai ELS, Ortin-Martinez A, Gurdita A, et al. Modeling of photoreceptor donor-host interaction following transplantation reveals a role for Crx, Muller glia, and Rho/ROCK signaling in neurite outgrowth. Stem Cells. 2019;37(4):529–41.
99. Imaizumi T, Kurosaka D, Tanaka U, Sakai D, Fukuda K, Sanbe A. Topical administration of a ROCK inhibitor prevents anterior subcapsular cataract induced by UV-B irradiation. Exp Eye Res. 2019;181:145–9.
100. Sanjari N, Pakravan M, Nourinia R, et al. Intravitreal injection of a Rho-kinase inhibitor (Fasudil) for recent-onset nonarteritic anterior ischemic optic neuropathy. J Clin Pharmacol. 2016;56(6):749–53.
101. Yu J, Luan X, Lan S, Yan B, Maier A. Fasudil, a Rho-associated protein kinase inhibitor, attenuates traumatic retinal nerve injury in rabbits. J Mol Neurosci. 2016;58(1):74–82.
102. Uchida T, Honjo M, Yamagishi R, Aihara M. The anti-inflammatory effect of ripasudil (K-115), a Rho kinase (ROCK) inhibitor, on endotoxin-induced uveitis in rats. Invest Ophthalmol Vis Sci. 2017;58(12):5584–93.
103. Yamada H, Yoneda M, Inaguma S, et al. A Rho-associated kinase inhibitor protects permeability in a cell culture model of ocular disease, and reduces aqueous flare in anterior uveitis. J Ocul Pharmacol Ther. 2017;33(3):176–85.
104. Yuan Y, Li M, To CH, et al. The role of the RhoA/ROCK signaling pathway in mechanical strain-induced scleral myofibroblast differentiation. Invest Ophthalmol Vis Sci. 2018;59(8):3619–29.
105. Wada Y, Higashide T, Nagata A, Sugiyama K. Effects of ripasudil, a Rho kinase inhibitor, on blood flow in the optic nerve head of normal rats. Graefes Arch Clin Exp Ophthalmol. 2019;257(2):303–11.
106. Liao JK, Seto M, Noma K. Rho kinase (ROCK) inhibitors. J Cardiovasc Pharmacol. 2007;50(1):17–24.
107. Chan W, Akhbanbetova A, Quantock AJ, Heard CM. Topical delivery of a Rho-kinase inhibitor to the cornea via mucoadhesive film. Eur J Pharm Sci. 2016;91:256–64.
108. Janes RG, Stiles JF. The penetration of C14-labeled atropine into the eye; a comparison of methods of application. AMA Arch Ophthalmol. 1959;62(1):69–74.
109. Asseff CF, Weisman RL, Podos SM, Becker B. Ocular penetration of pilocarpine in primates. Am J Ophthalmol. 1973;75(2):212–5.
110. Kiel JW, Kopczynski CC. Effect of AR-13324 on episcleral venous pressure in Dutch belted rabbits. J Ocul Pharmacol Ther. 2015;31(3):146–51.
111. Li G, Mukherjee D, Navarro I, et al. Visualization of conventional outflow tissue responses to netarsudil in living mouse eyes. Eur J Pharmacol. 2016;787:20–31.
112. Sit AJ, Lin SC, Kazemi A, McLaren JW, Pruet CM, Zhang X. In vivo noninvasive measurement of Young's modulus of elasticity in human eyes: a feasibility study. J Glaucoma. 2017;26(11):967–73.
113. Sturdivant JM, Royalty SM, Lin CW, et al. Discovery of the ROCK inhibitor netarsudil for the treatment of open-angle glaucoma. Bioorg Med Chem Lett. 2016;26(10):2475–80.
114. Bacharach J, Dubiner HB, Levy B, Kopczynski CC, Novack GD, Group A-CS. Double-masked, randomized, dose-response study of AR-13324 versus latanoprost in patients with elevated intraocular pressure. Ophthalmology. 2015;122(2):302–7.
115. Serle JB, Katz LJ, McLaurin E, et al. Two phase 3 clinical trials comparing the safety and efficacy of Netarsudil to Timolol in patients with elevated intraocular pressure: Rho kinase elevated IOP treatment trial 1 and 2 (ROCKET-1 and ROCKET-2). Am J Ophthalmol. 2018;186:116–27.
116. Pharmaceuticals A. Aerie Pharmaceuticals reports positive Roclatan (netarsudil/latanoprost ophthalmic solution) 0.02%/0.005% phase 3 topline efficacy results. 2017.
117. Pharmaceuticals A. Roclatan Mercury 1 phase 3 topline results. 2017.
118. Tanihara H, Inoue T, Yamamoto T, et al. One-year clinical evaluation of 0.4% ripasudil (K-115) in patients with open-angle glaucoma and ocular hypertension. Acta Ophthalmol. 2016;94(1):e26–34.
119. Williams RD, Novack GD, van Haarlem T, Kopczynski C, Group ARPAS. Ocular hypotensive effect of the Rho kinase inhibitor AR-12286 in patients with glaucoma and ocular hypertension. Am J Ophthalmol. 2011;152(5):834–841 e831.
120. Inoue T, Tanihara H, Tokushige H, Araie M. Efficacy and safety of SNJ-1656 in primary open-angle glaucoma or ocular hypertension. Acta Ophthalmol. 2015;93(5):e393–5.
121. Saito H, Kagami S, Mishima K, Mataki N, Fukushima A, Araie M. Long-term side effects including blepharitis leading to discontinuation of Ripasudil. J Glaucoma. 2019;28(4):289–93.
122. Dasso L, Al-Khaled T, Sonty S, Aref AA. Profile of netarsudil ophthalmic solution and its potential in

the treatment of open-angle glaucoma: evidence to date. Clin Ophthalmol. 2018;12:1939–44.
123. Hsu CR, Chen YH, Liu CP, et al. A highly selective Rho-kinase inhibitor (ITRI-E-212) potentially treats glaucoma upon topical administration with low incidence of ocular hyperemia. Invest Ophthalmol Vis Sci. 2019;60(2):624–33.
124. Kusuhara S, Katsuyama A, Matsumiya W, Nakamura M. Efficacy and safety of ripasudil, a Rho-associated kinase inhibitor, in eyes with uveitic glaucoma. Graefes Arch Clin Exp Ophthalmol. 2018;256(4):809–14.
125. Komizo T, Ono T, Yagi A, Miyata K, Aihara M. Additive intraocular pressure-lowering effects of the Rho kinase inhibitor ripasudil in Japanese patients with various subtypes of glaucoma. Jpn J Ophthalmol. 2019;63(1):40–5.
126. Claassen DA, Desler MM, Rizzino A. ROCK inhibition enhances the recovery and growth of cryopreserved human embryonic stem cells and human induced pluripotent stem cells. Mol Reprod Dev. 2009;76(8):722–32.
127. Hanson C, Arnarsson A, Hardarson T, et al. Transplanting embryonic stem cells onto damaged human corneal endothelium. World J Stem Cells. 2017;9(8):127–32.
128. Poosti F, Yazdani S, Dolman ME, et al. Targeted inhibition of renal Rho kinase reduces macrophage infiltration and lymphangiogenesis in acute renal allograft rejection. Eur J Pharmacol. 2012;694(1–3):111–9.
129. Chen W, Chen S, Chen W, Li XC, Ghobrial RM, Kloc M. Screening RhoA/ROCK inhibitors for the ability to prevent chronic rejection of mouse cardiac allografts. Transpl Immunol. 2018;50:15–25.
130. Meekins LC, Rosado-Adames N, Maddala R, Zhao JJ, Rao PV, Afshari NA. Corneal endothelial cell migration and proliferation enhanced by Rho kinase (ROCK) inhibitors in in vitro and in vivo models. Invest Ophthalmol Vis Sci. 2016;57(15):6731–8.
131. Tokushige H, Inatani M, Nemoto S, et al. Effects of topical administration of y-39983, a selective Rho-associated protein kinase inhibitor, on ocular tissues in rabbits and monkeys. Invest Ophthalmol Vis Sci. 2007;48(7):3216–22.
132. Isobe T, Mizuno K, Kaneko Y, Ohta M, Koide T, Tanabe S. Effects of K-115, a Rho-kinase inhibitor, on aqueous humor dynamics in rabbits. Curr Eye Res. 2014;39(8):813–22.
133. Kaneko Y, Ohta M, Inoue T, et al. Effects of K-115 (Ripasudil), a novel ROCK inhibitor, on trabecular meshwork and Schlemm's canal endothelial cells. Sci Rep. 2016;6:19640.
134. Dang Y, Wang C, Shah P, Waxman S, Loewen RT, Loewen NA. RKI-1447, a Rho kinase inhibitor, causes ocular hypotension, actin stress fiber disruption, and increased phagocytosis. Graefes Arch Clin Exp Ophthalmol. 2019;257(1):101–9.
135. Yamamoto K, Maruyama K, Himori N, et al. The novel Rho kinase (ROCK) inhibitor K-115: a new candidate drug for neuroprotective treatment in glaucoma. Invest Ophthalmol Vis Sci. 2014;55(11):7126–36.
136. Sagawa H, Terasaki H, Nakamura M, et al. A novel ROCK inhibitor, Y-39983, promotes regeneration of crushed axons of retinal ganglion cells into the optic nerve of adult cats. Exp Neurol. 2007;205(1):230–40.
137. Song H, Gao D. Fasudil, a Rho-associated protein kinase inhibitor, attenuates retinal ischemia and reperfusion injury in rats. Int J Mol Med. 2011;28(2):193–8.
138. Zhang XH, Feng ZH, Wang XY. The ROCK pathway inhibitor Y-27632 mitigates hypoxia and oxidative stress-induced injury to retinal Muller cells. Neural Regen Res. 2018;13(3):549–55.
139. Ni Y, Qin Y, Fang Z, Zhang Z. ROCK inhibitor Y-27632 promotes human retinal pigment epithelium survival by altering cellular biomechanical properties. Curr Mol Med. 2017;17(9):637–46.
140. Shaw PX, Sang A, Wang Y, et al. Topical administration of a rock/net inhibitor promotes retinal ganglion cell survival and axon regeneration after optic nerve injury. Exp Eye Res. 2017;158:33–42.
141. Kitaoka Y, Sase K, Tsukahara C, et al. Axonal protection by Ripasudil, a Rho kinase inhibitor, via modulating autophagy in TNF-induced optic nerve degeneration. Invest Ophthalmol Vis Sci. 2017;58(12):5056–64.
142. Kinoshita S, Koizumi N, Ueno M, et al. Injection of cultured cells with a ROCK inhibitor for bullous keratopathy. N Engl J Med. 2018;378(11):995–1003.
143. Boyle JE, Ghosh K, Gieser DK, Adamsons IA. A randomized trial comparing the dorzolamide-timolol combination given twice daily to monotherapy with timolol and dorzolamide. Ophthalmology. 1999;106(12 Suppl):10–6.
144. Craven ER, Walters TR, Williams R, et al. Brimonidine and timolol fixed-combination therapy versus monotherapy: a 3-month randomized trial in patients with glaucoma or ocular hypertension. J Ocul Pharmacol Ther. 2005;21(4):337–48.
145. Sherwood MB, Craven ER, Chou C, et al. Twice-daily 0.2% brimonidine-0.5% timolol fixed-combination therapy vs monotherapy with timolol or brimonidine in patients with glaucoma or ocular hypertension: a 12-month randomized trial. Arch Ophthalmol. 2006;124(9):1230–8.
146. Kopczynski C, Novack GD, Swearingen D, van Haarlem T. Ocular hypotensive efficacy, safety and systemic absorption of AR-12286 ophthalmic solution in normal volunteers. Br J Ophthalmol. 2013;97(5):567–72.
147. Lewis RA, Levy B, Ramirez N, et al. Fixed-dose combination of AR-13324 and latanoprost: a double-masked, 28-day, randomised, controlled study in patients with open-angle glaucoma or ocular hypertension. Br J Ophthalmol. 2016;100(3):339–44.
148. Pakravan M, Beni AN, Ghahari E, et al. The ocular hypotensive efficacy of topical Fasudil, a Rho-associated protein kinase inhibitor, in patients with end-stage glaucoma. Am J Ther. 2017;24(6):e676–80.

# Recent Advances in Endothelial Keratoplasty

19

Parnika Parashar and Soosan Jacob

Corneal diseases are one of the leading causes of significant vision impairment worldwide. Keratoplasty is one of the majorly performed procedures in such cases. However, the need for donor cornea exceeds the supply in many countries. It has been reported that almost 53% of the world's population lacks access to corneal transplantation, due to which there is only one cornea available for every 70 needed [1]. This necessitates the need for useful alternative corneal substitutes which can replicate the structure and function of cornea and reduce the dependency on human tissue. This is especially important in case of endothelial keratoplasty as the donor tissue pool of corneas with good quality endothelium is only a fraction of the total corneas harvested through eye donation.

## 19.1 Hemi- and Quarter DMEK (Descemet's Membrane Endothelial Keratoplasty), DWEK (Descemetorhexis Without Endothelial Keratoplasty)/DSO (Descemet's Stripping Only), DMET (Descemet Membrane Endothelial Transfer)

**Hemi- and quarter DMEK** [2–4]: These refer to usage of a full diameter DMEK graft as opposed to discarding the peripheral rim as is generally done. This gives a larger size graft which is then cut into two or four and used for two or four patients. An elliptical Descemetorhexis is created into which the half-moon or quarter shaped grafts

P. Parashar · S. Jacob (✉)
Dr. Agarwal's Refractive and Cornea Foundation, Chennai, India

Dr. Agarwal's Eye Hospital and Eye Research Centre, Chennai, India


S. Jacob (ed.), *Mastering DMEK and PDEK*, https://doi.org/10.1007/978-981-97-3469-6_19

are floated up. The technique is similar to DMEK otherwise. Though the central cornea clears rapidly, peripheral deturgescence is slow. Endothelial cell loss in the first month may also be higher.

**DWEK (Descemetorhexis Without Endothelial Keratoplasty)/DSO (Descemet's Stripping Only)** [5–8]: DWEK or DSO is used for patients with Fuchs' endothelial dystrophy and refers to the removal of diseased endothelium and Descemet's membrane without replacement with a graft. This is an option for patients with better peripheral endothelial cell count. The peripheral endothelium over time repopulates the central denuded cornea and clears the central corneal edema which results immediately after surgery secondary to intentional removal of the endothelium. Visual recovery is slow following this procedure but can be aided by adding topical ROCK inhibitors. In some cases, the central cornea may not clear at all with the resultant need of a thin membrane endothelial keratoplasty (TMEK) at this stage, and the patient should be counselled about this probability even before DSO surgery. The cut off for a secondary DMEK or PDEK is generally kept as 3 months. Advantages of this procedure are elimination of the risk of graft rejection as well as the need for long-term steroids.

**DMET** [9, 10]: Partially detached DMEK grafts can still result in corneal clearance. It is therefore thought that a partial contact of the graft with the host cornea can result in transfer of the endothelial cells from the donor to the recipient. DMET works on this principle and is used for patients with Fuchs' endothelial dystrophy. The surgery entails creation of a large Descemetorhexis followed by fixation of a donor Descemet roll within the corneo-scleral wound to ensure contact between the graft and the stroma. This can eliminate the need for difficult unrolling procedures, making the surgery quicker and easier while also removing the need for air within the anterior chamber. Disadvantages include prolonged post-operative edema, longer time to visual rehabilitation and the risk of the cornea not clearing at all.

For more details, see Chap. 15 [11].

## 19.2 ROCK Inhibitors

ROCK inhibitors were initially used to improve corneal endothelial cell survival, but they have now also been shown to have a role in corneal endothelial cell migration. It is therefore used in patients undergoing DSO, DMET, etc. and as we will soon read, together with intra-cameral endothelial cell injections [12]. For more details, see Chap. 15 [13].

## 19.3 Endo-in DMEK

Endo-in DMEK grafts allow spontaneous unfolding without significantly less cell loss. The graft is loaded with the endothelium on the inner side and the Descemet's membrane facing outwards. This configuration promotes correct side and easier unscrolling because the natural tendency of the graft is to curl towards the Descemet's membrane side. The graft is injected with the scrolls facing downwards. Since the Descemet's membrane is facing host stroma, it therefore has a tendency to unscroll with the DM facing upwards and the endothelium downwards. Therefore, the endo-in graft helps decrease surgical time and manipulation [14]. Cell loss may be less during its passage through the cartridge as the endothelium is facing inwards and thereby protected. It has a no-touch technique of graft unfolding and hence has decreased manipulation and rubbing maneuvers on the iris in the attempts to open the graft as compared to the classical DMEK technique. Rebubbling rate was reported to be higher in one study [15]. Others have reported no adverse effects on the visual outcomes or complication rates [16].

## 19.4 Corneal Endothelial Replacements

### 19.4.1 Intra-cameral Cultivated Allogeneic Endothelial Cell Injection

Injection of cultured human corneal endothelial cells (HCEC) into the anterior chamber together with a ROCK inhibitor after removing the abnormal extracellular matrix in the central 8 mm zone with a silicone needle has shown to give clinical and visual improvements in patients with bullous keratopathy [17]. The patient lies in the prone position for 3 h after injection to facilitate cell adhesion. Magnetic particles applied to HCEC culture followed by the use of a magnetic field to promote better localization and adhesion of injected HCEC to the back of the cornea as well as to increase the quantum of adhered cells is also another recent innovation [18]. Cadaveric HCEC, human embryonic stem cells, induced pluripotent stem cells, and corneal endothelial progenitors can be cultured for intra-cameral injections [19].

### 19.4.2 Ex Vivo Expanded Endothelial Keratoplasty

Guttae or breaks or unevenness of the Descemet membrane may hinder migration of HCEC. Cells seeded on to a thin basement membrane or other scaffold may have advantages. Implants of high density ex vivo expanded HCEC supported on a sheet of porcine Descemet's membrane [20], human amniotic membrane, thin human corneal stromal sheets, [21] or human collagen [22] ready to be implanted using a technique similar to DMEK and PDEK are being researched on. Advanced polymeric bioscaffolds delivery systems as well as scaffold-free cell sheets are also being studied [23, 24]. Ex vivo expansion ensures high supply of high quality and quantity of endothelial cells. Precise Bio, Israel manufactures PVEK (Precise Vision Endothelial Keratoplasty)™ by using 3D-printed ex vivo expanded EK [22]. Animal trials led by Michael Mimouni, MD, have shown good outcomes. Human clinical trials are still awaited. PVEK and other ex vivo expansion techniques have the advantage of obtaining a huge number of implants from a single donor cornea.

### 19.4.3 EndoArt

Made out of a biosynthetic acrylic hydrophobic material, the EndoArt (EyeYon Medical) is a form of artificial acellular endothelium [25]. It seals the posterior stroma off from the aqueous preventing fluid from entering and hydrating the cornea. The implant's diameter however has to be limited in order to allow passage of nutrition through the peripheral cornea. Patients who are not suitable for standard corneal transplantation such as those with multiple failed grafts, rejections can be candidates for this implant. An advantage is that it does not require continued usage of steroids in the post-operative period.

### 19.4.4 Stem Cells

Reprogrammed stem cells from other sources such as human embryonic stem cells [26], adipose-derived stem cells [27], etc. may also be used. Adult stem cells for the corneal endothelium may be available in the extreme periphery of the cornea and may be a source for CEC [28].

## 19.5 Nanoparticles

Nanoparticles can be used to enhance growth and function of stem cells [29]. Nanocarrier delivery systems can enhance efficient delivery of therapeutic molecules to the scaffolds delivering antibiotics and other antimicrobials if required [29]. Gold, silver, and magnetic nanoparticles are modified to enable them to be therapeutic carriers. They are also used to improve penetration, distribution, uptake, and half-life of drugs while decreasing toxicity by targeted delivery. Enhanced biocompatibility is another advantage.

## 19.6 Gene Therapy in Keratoplasty

The avascular, transparent, and immunologically immune nature of cornea has enabled researchers worldwide to explore the concept of gene therapy in the treatment of various genetic disorders of cornea. This involves direct deliverance of therapeutic genes into the corneal cells, thereby targeting the specific genetic mutations, associated with corneal dystrophies [30, 31]. A variety of vectors, techniques, and strategies have been identified and tested for delivering gene therapy in the cornea. This novel genetic approach carries the potential of rectifying underlying genetic defects, thus arresting the progression of the disease [32–35].

## 19.7 Conclusion

The above discussed emerging technologies offer tremendous potential in improving the future of keratoplasty worldwide. Synthetic corneas, bioengineered constructs, nanotechnology, and artificial intelligence systems may revolutionize the face of transplantation in a significant way, offering a better and more advanced approach to keratoplasty surgeries.

## References

1. Gain P, Jullienne R, He Z, Aldossary M, Acquart S, Cognasse F, Thuret G. Global survey of corneal transplantation and eye banking. JAMA Ophthalmol. 2016; 134:167–73. https://doi.org/10.1001/jamaophthalmol.2015.4776.
2. Lam FC, Baydoun L, Dirisamer M, et al. Hemi-Descemet membrane endothelial keratoplasty transplantation: a potential method for increasing the pool of endothelial graft tissue. JAMA Ophthalmol. 2014;132(12):1469–73.
3. Lie JT, Lam FC, Groeneveld-van Beek EA, et al. Graft preparation for hemi-Descemet membrane endothelial keratoplasty (hemi-DMEK). Br J Ophthalmol. 2016;100:4204.
4. Gerber-Hollbach N, Parker JS, Baydoun L, et al. Preliminary outcome of hemi-Descemet membrane endothelial keratoplasty for Fuchs endothelial dystrophy. Br J Ophthalmol. 2016;100(11):1564–8.
5. Moloney G, Chan UT, Hamilton A, et al. Descemetorhexis for Fuchs' dystrophy. Can J Ophthalmol. 2015;50(1):68–72.
6. Moloney G, Petsoglou C, Ball M, et al. Descemetorhexis without grafting for Fuchs endothelial dystrophy—supplementation with topical ripasudil. Cornea. 2017;36:642–8.
7. Huang MJ, Kaine S, Dhaliwal DK. Descemetorhexis without endothelial keratoplasty verses DMEK for treatment for Fuchs endothelial corneal dystrophy. Cornea. 2018;37(12):1479–983.
8. Macsai MS, Shiloach M. Use of topical rho kinase inhibitors in the treatment.
9. Balachandran C, Ham L, Verschoor CA, et al. Spontaneous corneal clearance despite graft detachment in Descemet membrane endothelial keratoplasty. Am J Ophthalmol. 2009;148(2):227–34.
10. Dirisamer M, Ham L, Dapena I, et al. Descemet membrane endothelial transfer: "free-floating" donor Descemet implantation.
11. Dockery PW, Parker J, Melles GRJ. New frontiers of corneal endothelial regeneration: Descemet membrane endothelial transfer, descemetorhexis without endothelial keratoplasty, hemi-DMEK, quarter-DMEK, and cultured corneal endothelial cells. In: Jacob S, editor. Mastering DMEK/PDEK: A video textbook on thin membranous endothelial Keratoplasty. Chapter 15. Springer; 2025.
12. Parekh M, Miall A, Chou A, Buhl L, Deshpande N, Price MO, Price FW, Jurkunas UV. Enhanced migration of Fuchs corneal endothelial cells by rho kinase inhibition: a novel ex vivo Descemet's stripping only model. Cells. 2024;13(14):1218.
13. Singh A. ROCK inhibitors. In: Jacob S, editor. Mastering DMEK/PDEK: a video textbook on thin membranous endothelial Keratoplasty. Chapter 18. Springer; 2025.
14. Parekh M, Ruzza A, Ferrari S, Ahmad S, Kaye S, Ponzin D, Romano V. Endothelium-in versus endothelium-out for Descemet membrane endothelial keratoplasty graft preparation and implantation. Acta Ophthalmol. 2017;95(2):194–8.
15. Kronschläger M, Ruzza A, Zeilinger J, Schlatter A, Ruiss M, Findl O. Comparison of rebubbling rate between preloaded endothelium-in and preloaded no-touch endothelium-out Descemet membrane endothelial keratoplasty transplantation. BMC Ophthalmol. 2024;24(1):301.
16. Busin M, Leon P, D'Angelo S, Ruzza A, Ferrari S, Ponzin D, Parekh M. Clinical outcomes of preloaded Descemet membrane endothelial keratoplasty grafts with endothelium tri-folded inwards. Am J Ophthalmol. 2018;193:106–13.
17. Kinoshita S, Koizumi N, Ueno M, et al. Injection of cultured cells with a ROCK inhibitor for bullous keratopathy. N Engl J Med. 2018;1:995–1003.
18. Park JH, Lee K, Park CY. Effect of magnetic microparticles on cultivated human corneal endothelial cells. Transl Vis Sci Technol. 2023;12(2):14.

19. Wong EN, Mehta JS. Cell therapy in corneal endothelial disease. Curr Opin Ophthalmol. 2022;33:275–81.
20. Lu Q, Peng RM, Feng N, Wen MD, He LH, Hong J. Evaluation of reconstructed human corneal endothelium sheets made with porcine Descemet's membrane in vitro and in vivo. Exp Eye Res. 2020;197:108125.
21. Mimura T, Yamagami S, Amano S. Corneal endothelial regeneration and tissue engineering. Prog Retin Eye Res. 2013;35:1–17.
22. Mimouni M. 3D-printed ex vivo-expanded endothelial keratoplasty. Corneal Physician, Nov 2024. https://www.cornealphysician.com/issues/2024/november/3d-printed-ex-vivo-expanded-endothelial-keratoplasty/. Accessed 9 Nov 2024.
23. Wu KY, Belaiche M, Wen Y, Choulakian MY, Tran SD. Advancements in polymer biomaterials as scaffolds for corneal endothelium tissue engineering. Polymers (Basel). 2024;16(20):2882.
24. Mahdavi SS, Abdekhodaie MJ, Mashayekhan S, Baradaran-Rafii A, Djalilian AR. Bioengineering approaches for corneal regenerative medicine. Tissue Eng Regen Med. 2020;17(5):567–93.
25. Auffarth GU, Son HS, Koch M, Weindler J, Merz P, Daphna O, Marcovich AL, Augustin VA. Implantation of an artificial endothelial layer for treatment of chronic corneal edema. Cornea. 2021;40(12):1633–8.
26. Lovatt M, Yam GH, Peh GS, Colman A, Dunn NR, Mehta JS. Directed differentiation of periocular mesenchyme from human embryonic stem cells. Differentiation. 2018;99:62–9.
27. Dai Y, Guo Y, Wang C, et al. Non-genetic direct reprogramming and biomimetic platforms in a preliminary study for adipose-derived stem cells into corneal endothelia-like cells. PLoS One. 2014;9:e109856.
28. McGowan SL, Edelhauser HF, Pfister RR, Whikehart DR. Stem cell markers in the human posterior limbus and corneal endothelium of unwounded and wounded corneas. Mol Vis. 2007;13:1984–2000.
29. Mijanović O, Pylaev T, Nikitkina A, et al. Tissue engineering meets nanotechnology: molecular mechanism modulations in cornea regeneration. Micromachines (Basel). 2021;12:1336.
30. Sarkar S, Panikker P, D'Souza S, Shetty R, Mohan RR, Ghosh A. Corneal regeneration using gene therapy approaches. Cells. 2023;12:1280.
31. Kostenko A, Swioklo S, Connon CJ. Alginate in corneal tissue engineering. Biomed Mater. 2022;17(2):022004. https://doi.org/10.1088/1748-605X/ac4d7b.
32. Guérin LP, Le Bel G, Desjardins P, Couture C, Gillard E, Boisselier É, et al. The human tissue-engineered cornea (hTEC): recent progress. Int J Mol Sci. 2021;22:1291.
33. Qazi Y, Hamrah P. Gene therapy in corneal transplantation. Semin Ophthalmol. 2013;28:287–300.
34. Amador C, Shah R, Ghiam S, Kramerov AA, Ljubimov AV. Gene therapy in the anterior eye segment. Curr Gene Ther. 2022;22:104–31.
35. Mohan RR, Rodier JT, Sharma A. Corneal gene therapy: basic science and translational perspective. Ocul Surf. 2013;11(3):150–64. https://doi.org/10.1016/j.jtos.2012.10.004. Epub 2013 Feb 13.

GPSR Compliance

*The European Union's (EU) General Product Safety Regulation (GPSR) is a set of rules that requires consumer products to be safe and our obligations to ensure this.*

*If you have any concerns about our products, you can contact us on ProductSafety@springernature.com*

In case Publisher is established outside the EU, the EU authorized representative is:

Springer Nature Customer Service Center GmbH
Europaplatz 3
69115 Heidelberg, Germany

**Batch number: 08179696**

Printed by Printforce, the Netherlands